Grasping
the
Wind

— by —

Andrew Ellis, Nigel Wiseman, Ken Boss

Paradigm Publications • *Brookline, Massachusetts*

— 1989 —

Grasping the Wind

Published by

Paradigm Publications
44 Linden Street
Brookline, Massachusetts, 02146, U.S.A.

ISBN 0-912111-19-4

Library of Congress Cataloging in Publication Data:

Grasping the Wind / by Andrew Ellis, Nigel Wiseman, Ken Boss
p.   cm.
Bibliography: p. 456
Includes index.
ISBN 0-912111-19-4 : $24.95
1. Acupuncture -- Popular works I. Wiseman, Nigel.
II. Boss, Ken, 1959- . III. Title.
RM184.E443   1989
615.8'92--dc19

Paradigm Publications

Publisher: Robert L. Felt
Editor: Martha Lee Fielding

Chinese Character Typesetting:
Leadtech, Taipei, R.O.C.

Additional Software and Distribution
provided by
Redwing Book Company, Brookline, Massachusetts

Cover Painting: The Cleveland Museum of Art, John L. Severance Fund, 70.76
River Village in a Rainstorm, Lu Wen-Ying, Ming Dynasty

Preface

"The names of the points are not merely nominal; each has a profound meaning."

Sun Si Miao

For Western students of Chinese acupuncture, who have only to memorize a numbered sequence channel by channel, recognition of the significance and usefulness of the names of the acupuncture points is easy to miss. In comparison with what the Chinese student must cope, the Western system is convenient, logical and easy to learn. Yet alphanumeric codes deprive Western students of a great advantage, both in possible insights into Chinese culture and medicine, and in learning about the points themselves. It is to aid this perceived lack that we set about the task of translating and compiling.

Readers may note that all the material presented in this text has been drawn solely from Chinese sources. The explanations of the point names are those expressed by Chinese authors, both ancient and modern. Each point name is presented in Chinese, English translation, alphanumeric code and pinyin. Alternate names that may be encountered are listed, as are relevant translations for each character in the point name. **Appendix A, The Glossary of Single Characters** provides more extensive character definitions.

Because the point's location, as expressed in the classics, will often shed light on the name of the point, the classical location is given for each point name. This information is largely drawn from the *Great Compendium of Acupuncture*, except where other sources were more revealing.

Often, a point name will contain either a direct or veiled reference to the point's function in the context of point associations. These special groupings are included where applicable. **Appendix B** contains further discussion of special point groupings and the characters that are used to denote them.

Explanations of point names constitute the major portion of the text. More than one explanation for a point name is given where it adds to the reader's understanding of function, location, or context.

A work such as this is inevitably the work of many people. No list could include all the individuals who have made this book possible. Special thanks go to Bev Cubbage for her typing of the original draft, Huang Sheng-Jing for her patient explanations of the difficult passages and her proficient typing of Chinese characters, James Cleaver for his carefully considered comments on parts of the manuscript, Fan Shi Lei for her willingness to be a walking Chinese reference, and Hsü Fu-Shu, Shi Neng-Yun, Chen Jun-Chao, and Doctor James Tin Yau So, the teachers who have nurtured my interest in Chinese medicine.

Two main styles of Chinese characters are used in this text. *Kai Shu,* a font that preserves the strokes used to form the characters when hand written, is used for headings. Students interested in writing Chinese may thus see something of their construction. The text characters are *Zhong Ming,* a modern style designed for readability when printed. There are stylistic differences. *Shū,* for example, when printed in *Zhong Ming* appears as: 俞 . When printed in *Kai Shu* it is: 俞 . See **Appendix A** and **Appendix B** for further discussion of *shū*.

Table of Contents

PART I
Characters

Introduction

Influences on

the Development of

Point Names

The cultural milieu in which Chinese point nomenclature evolved reflects the pervasive philosophical and metaphysical world view supported by the pillars of Taoism and Confucianism. It includes a veneration for custom and history, a propensity to observe and correlate the phenomena of nature, and a long medical tradition of apprenticeship and secret teaching.

The Taoist view of man as a microcosmic representation of the universe, the Confucian edicts of social form and propriety, and the observation of and dependence on nature characteristic of China's agrarian society are reflected in Chinese medicine as a whole, and specifically in the selection of point names. The careful observation of the geophysical characteristics of the earth, the cycles of the seasons, the stars, the heavens, helped develop a medical language of metaphor and imagery replete with words that mirrored these cosmologic, geographic, and sociologic phenomena: pathogens termed wind, cold, heat, dryness, damp, fire and summerheat perturb a body that is described in terms of seas, valleys, rivers, channels. Stars and constellations serve as guideposts, and divinities haunt each region. Emperors and ministers rule the land, distributing grain and protecting the borders. With heaven above and earth below, man was viewed as a flowing intercourse of yin and yang subject to the influences of the five phases and inseparable from the Tao itself.

Even the Chinese concept of an acupuncture point is different from a Westerner's, a difference manifest in the words used to express the concept. The word "point" indicates a linear coordinate, i.e., the intersection of two lines, a dot on the skin suitable for the insertion of needles or the application of some other stimulation. The Chinese character for acupuncture point, 穴 *xuè*, brings to mind an altogether different picture. This character means "cave" or "hole." The meaning is clear from the two parts of the character: the top portion represents a roof, while the bottom portion is a character in its own right, meaning to divide or remove. The combined meaning of the two parts is a dwelling that is made by removing dirt or rocks, i.e., a cave, a hole, a den. Thus we can see that in this case, as in many others, the meanings of Chinese characters bring us to a greater understanding of the concepts of acupuncture.

Traditionally, knowledge of Chinese medicine was handed down from father to son, teacher to apprentice. Memorization of the classics was required, and point names containing mnemonic symbols aided the retention of important information about the point. Point names might also contain hidden meanings known only to students or apprentices of a particular master. In this way, the point names helped to keep a master's secrets safe from other practitioners, and thus protected his income. Though it is not always possible to determine with great surety the reason for the choice of a point name, hints about the location and function of the point were embedded in the name. The point names are thus poetic; they are only fully understood through patient effort to assimilate the intricacies of their veiled meanings. With time and study the point names become more than labels; they become guides to the understanding of the points and the system of medicine that named them.

Chinese point names, as they evolved over the centuries, did provide particular benefits. They allowed the point-channel system to grow and change without fundamentally changing the names and principles set down in the classics, and thus satisfied the conservative nature of the culture. The inherent ambiguity of the point names lent an air of mystery to the healing arts and aided in preserving the secrets of the masters. In addition, the point names revealed important information about the points and imbued them with a poetic spirit that evoked a multitude of valuable associations.

Point Name Taxonomy

For the clinician, much of the value of the point names lies in their didactic and mnemonic qualities. The point names either tell us something about the points or remind us of something that we already know. This information is conveyed through the name in either a concrete or abstract manner, and generally falls into one of four categories: function, location, five-phase, yin-yang association, or channel relationship.

Point names categorized by function include names that refer directly to the function of a point and names that imply function by indicating the special point grouping to which a point belongs. When referring directly to the function of a point, the reference can be concrete, as in Tear Container (ST-1), or more abstract, as in Four Whites (ST-2). The names that indicate special point groupings can also be either concrete or abstract, as exemplified in the names Yin Cleft (HT-6, cleft-xi point of the heart channel), or Woodworm Canal (LV-5, connecting-luo point of the liver channel).

Locational point names, by far the most common, may refer either to the area where a point is located or the position that the patient must assume for treatment. For example, Wrist Bone (SI-4) is a reference to the precise location of a point. Crouching Rabbit (ST-32) refers to the location of the point on the part of the thigh where the bulging muscle resembles a crouching rabbit.

Reference to yin and yang in a point name is straightforward, such as Instep Yang (BL-50). Concrete reference may also be given to a five-phase relationship, such as Water Spring (KI-5). More abstract are point names that imply a five-phase association through reference to a color associated with a phase, such as Guarding White (LU-4).

Point names may often serve to remind the practitioner of the channel to which a point belongs. Earth Granary (ST-4), for example, recalls the stomach channel because the stomach is the "granary organ" and is associated with the earth phase. In a more abstract manner the name Central Treasury (LU-1) indicates that the point is the intersection-jiaohui point of the lung (treasury) and stomach (center) channels. Point names may have other functions such as recalling prohibitions for a point, as in Arm Five Li (LI-13), which, if needled, damages the qi of the five wards or interiors (viscera).

Usually two or more functions can be cited for a given point name. For example, the name Ear Gate (TB-21) is both functional and locational because it refers to the point's effectiveness in the treatment of ear disease, as well as the point's location at the front of the ear. The name Yin Cleft (HT-6) recalls that the point is located on the yin side of the arm, that it belongs to the shao yin channel, and that it is in the cleft-xi point of that channel. This point name is thus locational and functional and at the same time recalls the point's relationship to its home channel.

Though Chinese sources disagree on the number of classifications of point names, many texts do make an effort to categorize the names. The fourteen categories that follow are representative of the Chinese system, and include clarifying examples. Readers may note that further information may be gleaned by reference to **Appendix A, Glossary of Single Characters.**

Sample Categorizations	
Yin, Yang & Five Phases	
Yin	Yin Intersection (CV-7)
	Yin Market (ST-33)
Yang	Yang Valley (SI-5)
	Yang Mound Spring (GB-34)
Five Phases	Yellow Emperor (SP-4)
	Lesser Shang (LU-11)
Organs, Qi and Blood	
Organ names	Heart Shu (BL-15)
	Gallbladder Shu (BL-19)
Organ functions	Spirit Hall (BL-44)
Qi	Sea of Qi (CV-6)
	Origin Pass (CV-4)
Blood	Sea of Blood (SP-10)
Channels	
Channel Pathway	Eyebrow Ascension (BL-3)
Channel Intersections	Hundred Convergences (GV-20)
	Three Yin Intersection (SP-6)
Channel Name	Girdling Vessel (GB-26)
Periodic Qi Flow	Extending Vessel (BL-62)
Location & Function	
Point Function	Wind Pool (GB-20)
	Bright Eyes (BL-1)
Anatomy	Breast Center (ST-17)
	Jade Pillow (BL-9)
Locational Hints	Winnower Gate (SP-11)
	Standing by White (LU-4)
Body Measurements	Cubit Marsh (LU-5)
	Foot Three Li (ST-36)
Astronomic, Meteorologic & Geographic Associations	
Astronomic	Sun and Moon (GB-24)
	Celestial Pivot (ST-25)
Meteorologic	Wind Mansion (GV-16)
	Cloud Gate (LU-2)
Geographic	Mountain Support (BL-57)
	Outer Mound (ST-26)
Water-related phenomenon	Branch Ditch (TB-6)
	Shining Sea (KI-6)
Place names	Metal Gate (BL-63)
	Shang Hill (SP-5)

Numeric & Trigrammatic Relationships	
Numeric	Second Space (LI-2)
	Fifth Place (BL-5)
Trigrammatic	Severe Mouth (ST-45)
Architectural Structures	
Gate Tower	Great Gate Tower (CV-14)
Palace	Purple Palace (CV-19)
Storeroom	Storeroom (ST-14)
Granary	Stomach Granary (BL-50)
Abode	Qi Abode (ST-11)
	Bowel Abode (SP-13)
Hall	Jade Hall (CV-18)
Chamber	Will Chamber (BL-52)
Corridor	Corridor Walk (KI-22)
Court (Courtyard)	Spirit Court (GV-24)
	Central Courtyard (CV-16)
Window	Eye Window (GB-16)
	Celestial Window (SI-16)
Gate	Wind Gate (BL-12)
	Spirit Gate (HT-7)
Door	Qi Door (ST-13)
Space	Unyielding Space (GV-18)
	Second Space (LI-2)
Places of Activity	
Metropolises	Great Metropolis (SP-2)
	Yin Metropolis (KI-19)
Markets	Wind Market (GB-31)
	Yin Market (ST-33)
Countryside (Village)	Chest Village (SP-19)
Li (Ward or District)	Foot Three Li (ST-36)
	Connecting Li (HT-5)
Path	Spirit Path (GV-11)
	Linking Path (GB-28)
Pass	Yang Pass (GB-3)
	Outer Pass (TB-5)
Plants, Animals & Objects	
Plants	Grain Bone-Hole (LI-19)
Animals	Crouching Rabbit (ST-32)
Objects	Celestial Tripod (LI-17)
Characters	Celestial Pivot (ST-25)
	Inner Courtyard (ST-44)

The reader should note that alternate point names usually come from schools and traditions whose practice styles have faded from use in modern China. The main point names used in this book are a standard set of names adopted by most Chinese texts. GV-2 and GB-39 are the only points that have more than one name in most modern books. In contrast, the *Great Compendium of Acupuncture and Moxibustion* (1601), in a chapter entitled "Points that have Various Names" lists 88 points that have two names, 26 points that have three names, eight points that have four names, two points that have five names and two points that have six names. The listing in that book was compiled from the *Glorious Anthology of Acupuncture* and reflects only the alternate names from certain books and traditions. If all the alternate names ever coined were included, the list would be considerably longer.

Frequently, alternate names were the result of erroneous written transcription. Mistranscriptions due to printer error, for example, are not uncommon. In the *Thousand Gold Piece Prescriptions,* the author, Sun Si Miao, calls LI-14 頭沖 *tóu chōng,* Head Surge. In the book he wrote fifty years later, the *Supplemented Thousand Gold Piece Prescriptions,* LI-14 is named 頸沖 *jǐng chōng,* Neck Surge. Presumably, the latter name was the result of a mistranscription by the printer owing to the similarity of the characters for neck and head, 頸 and 頭 , although it is also possible that the former name was incorrect and Sun Si Miao corrected the error in the latter book. Alternate names that resulted from this type of mistranscription are easy to recognize because the characters of various names for the same point are similar in appearance.

Mistranscriptions due to mistakes in verbal transmission also occurred. Some were attributable to the scribe who, while recording the words of the teacher, mistook the teacher's intended word for a homophone. This resulted in point names of the same pronunciation represented by different characters and therefore different meanings. The second type resulted when a scribe understood what word the teacher was saying but couldn't remember how to write the proper character. He then substituted a character that was similar in either sound or construction to the correct one. The alternate names that resulted from this type of mistranscription are similar to the original name in pronunciation and/or appearance.

Some schools of acupuncture gave the points different names either to distinguish the school or to maintain secret traditions. These point names are recognizable by their lack of resemblance to the other names for the same point. They are found in books that expound a particular school of thought. Perhaps most obvious among this type of point name are the thirteen ghost points. The earliest extant recording of these points as a group is that given by Sun Si Miao in the *Thousand Gold Piece Prescriptions*. They were based on an earlier list from the Song Dynasty and were specifically intended for the treatment of ghost diseases, i.e. diseases where the patient behaves as if possessed by a ghost. Each of the ghost points thus has an alternate name that includes the word "ghost," for example, Ghost Heart (PC-7) and Ghost Pillow (GV-14).

Other alternate names come directly from the classics. An alternate name for ST-25, Large Intestine Mu, owes its existence to a passage in the *Classic of Difficult Issues* that describes ST-25 as being the alarm-mu point of the large intestine. Because the Chinese revered classical texts, later writers adopted this description as a name for the point.

Readers who wish to discover the origins of alternate names may compare the pinyin and the characters, thus discerning similarities and connections. This type of investigation often reveals a great deal about the primary point name or about the point itself, especially if studied in conjunction with the function, treatment scope and location of the point. Study of the alternate names provides a broader terrain in which to explore the primary point names as a means to understanding the points themselves.

A Brief Discussion
of Chinese Characters

Before embarking on an exploration into the Chinese names of the acupuncture points, it is best that the reader have some familiarity with the construction of Chinese characters. Certain characters and parts of characters should be recognizable in order to derive the greatest benefit from the text. The following discussion is intended to provide the reader with enough information to make reading the explanations of point names a richer and more satisfying experience.

The simplest Chinese characters are stylized images of the things they represent. For example, the Chinese character 日 *rì*, which means the sun, was originally written as a circle with a dot in the middle. It was later squared for ease of writing and the dot extended to a line for clarity. The character 月 *yuè,* meaning moon, similarly derives from a picture of the crescent moon.

The vast majority of characters are not composed of one element as in the examples above, but of two or more. For instance, the characters 日 and 月 are combined to form 明 *míng,* meaning bright, clear or light.

In characters consisting of more than one element, one element is the radical while the other element or elements are additional meaning components or characters borrowed only for their sound. Characters that are used as sound elements within other characters are called phonetic elements. Returning to the example of 明 *míng,* 日 is the radical while 月 is an additional meaning component. In 灸 *jiǔ,* meaning moxibustion, 火 is the radical while the element 久 simply represents the sound *jiŭ*. As a character in its own right, 久 *jiŭ* means "for an extended period of time," a notion that has little or nothing to do with moxibustion. The fact that it shares the same sound as 灸 suggests that it was incorporated for its sound rather than its meaning.

Radicals

Each character has one element that is called its radical, comprising the essential category of meaning. The term "radical," which means literally "of the root," is of primary importance in the discussion of the structure of Chinese characters. The ability to recognize some of the more common radicals will greatly enhance the benefit that the student derives from the study of the acupuncture point names. There are 214 radicals all told. Following is a discussion of 22 that occur frequently in characters relating to Chinese medicine.

The fire radical, 火 *huŏ*

This radical is a character in its own right and is a picture of a flame. As might be expected, this radical lends a meaning of heat to characters of which it is a part. It is sometimes written as four dots at the bottom of a character. In some such cases, it originally represented not fire but the legs of an animal. Examples of characters with the fire radical are 炮 *pào*, to roast; 熱 *rè*, heat; 煩 *fán*, annoyed, vexed; 烏 *wū*, a crow, or black; 烤 *kǎo*, to bake or roast; 燒 *shāo*, to burn; and 灸 *jiŭ*, moxibustion. The character 火 *huŏ* represents the fire phase of the five phases.

The earth radical, 土 *tǔ*

This radical is also its own character and represents earth in the five phases. It also means land or soil. The top horizontal line represents the surface of the earth while the bottom line is the rock below the earth. The vertical line is a symbol for the life that the earth produces. Examples of characters with the earth radical include: 堅 *jiān,* durable; 增 *zēng,* to increase; and 墟 *xū,* ruins.

The metal radical, 金 *jīn*

This radical is its own character and represents the metal phase of the five phases. It can refer specifically to gold or to metal in general. The top portion of the character is a modified form of the character 今 *jīn* and is in this case a phonetic element. The lower portion is a pictograph of two nuggets of gold lying beneath the earth (土). Characters that contain this radical are usually related to metal in some way: 針 *zhēn,* needle; 銅 *tóng,* copper or bronze; and 錢 *qián,* money.

The water radical, 水 *shuǐ*

This character represents the water phase of the five phases. In its radical form it generally appears as three dots on the left side of characters that represent bodies of water or are related to water or fluids in some way. Examples include: 池 *chí* , pool or pond; 海 *hǎi,* sea; and 漿 *jiāng,* thick liquid.

The wood radical, 木 *mù*

This character is a pictograph of a tree and represents the wood phase of the five phases. Most characters that contain a wood radical are related to wood or trees, but in some cases the connections are more abstract. This radical is usually found on the left of a character, but is sometimes printed underneath. The following characters contain the wood radical: 根 *gēn,* root; 森 *sēn,* forest; 樞 *shū,* pivot; 橫 *héng,* horizontal; and 榮 *róng,* glorious or luxuriant.

The hand radical, 手 *shǒu*

This radical is most often seen in its alternate form with only two crosswise strokes, as in the left-hand portion of the character 扶 *fú*, to support. It is a pictorial representation of a hand and is thus a part of characters that relate to the hand itself or to actions that can be performed by the hand. Examples of this radical are: 找 *zhǎo*, to search; 打 *dǎ*, to hit; 推 *tuī*, to push; and 掌 *zhǎng*, the palm of the hand. Note that in the last example the primary form of the radical is used.

The mouth radical, 口 *kǒu*

This character is usually found on the left or in the middle of characters in which it is a radical. Because it is a picture of a mouth it often implies a relationship to speaking, eating, or making sounds. Examples include: 句 *jù*, a sentence; 問 *wèn*, to ask; 吃 *chī*, to eat; 吐 *tù*, to vomit, to spit up; and 叫 *jiào*, to call out.

The heart radical, 心 *xīn*

This character is a stylized pictograph of a heart. Characters in which 心 is a radical carry meanings that relate to the heart, mind and emotions. This radical is usually found on the left side of the character in its altered form, as the following examples show: 情 *qīng*, feeling, emotion; or 怕 *pà*, to fear. When in its unaltered form it is generally found at the bottom of a character. Examples of characters containing the heart radical are: 思 *sī*, to contemplate; 恨 *hèn*, to hate; 悶 *mēn*, feeling of oppression; 怒 *nù*, anger; 意 *yì*, thought or meaning; 念 *niàn*, to ponder; 忘 *wàng*, to forget; and 志 *zhì*, will.

The person radical, 人 *rén*

This character is a stick picture of a person. As a radical it is generally found on the left of the character in its alternate form as seen in the examples below. Though it often brings a connotation of person to characters for which it is a radical, the simplicity of the character has led to it becoming a derived form of what were once other elements. This radical is also used to indicate male as opposed to female in characters that require gender clarification. The characters that follow contain the person radical: 他 *tā*, he; 仁 *rén*, benevolence; 什 *shé*, what; 便 *biàn*, convenient; and 住 *zhù*, to reside.

The sun radical, 日 *rì*

The character 日 *rì* is a pictograph of the sun. It is often found as a radical in words that are related to the sun or, by extension, time or brightness. Some examples are: 星 *xīng*, star; 暫 *zhàn*, temporarily; 暮 *mù*, sunset; 早 *zǎo*, early; and 明 *míng*, bright, clear or light.

The moon radical, 月 *yuè*

This character is a pictograph of a crescent moon. It is found in characters that have to do with moonlight or the passage of time (months). It is not a common radical but is included here to differentiate it from the flesh radical discussed next. An example of the moon (or month) radical is 期 *qí*, time period.

The flesh radical, 肉 *rù*

This character represents meat or muscle. When functioning as a radical it is usually written as 月 and is thus easily confused with the moon radical. Since only a few characters contain the moon radical it is usually safe to assume that most characters that involve 月 as an element are related to flesh in some way. Furthermore, the moon radical is found on the right of a character while the flesh radical is found on the left or bottom. Characters containing this radical include: 胃 *wèi,* stomach; 肝 *gān,* liver; 腕 *wàn,* wrist; 脊 *jí ,* spine; and 肩 *jiān,* shoulder.

The disease radical, 疒 *chuāng*

This radical was originally a pictorial representation of a person in bed. It is found on the outside of most characters relating to illness. Some examples are: 病 *bìng,* disease; 痹 *bì ,* bi (blockage and pain); 瘡 *chuāng,* sore or ulcer; 療 *liáo,* to cure; and 疤 *bā,* a scar. The disease radical is not used as a character itself, it is always combined with other components.

The gate radical, 門 *mén*

This character is a picture of a double door that opens in the middle. It is used as a radical in many characters that have meanings related to gates or openings or extended meanings such as to open or close. Some examples are: 關 *guān,* a pass, to shut, relationship; 開 *kāi,* to open, to start; 闕 *què,* gate tower, a mistake; and 間 *jiān,* a space, between.

The bone radical, 骨 *gǔ*

This character means bone and is often used as a radical in characters that relate to the skeleton. It is almost always on the left of the character. Examples include: 體 *tǐ,* body; and 髎 *liáo,* bone-hole;

The head radical, 頁 *yè*

When used alone this character means a page of a book, but as a radical it represents the head. It usually occurs on the right side of characters. Examples of characters containing this radical are: 頂 *dǐng,* a summit; 頭 *tóu,* head; 顱 *lú,* skull; and 額 *è,* forehead.

The bamboo radical, 竹 *zhú*

This character appears as a radical at the top of characters in slightly altered form. 筆 *bǐ,* pen; and 管 *guǎn,* tube or pipe are examples of this radical.

The silk radical, 糸 *mì*

This character, when used as a radical, appears generally on the left of characters, although it is sometimes printed underneath. Examples are: 細 *xì,* fine, minute, detailed; 素 *sù,* plain, simple.

The grass radical, 艸 *cǎo.*

This character appears as a radical in altered form at the top of characters, much like two "+" signs side by side. Examples are: 艾 *ài,* moxa; 芽 *yá,* a sprout; 茶 *chá,* tea.

The ear radical, 耳 *ěr*

This character appears as a radical either on the left or at the bottom of characters. Examples are: 聯 *lián,* to unite, to connect; 聽 *tīng,* to listen; 聲 *shēng,* sound, voice.

The word radical, 言 *yán*

This character appears as a radical most commonly on the left side of characters, though it is sometimes found underneath. Examples are: 説 *shuō,* to speak, to say; 請 *qǐng,* to invite; 警 *jǐng,* to alert, to warn.

The rock radical, 石 *shí*

This character appears as a radical most often at the left of and sometimes underneath characters. 砂 *shā*, sand, gravel; 破 *pò*, to break, are examples.

The student of Chinese medicine will find that these twenty-two radicals provide a good basis for approximating meanings or achieving general associations for unfamiliar characters.

Character Categories

When studying Chinese characters it is helpful to be familiar with the six categories of characters. The reader who wishes to gain a deeper understanding of the origins and relations of the various alternate names for the acupuncture points will find these categories especially useful. These include imitative symbols, indicative symbols, logical combinations, phonetic components, false borrowing and extended interpretation. Each is discussed separately below.

Imitative Symbols

Characters that resemble in form the thing that they represent are called imitative symbols. Examples are: 木 *mù*, tree; 門 *mén*, door; and 弓 *gōng*, archer's bow.

Indicative Symbols

These are characters that represent concepts or actions. For example, the character 旦 *dàn*, meaning sunrise, is a picture of the sun, (日) rising over the horizon (一). The characters 上 *shàng* and 下 *xià* are also indicative symbols, deriving their respective meanings of above and below by depicting objects above and below the horizon.

Logical Combinations

Characters in this category are formed by combining characters from the above two categories in such a way that a new concept or object is expressed. The character 男 *nán*, meaning man, is a good example. It is made up of the characters 田 *tián,* meaning field, and 力 *lì,* meaning strength. 男 *nán* then comes to mean man through the idea that a man is one who uses his strength working the fields. Examples of logical combinations include: 林 *lín,* which is formed of two wood (木 *mù*) radicals side by side and means forest, and 炎 *yán,* two fires (火 *huǒ*) one atop the other, meaning burning hot.

Phonetic Compounds

These are characters made up of a radical combined with an element that provides a cue for the pronunciation of the character. The character 揚 yáng, which means to raise up, is composed of the hand radical (手 *shǒu*) on the left and the character 易 *yáng,* which means bright or glorious, on the right. The hand radical provides the meaning for the character, as the hand is often the motivating force behind a lifting action. The addition of 易 *yáng* on the right side serves only to lend its sound to the character and has no bearing whatsoever on its meaning.

Often a phonetic element contributes only the final part of its sound to a character. Therefore, in the characters 腸 *cháng* (intestine) and 湯 *tāng* (soup, decoction), the phonetic 易 *yáng* represents only the final sound "ang" of the characters, while the initial "y" sound in 易 *yáng* has been changed to the sound "ch" in 腸 *cháng* and "t" in 湯 *tāng.*

In rarer cases a phonetic element contributes meaning as well as sound to a character. For example, the character 陽 *yáng,* the complement of *yīn,* is composed of the radical that means a pile of earth on the left and the phonetic element 易 *yáng* on the right. As stated above, 易 , when standing alone as a character, can mean bright. Thus it can be seen that 易 lends meaning as well as sound to the character 陽 , which originally meant the sunny side of a hill.

Secondly, sound changes, which occur in all languages with the passage of time, have wreaked considerable havoc on the Chinese phonetic system. Unfortunately, this damage is most pronounced in the Mandarin dialect of northern China, which pinyin romanization transcribes. The student who is unaware of this problem may wonder why 河 is pronounced *hé* when the character that acts as its phonetic component, 可, is pronounced *kě*. The answer lies in the assumption that the two characters were originally pronounced in the same way, and that the pronunciation of one has changed. The original identity of sound, partially destroyed in Mandarin, has nevertheless been preserved by Cantonese, in which both characters are pronounced *hé*. In many instances, the sound changes that have occurred in northern China, while affecting initial sounds, have spared the final sounds. Focusing attention on the final sounds will often reveal this, as the above example shows: the "k" and "h" indicate a sound change, though the final sound "e" is preserved.

The above four categories explain the composition of original characters. The following two categories relate to the expression of new ideas using already established characters.

False Borrowing

When a character takes on a meaning that was not originally its own, it is referred to as false borrowing. This can occur through erroneous substitution of one character for another, or by the intentional use of an already existing character to express the meaning of a word that previously existed only in the spoken language. In the latter case characters of the same pronunciation as the spoken words were borrowed to represent new meanings.

Extended Interpretation

A character whose meaning is derived, metaphorical, adapted or figurative belongs to the category of extended interpretation. For example, the character 尊 *zūn* was originally a pictorial representation of two hands offering forth some wine. By extension it has come to mean to honor or respect.

Characters and Meaning

Certain aspects of the Chinese language make the interpretation of ancient Chinese writings, including the point names, particularly difficult. The two aspects of Chinese that prove most troublesome in this respect are the numerous grammatical roles that single characters can assume and the multitude of meanings inherent in a given character.

In Chinese, unlike European languages, parts of speech are not clearly distinguished. Take for example the character 中 *zhōng*. As an adjective this character means central, as a noun it means center, and as a verb, to strike (i.e., in the center). The grammatical function of characters and the relationships between the concepts they represent are determined largely by context. This presents particular problems in terms of the point names, as they are presented with no context other than that we know they are names of points. Take for example Lung One, which in Chinese is called 中府 *zhōng fǔ*. Owing to lack of context, the intended grammatical function of the character 中 *zhōng* is unclear. It could conceivably be an adjective, a noun or a verb. Thus, the name could be interpreted as meaning "central treasury," "center's treasury," "center of the treasury," or even "strike the treasury." While the last possibility can be eliminated due to illogic, plausible explanations can be offered for each of the other three.

A character can take on not only numerous grammatical roles, but numerous meanings and nuances as well. This is a result of the long history of the Chinese language and the tendency of the characters to take on extended meanings. The looseness of Chinese syntax and the wide range of meanings associated with a given character mean that almost any point name could be rendered in a host of different ways in English. Take again the example of Lung One, 中府 *zhōng fǔ*. The character 府 *fǔ*, though always used as a noun, can take on meanings as various as "treasury," "storehouse," "mansion," or "prefecture." This name could be rendered as Central Treasury, Central Storehouse, Central Mansion, Center's Prefecture, Center's Treasury, Center's Storehouse, Center's Mansion, Center's Prefecture etc.

In many cases, it is difficult to decide which rendering comes closest to the meaning originally intended. It is sometimes impossible to find a phrase in English that will cover more than one of the completely different possible interpretations. For example, in the Chinese point name for Liver Five, 蠡溝 *lí gōu,* the character 蠡 (pronounced both *lí* and *lǐ*) can represent either a wood-boring insect or a gourd, and the character 溝 *gōu* can mean a ditch, a canal or a gutter. Since no single English word expresses the many meanings implied by the two Chinese characters, renderings as different as Woodworm Canal and Gourd Ditch can be equally justified.

Since innumerable interpretations of the point names are possible, the reader is encouraged to explore the various possibilities and create renderings that meet his or her own needs. By no means should the renderings given in this or any other text be taken as the only correct interpretations. Attempts to translate or to learn a "one and only" rendering will result in the loss of insight, information, and understanding.

PART

II

Point Names

The Lung Channel
(Hand Tai Yin)

手太陰肺經

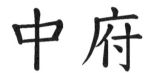

Central Treasury

LU-1 *(zhōng fǔ)*

中 *zhōng:* central, center
府 *fǔ:* treasury, storehouse; mansion

Alternate Names

Treasury Center Shu	府中俞	*fǔ zhōng shū*
Breast Center Shu	膺中俞	*yīng zhōng shū*
Breast Shu	膺俞	*yīng shū*
Lung Mu	肺募	*fèi mù*

Classical Location: One inch and six fen below Cloud Gate (LU-2), above the breast in the third intercostal space, six body inches lateral from Florid Canopy (CV-20), in a depression where a pulsating vessel can be felt.
(Great Compendium)

Point Associations: Alarm-mu point of the lung; intersection-jiaohui point of the hand tai yin lung and foot tai yin spleen channels.

Explanation of Point Name

This point is the intersection-jiaohui point of the lung and spleen channels, and its name reflects the lung's relationship to the spleen and stomach as a "treasury" for center (i.e., spleen-stomach) qi. *The Systematized Canon* asserts that "central qi resides in the chest [i.e., the lung]." (中氣舍于胸中). This is traditionally explained as referring to the spleen's function of extracting the essence of digesta and sending it to the lung, where it is combined with celestial qi (air) to form channel qi, and to the fact that the lung channel originates in the stomach: two manifestations of earth (spleen) engendering metal (lung) in five-phase theory.

LU-1 is also the alarm-mu point of the lung, alarm-mu points being places where the qi of the associated organ gathers. Lung qi collects at this point just as taxes are collected at the central treasury.

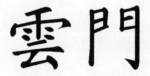

Cloud Gate

LU-2 *(yún mén)*

雲 *yún:* cloud
門 *mén:* gate, door

Classical Location: Below the clavicle, in the depression two inches to the side of Qi Door (ST-13), six inches from the midline of the chest, where a pulsating vessel can be felt. The point is located with the arm raised.
(Great Compendium)

Explanation of Point Name

The *Inner Canon* describes the fluids in the upper burner as a fog or mist. The lung is in the upper burner amongst the mist of the heavens or "clouds." Furthermore, the lung distributes fluids throughout the body (and is the origin of the qi cycle, which nourishes the whole body) and may therefore be likened to clouds giving rain and nourishment to the earth.

LU-2 is the point where the channel qi cycle begins. The cycle goes through the 12 channels until it reaches LV-14. From there the cycle begins anew via a branch that reconnects with LU-2. Because it is the entry point of the channel qi, it is called a gate.

As is true of Central Treasury (LU-1), the name Cloud Gate implies a relationship with the qi of the earth. *Essential Questions* points this out in the following phrase: "Earth's qi ascends as clouds; heaven's qi descends as rain." (素問: 陰陽應象大論 "地氣上爲雲， 天氣下爲 雨.") 地 *dì* , the character used for earth in this quote, is the counterpart of heaven, and not the earth of the five phases, 土 *tǔ*. In older texts these two characters often imply each other.

The derivation of this name may also have some relation to 雲門 *yún mén,* the name of an ancient piece of music.

天府

Celestial Storehouse

LU-3 *(tiān fǔ)*

天 *tiān:* celestial, of the heavens; sky; Nature; heaven
府 *fǔ:* storehouse, treasury; mansion

Classical Location: Located at a pulse three inches below the armpit and five inches above the elbow. The tip of the nose can just reach this point; dab the nose with ink to mark the spot. *(Great Compendium)*

Explanation of Point Name

Because it is the gathering place of celestial qi the lung is, in a sense, a Celestial Storehouse. The *Spiritual Axis* states, "from the waist up is celestial, and from the waist down is earthly." (腰以上爲天,腰下爲地.) This analogy applies not only to position, but also to function. The lung receives qi from the earth and nourishes the body just as a storehouse receives produce from the land and nourishes the people, or as a treasury receives income and supports the country.

The character combination 天府 *tiān fǔ* is a star name, a place name and a government position. It is also an ancient expression for the breasts, the place in the upper body (天) where milk is "stored." This point is located on the arm at the level of the breasts, and its name is helpful in reminding us of this fact.

俠白

Guarding White

LU-4 *(xiá bái)*

俠 *xiá:* to protect, to guard; hero (someone who performs heroic deeds such as protecting the weak)
白 *bái:* white

Alternate Name

Pinching White 夾白 *jiā bái*

Classical Location: Below Celestial Storehouse (LU-3) at a pulsating vessel five inches from the elbow.
(Great Compendium)

Explanation of Point Name

The character 俠 *xiá* has the meaning "to protect." White, the color associated with metal in five phase theory, is often used to represent the lung. Therefore the point name conveys a sense of protecting the lung, while at the same time it serves as a reminder that the point is on the lung channel.

Sometimes the character 俠 *xiá* is explained as meaning 夾 *jiā* because these two characters were not clearly distinguished in classical Chinese. 夾 *jiā* carries the meaning of to pinch (or be pinched) from both sides. Thus, because LU-4 is "pinched" between the white skin of the arm and the chest, or between the red and white skin of the arm, it could be considered to be "pinched by white." In fact, 夾

-27-

白 *jiā bái* , Pinching White, is the alternate name for this point. The name Guarding White can reflect this interpretation as well if one considers that a guarded object is often "pinched" between those who guard it.

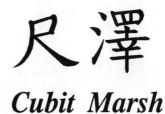

Cubit Marsh

LU-5 *(chǐ zé)*

尺 *chǐ:* a Chinese measure (about one foot)
澤 *zé:* marsh; dregs

Alternate Names

Ghost Endurance	鬼受	*guǐ shòu*
Ghost Hall	鬼堂	*guǐ táng*

Classical Location: Where a pulsating vessel can be felt on the elbow crease, in the depression between the sinew and bone, felt with the elbow flexed. *(Great Compendium)*

Point Associations: Uniting-he (water) point.

Explanation of Point Name

Each transporting-shu point of the regular channels has a five-phase correspondence. The uniting-he points on the yin channels are water points. The character 澤 *zé*, marsh, is a reference to its designation as the water point of the lung channel. The point is located in a depression one foot (cubit) away from the pulse of the hand and is therefore named Cubit Marsh. By giving the point this name the ancients included references to both the location and the five-phase relationship of the point.

The word marsh in the point name also can serve to recall that LU-5 is the uniting-he point of the channel. A marsh often exists where rivers unite with the sea and the qi at uniting-he points is said to resemble the water of a river as it joins the sea.

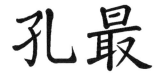

Collection Hole

LU-6 *(kŏng zuì)*

孔 *kŏng:* hole, aperture
最 *zuì:* to collect, to gather; a superlative adverb, that
is equivalent to "most" or the suffix "-est"

Classical Location: Below Cubit Marsh (LU-5), seven inches from the wrist crease, in the depression between the two bones. *(Golden Mirror)*

Point Associations: Cleft-xi point of the lung channel.

Explanation of Point Name

Being the cleft-xi point of the lung channel, LU-6 is, by definition, located in a fissure-like depression. The character 最 *zuì* in this name refers to the depth of the hole and the point's subsequent ability to collect qi and blood. The character 孔 *kŏng,* meaning hole, further serves to remind the practitioner of the point's ability to treat diseases of the mouth and throat such as loss of voice, spitting of blood and sore throat.

列缺

Broken Sequence

LU-7 *(liè quē)*

列 *liè:* sequence; to arrange, to place
缺 *què:* imperfect, incomplete, deficient; vacant

Alternate Names

Child Mystery	童玄	*tóng xuán*
Wrist Taxation	腕勞	*wàn láo*

Classical Location: One and a half inches from the wrist. When the thumb and index finger of one hand are interlocked with those of the other, the point lies on the edge of the index finger, in a depression between the sinew and bone. *(Great Compendium)*

Point Associations: Connecting-luo point of the lung channel connecting to the large intestine channel; one of the four command points (it treats the head and neck).

Explanation of Point Name

The name of this point may be understood in terms of the path of the lung channel. At LU-7 the path splits to join the large intestine channel at LI-4. This splitting can be seen as a break in the sequence of points on the lung channel. This argument may also be understood as a break in the general sequence of the channel system. In most cases qi is transferred from the last point of one channel to the first point of the following channel. Here LU-7, and not the last lung channel point, LU-11, is the issue point of the lung channel (qi flows from LU-7 to LI-4), creating, in effect, a deviation from the basic sequential pattern of qi flow through the channels.

The character 列 *liè,* meaning "sequence," may have been a transcription of its homophone 裂 *liè,* meaning "burst." The qi of the lung channel is gathered at LU-6, the cleft-xi point, and from there like a river breaking open a dam the qi bursts forth and forks at LU-7. If we combine the meaning of 列 with that of 裂 we can interpret the name as "bursting forth and breaking sequence," which is a description of the flow of qi at this point.

Ma Dan Yang describes LU-7, one of his twelve heavenly star points, as a "thunderhead spitting fire." This description refers to both the fork in the pathway, which is similar to a fork in a bolt of lightning, and to the nature of the qi at this point. It further carries out the analogy of the lung and heaven exemplified in the names Cloud Gate (LU-2) and Celestial Treasury (LU-3). Interpreting the point name in line with Ma Dan Yang's description is justified by the fact that 列缺 is an ancient expression for lightning.

LU-7 may be located by interlocking the two tigers' mouths (the tiger's mouth is the space between the index finger and the thumb) and placing the forefinger on the hollow in the bone (radius). The character 列 *liè* can mean "to place" and 缺 *què* may indicate an empty place or a hollow. Viewed in this way the name then becomes a mnemonic device for remembering the method of location; i.e., placing the finger on the hollow.

經渠

Channel Ditch

LU-8 (jīng qú)

經 *jīng:* channel, river; warp (as in the warp and woof
      of weaving)
渠 *qū:* gutter, ditch, canal

Classical Location: In the depression at the inch pulse.
(Great Compendium)

Point Associations: River-jing (metal) point.

Explanation of Point Name

Essential Questions states that the qi and blood at river-jing
points "move and do not dwell." As LU-8 is the river-jing
point of the channel the qi is said to flow unceasingly here.
The character 經 *jīng* is used in Chinese medicine to denote not only the channels, but also the river-jing points,
because the original meaning of the character 經 *jīng* had
to do with the flow of water, implying the flow at the
point. The character 渠 *qū* made reference to the location
of the point in the ditch-like depression between the radius
and the flexor carpi radialis tendon.

The point name is therefore a reminder both that LU-8 is
the river-jing point and that it is located in a ditch-like depression.

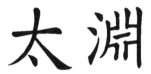

Great Abyss

LU-9 *(tài yuān)*

太 *tài:* great, very
淵 *yuān:* abyss, deep source (of water)

Alternate Names

Ghost Heart	鬼心	*guǐ xīn*
Great Spring	太泉	*tài quán*

Classical Location: At the pulsating vessel, at the inner extremity of the crease, behind the hand. *(Great Compendium)*

Point Associations: Meeting-hui point of the vessels; stream-shu (earth) point; source-yuan point of the lung.

Explanation of Point Name

The three dots on the left side of the character 淵 *yuān* indicate that it represents an abyss from which water flows (the three dots are an abbreviated form of the character for water). In this sense it is much the same as the characters 源 and 原 , both of which are pronounced *yuān* and can mean source or origin. LU-9 is the source-yuan point of the lung channel and the meeting-hui point of the vessels, thus the qi here is plentiful and deep like an abyss. The 淵 (abyss) portion of the point name underscores the relationship between LU-9 and source qi, describes the nature of the qi at the point and brings to mind the point's location in a depression. LU-9 is a "great" abyss because it is more than simply the source-yuan point of the lung channel; it is also the earth point of the metal channel, and since in the five phases earth engenders metal, LU-9 can be said to be the source of metal qi on the lung channel.

A spring (i.e., a mountain spring) is an origin or source and an alternate name for LU-9 is Great Spring. The two names thus return to the same meaning.

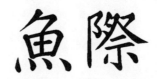

Fish Border

LU-10 (yú jì)

魚 yú: fish
際 jì: border

Classical Location: Behind the base joint of the thumb, in the depression on the inside border of the red and white flesh. *(Great Compendium)*

Point Associations: Spring-ying (fire) point.

Explanation of Point Name

The fleshy portion of the hand where LU-10 is located reminded the Chinese of the belly of a fish. Border, in this case, refers to the border of the red and white flesh, the yang and yin aspects of the body's exterior.

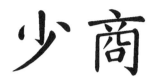

Lesser Shang

LU-11 *(shào shāng)*

少 *shào:* few, little
商 *shāng:* 5th sound of the Chinese musical scale;
merchant, trader

Alternate Name

Ghost Sincerity 鬼信 *guǐ xìn*

Classical Location: On the inside of the thumb, about the width of a Chinese leek leaf from the corner of the nail. *(Great Compendium)*

Point Associations: Well-jing (wood) point. The second of the thirteen ghost points.

Explanation of Point Name

The 商 *shāng* sound is the note related to metal and thus the lung. LU-11, which is located on a yin channel, is referred to as Lesser Shang because the five sounds are divided into greater and lesser aspects, and the yin aspect of each sound is called lesser.

Shang may be qualified by 少 *shào* because this is the well-jing point of the channel, where the channel is a mere trickle, i.e., has little qi. If that is the case the translation Small Shang would be appropriate.

Large Intestine Channel
(Hand Yang Ming)

手陽明大腸經

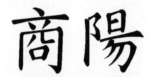

Shang Yang

LI-1 *(shāng yáng)*
商 *shāng:* 5th note of Chinese musical scale; merchant
陽 *yáng:* yang, the complement of yin

Alternate Name

Extreme Yang   絶陽   *jué yáng*

Classical Location: On the inside of the index finger, the width of a Chinese leek leaf from the corner of the nail. *(Great Compendium)*

Point Associations: Well-jing (metal) point.

Explanation of Point Name

The character 商 *shāng* represents the sound associated with metal in five phase theory. LI-1 is the metal point of the yang metal channel, thus it is called Shang Yang. It is not entirely clear why the *shāng* sound is represented at LI-1 and LU-11 and not at other points of the metal channels. It may be because these two points are effective in treating disorders of the throat, the organ that produces the five sounds.

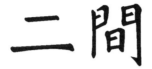

Second Space

LI-2 *(èr jiān)*

二 *èr:* two, second
間 *jiān:* space, gap, crevice

Alternate Names

Space Valley	間谷	*jiān gǔ*
Whole Valley	周谷	*zhōu gǔ*

Classical Location: On the inner side of the index finger, in the depression in front of the base joint.
(Great Compendium)

Point Associations: Spring-ying (water) point.

Explanation of Point Name

"Second space" refers to the "space," i.e., the depression on the distal side of the metacarpal phalangeal joint, at which the second point of the large intestine channel is located.

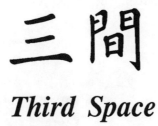

Third Space

LI-3 *(sān jiān)*

三 *sān:* three, third

間 *jiān:* space, crevice, gap

Alternate Names

Lesser Valley	少谷	*shào gǔ*
Small Valley	小谷	*xiǎo gǔ*

Classical Location: On the inner side of the index finger, in the depression behind the base joint of the index finger. *(Great Compendium)*

Point Associations: Stream-shu (wood) point.

Explanation of Point Name

The character 三 *sān,* meaning third, refers to LI-3 being the third point on the channel, while the character 間 *jiān,* which means space, refers to the depression proximal to the head of the second metacarpal bone.

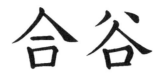

Union Valley

LI-4 *(hé gǔ)*

合 *hé:* a union; to meet
谷 *gǔ:* valley

Alternate Names

Tiger's Mouth	虎口	*hǔ kǒu*
Uniting Bones	合骨	*hé gǔ*
Holding Mouth	含口	*hán kǒu*

Classical Location: In the depression where the index finger and thumb bones part. *(Great Compendium)*

Point Associations: Source-yuan point; the command point of the face and mouth; one of the nine needles for returning yang.

Explanation of Point Name

This point is found in a valley-like depression at the union of the first and second metacarpal bones. Because the Chinese words for valley (谷 *gǔ*) and bone (骨 *gǔ*) are homophonic, the name serves as a particularly poetic mnemonic device.

The name of this point is also the name of a mountain. The flesh that protrudes at LI-4 when the thumb and forefinger are pressed together resembles a mountain.

The alternate names applied to LI-4 are particularly illuminating. Tiger's Mouth is a reference to the ability of the thumb and forefinger to open wide like a tiger's mouth. Holding Mouth is most likely a description of the point's location in the Tiger's Mouth, though it is possible that the character 含 *hán,* to hold or contain, is a mistranscription of the character 合 *hé* because the two characters are so similar. The name 合骨, Uniting Bones, is an intentional or unintentional variation based on the similar pronunciation of the characters 谷 *gǔ* and 骨 *gǔ.*

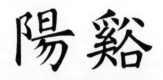

Yang Ravine

LI-5 *(yáng xī)*

陽 *yáng:* yang, the complement of yin
谿 *xī:* ravine, mountain creek gully, gorge

Alternate Name

Central Eminence   中魁   *zhōng kuí*

Classical Location: In the depression between the two sinews on the upper face of the wrist. *(Great Compendium)*

Point Associations: River-jing (fire) point.

Explanation of Point Name

This name is a reference to the location of the point on the yang aspect of the hand between the two tendons. The tendons represent the two walls of the ravine.

偏歷

Veering Passageway

LI-6 *(piān lì)*

偏 *piān:* inclined to one side; partial
歷 *lì:* to pass through; order, sequence

Classical Location: Moving upward from Yang Ravine (LI-5), three inches behind the wrist, located with the thumb and forefinger stretched out. *(Golden Mirror)*

Point Associations: Connecting-luo point of the hand yang ming large intestine channel connecting to the hand tai yin lung channel.

Explanation of Point Name

This point name is a reference to the connecting channel that veers from the main channel at LI-6 and travels to the lung channel.

溫溜

Warm Dwelling

LI-7 *(wēn liù)*

溫 *wēn:* warm
溜 *liū:* to flow; to slide, glide; slippery

Alternate Names

Snake Head	蛇頭	*shé tóu*
Pool's Head	池頭	*chí tóu*
Counterflow Pouring	逆注	*nì zhù*

Classical Location: Back from the wrist five inches on a tall person and six inches on a short one.
(Great Compendium)

Point Associations: Cleft-xi point of the hand yang ming large intestine channel.

Explanation of Point Name

The character 溜 *liū*, meaning to flow, and the character 留 *liú*, meaning to remain or stay, though clearly distinguished in modern writing, were much less so in classical Chinese. Without the three dots that indicate water the character can mean "to remain or stay." The yang ming channel is said to have copious qi (yang), and if the latter character is substituted in the name of this cleft-xi point it may then be taken as a reference to the warming yang qi that gathers at this location. Thus the name can be rendered as Warm Dwelling.

The *Essential Questions* says that the phenomenon of yin and yang existing simultaneously is called flowing (溜 *liū*). Although this is usually taken to refer to the quality of the pulse in the Spring (when yin and yang both exist), it can also be a description of the hand yang ming large intestine channel where both yin (blood) and yang (qi) are found in abundance. The point name can be seen as a reference to the warming flow of qi and blood through the yang ming channel.

The alternate name Snake Head is a reference to the point's location. The muscle at LI-7 parts and resembles a snake's head when a fist is made.

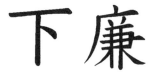

Lower Ridge

LI-8 *(xià lián)*
下 *xià:* lower, below
廉 *lián:* ridge, edge; sincere, honest

Alternate Name

Lower Ridge of the Arm　　手之下廉　*shǒu zhī xià lián*

Classical Location: One inch from Upper Ridge (LI-9), under the assisting bone [i.e., the radius] and in the parting of the protuberant flesh that covers it. *(Great Compendium)*

Explanation of Point Name

LI-8 is located on the forearm four body inches below the elbow. The point name refers to the location of the point on the "ridge" of the arm (i.e., the inner edge of the radius) below the elbow. "Lower" simply indicates that this is the lower of two points (LI-8 and LI-9) that are both named "ridge."

上廉

Upper Ridge

LI-9 *(shàng lián)*
上 *shàng:* upper, above
廉 *lián:* ridge, edge; honest, sincere

Alternate Name

Upper Ridge of the Arm   手之上廉 *shǒu zhī shàng lián*

Classical Location: One inch below Arm Three Li (LI-10). *(Great Compendium)*

Explanation of Point Name

This point is located along the ridge of the radius, above the Lower Ridge (LI-8).

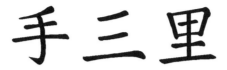

Arm Three Li

LI-10 *(shǒu sān lǐ)*

手 *shǒu:* arm, hand
三 *sān:* three
里 *lǐ:* ward (as in a city), a measure of distance equal
to approximately one third of an English mile

Alternate Names

| Upper Three Li | 上三里 | *shàng sān lǐ* |
| Ghost Evil | 鬼邪 | *guǐ xié* |

Classical Location: At the end of the protuberant flesh two
inches below Pool at the Bend (LI-11); the flesh bulges
when pressure is applied. *(Golden Mirror)*

Explanation of Point Name

The name of this point is closely related to that of ST-36,
Leg Three Li. Both are on yang ming channels located just
below the joint (elbow and knee, respectively, for hand and
foot yang ming). LI-10 derives its name from its location
three body inches below the prominent bone of the elbow.

In classical Chinese the character 里 *lǐ* was often employed
to express the meaning associated with the homophone 理,
which means to rectify or regulate. In this sense, the name
may be a reference to this point's ability to rectify the three
burners.

The modern character 裡 *lǐ,* which carries the meaning of
inner or inside, was often represented by the character 里

lǐ in classical Chinese (as it always is nowadays in the simplified script of mainland China). If 里 is considered to hold this connotation, then this point name could be rendered as Three Interiors, also a reference to the triple burner. The same holds true if 里 *lǐ* is taken in its original sense of a small administrative section of a village: a ward or precinct.

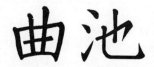

Pool at the Bend

LI-11 *(qū chí)*
曲 *qū:* bent, crooked, curved
池 *chí:* pool, pond

Alternate Names

Yang Marsh	陽澤	*yáng zé*
Ghost Minister	鬼臣	*guǐ chén*
Ghost Leg	鬼腿	*guǐ tuǐ*

Classical Location: On the outer side of the assisting bone [i.e., the radius] at the elbow. When the hand is placed on the chest, the point is in the depression at the end of the elbow crease. *(Great Compendium)*

Point Associations: Uniting-he (earth) point; twelfth of the thirteen ghost points.

Explanation of Point Name

LI-11 may be named after its location; it is found at the crook of the elbow in a depression that resembles a shallow pool. This point name could also be considered as a description of qi as it pours into the uniting-he point, which is like water pouring into a pool. This pool is located at the crook of the elbow, so it is the "pool at the bend." For similar reasons, and because it is located on a yang channel, an alternate name for this point is Yang Marsh (see Cubit Marsh, LU-5).

Additionally, 曲池 *(qū chí)* was a place name in ancient China.

肘髎

Elbow Bone-Hole

LI-12 *(zhǒu liáo)*
肘 *zhǒu:* elbow
髎 *liáo:* bone-hole

Alternate Name

Elbow Tip   肘尖   *zhǒu jiān*

Classical Location: In the depression at the outer corner of the large elbow bone. *(Great Compendium)*

Explanation of Point Name

This point is named for its location in a bony depression one body inch above the elbow.

手五里

Arm Five Li

LI-13 *(shǒu wǔ lǐ)*

手 *shǒu:* arm, hand
五 *wǔ:* five
里 *lǐ:* ward or district (as in a city), a measure of distance
equal to approximately one third of an English mile

Alternate Names

Five Li of the Arm	手之五里	*shǒu zhī wǔ lǐ*
Five Li of the Cubit	尺之五里	*chǐ zhī wǔ li*
Great Prohibition	大禁	*dà jìn*

Classical Location: At the pulsating vessel, three inches above the elbow and slightly inward. *(Great Compendium)*

Explanation of Point Name

The character 里 *lǐ*, by extension of its original meaning of a city ward or district, has come to have the additional meaning "to reside." This point resides at a pulse about five body inches above the elbow and five body inches below the Celestial Treasury (LU-3). In this interpretation of the point name, 里 *lǐ* means "to reside" and at the same time represents a unit of distance.

Classical Chinese texts often make reference to "the five positions", i.e., east, west, south, north, and center. The number five is associated with the center. The old writing of 五 consisted of an "X" placed between two lines 二. It had the meaning of center, or as we say in English, "X marks the spot." Each of the four lines in the X represents a position and the intersection represents the fifth position, the center. The depiction of the five positions (pictured between heaven and earth, which are delineated by the two lines 二), gives the character the meaning of "five."

The *Spiritual Axis* states that needling Five Li (LI-13) damages the qi of the five viscera. The point name, if interpreted as Five Li (wards) or Five Interiors, could be a reminder that needling of this point is forbidden.

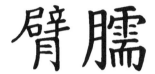

Upper Arm

LI-14 *(bì nào)*

臂 *bì:* arm, forearm
臑 *nào:* upper arm, humerus

Alternate Names

Head Surge	頭沖	*tóu chōng*
Head Thoroughfare	頭衝	*tóu chōng*
Neck Surge	頸沖	*jǐng chōng*
Neck Thoroughfare	頸衝	*jǐng chōng*

Classical Location: Up four inches from Five Li (LI-13), in the depression between the two sinews and bone, felt when the arm is raised and the hand is held flat.
(Golden Mirror)

Point Associations: Intersection-jiaohui point of the hand tai yang small intestine, hand yang ming large intestine and foot tai yang bladder channels, and the yang linking vessel.

Explanation of Point Name

Since this point is located on the upper arm and is used to treat arm disorders, the name serves as a reminder of both the location and function of the point.

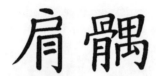

肩髃

Shoulder Bone

LI-15 *(jiān yú)*

肩 *jiān:* shoulder
髃 *yú:* clavicle

Alternate Names

Collarbone	髃骨	*yú gǔ*
Shoulder Tip	肩尖	*jiān jiān*
Shoulder Bone	肩骨	*jiān gǔ*
Flat Shoulder	扁肩	*biǎn jiān*
End Bone	偏骨	*piān gǔ*
Central Shoulder Well	中肩井	*zhōng jiān jǐng*

Classical Location: In the depression between the sinew and bone at the end of the humerus where it meets the shoulder bone. A hollow appears at the point when the arm is lifted. *(Great Compendium)*

Point Associations: Intersection-jiaohui point of the hand tai yang small intestine and hand yang ming large intestine channels and the yang motility vessel.

Explanation of Point Name

All the names for this point refer to its location at the junction of the humerus and acromium.

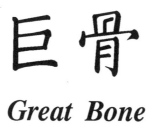

Great Bone

LI-16 *(jù gǔ)*

巨 *jù:* great, large, giant
骨 *gǔ:* bone

Classical Location: Up from the tip of the shoulder, in the depression that lies between the two forking bones.
(Great Compendium)

Point Associations: Intersection-jiaohui point of the hand yang ming large intestine and the yang motility vessel.

Explanation of Point Name

This point name is locational in nature, referring to the obvious prominence at the articulation of the clavicle and scapula. It is also an ancient name for the clavicle.

天鼎

Celestial Tripod

LI-17 *(tiān dǐng)*

天 *tiān:* heaven; celestial, of the heavens; Nature
鼎 *dǐng:* an ancient Chinese sacrificial or cooking vessel

Alternate Names

Celestial Nape	天項	*tiān xiàng*
Celestial Summit	天頂	*tiān dǐng*

Classical Location: Above the supraclavicular fossa, one body inch below Protuberance Assistant (LI-18).
(Great Compendium)

Explanation of Point Name

The character 鼎 *dǐng* is a pictographic representation of an ancient Chinese sacrificial cooking vessel that had two ear-like extensions for handles and was supported on a stand with three legs. Here it serves as a metaphor for the neck, which supports the head just as the tripod supports the vessel. It is especially suitable for the head to be portrayed as a precious vessel because it houses the brain, the "storehouse of the original spirit." (李時珍:"腦爲元神中府.") The name Celestial Tripod brings to mind both the location and function of LI-17, which is located at the base of the neck and treats neck and throat disorders. Many points in the upper body are entitled Celestial (天 *tiān*), but that appellation is particularly appropriate here because the Celestial Tripod supports the absolute top of the body, the head. A more direct expression of this image is given by the alternate name, Celestial Nape.

The alternate names for LI-17 are interesting. The name 天頂, Celestial Summit, is homophonic with 天鼎 (Celestial Tripod). The character 頂 *dǐng,* meaning summit, differs by only one stroke from 項 *xiàng,* meaning neck, which occurs in the alternate name 天項 *tiān xiàng,* meaning Celestial Nape. Although 頂 and 項 may be the result of mistranscriptions, both contribute toward meaningful alternate names because of the location of the point.

扶突

Protuberance Assistant

LI-18 *(fú tú)*
扶 *fú:* to assist, to aid
突 *tú:* protuberance; sudden, abrupt

Alternate Name

> Water Hole 水穴 *shuǐ xuè*

Classical Location: Going up from Celestial Tripod (LI-17), Protuberance Assistant is one inch below the corner of the jaw, and one inch and five fen behind ST-9, Man's Prognosis. LI-18 is found in supine posture. *(Golden Mirror)*

Explanation of Point Name

LI-18 is located lateral to the laryngeal prominence. It assists the functioning of this area by treating such ailments as cough, hoarseness and difficulty in swallowing; and thus derives its name, Protuberance Assistant.

A further explanation is found in the fact that the width of four fingers is equal to three body inches and is termed 扶 *fú* (also written 夫). LI-18 is located three body inches lateral from the prominence of the larynx, so its name is also a convenient device for remembering the location of the point, i.e., one 扶 *fú* from the laryngeal prominence.

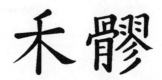

Grain Bone-Hole

LI-19 *(hé liáo)*
禾 *hé:* grain, rice, corn
髎 *liáo:* bone-hole

Alternate Names

Long Shore	長頻	*cháng pín*
Long Cheek	長頰	*cháng jiá*
Long Plate	長顪	*cháng huì*
Long Cheek	長頰	*cháng jiá*
Long Bone-Hole	長窌	*cháng liáo*
Long Bone-Hole	長窌	*cháng liáo*

Classical Location: Below the nostril, five fen from the philtrum [or Water Trough (GV-26)]. *(Great Compendium)*

Explanation of Point Name

LI-19 is located below the lateral edge of the nostril, level with GV-26. Palpation at this point will reveal a depression (actually, the space between the teeth at gum level) about the size of a grain of rice. Since rice is the grain associated with the metal phase (and thus the large intestine), the point name could be translated as either Grain Bone-Hole or Rice Bone-Hole.

Note that *jī* was long ago mistranscribed as the more familiar 禾 *hé*. Thus the point name should be *jī liáo* and not
禾髎 *hé liáo*. 禾 is a pictograph of a tree that serves as a
map to the point. The trunk (philtrum) bends into the bone-
hole.

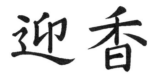

Welcome Fragrance

LI-20 (*yíng xiāng*)
迎 *yíng:* to welcome, to receive
香 *xiāng:* fragrance

Alternate Names

Surging Yang	沖陽	*chōng yáng*
Thoroughfare Yang	衝陽	*chōng yáng*

Classical Location: Up one body inch from Grain Bone-
Hole (LI-19), five fen to the side of the nostril.
(Great Compendium)

Point Associations: Intersection-jiaohui point of the hand
yang ming large intestine and foot yang ming stomach
channels.

Explanation of Point Name

This point has the function of opening the nasal passages,
allowing the patient to welcome in fragrance. Fragrance (香
xiāng) is the aroma associated with the earth phase. The
point name serves to demonstrate that LI-20 is where the
stomach channel (earth) intersects the large intestine channel.

The Stomach Channel
(Foot Yang Ming)

足陽明胃經

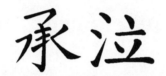

Tear Container

ST-1 (chéng qì)

承 chéng: to contain, to hold, to carry; to receive
泣 qì: tears

Alternate Names

Face Bone-Hole	面髎	miàn liáo
Face Bone-Hole	面窌	miàn liáo
Brimming Tears	羕泣	yàng qì
Mouse Hole	蹊穴	xī xuè
Ravine Hole	谿穴	xī xuè

Classical Location: In the depression seven fen below the eye, level with the pupil [when the eye looks straight forward]. *(Great Compendium)*

Point Associations: Intersection-jiaohui point of the foot yang ming stomach channel and the yang motility and conception vessels.

Explanation of Point Name

ST-1 is located just below the orbit, in a depression that can catch and contain the tears that fall from the eye. It is used to treat excessive lacrimation due to wind or other causes, and helps the body to "contain tears;" hence the name.

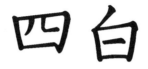

Four Whites

ST-2 *(sì bái)*
四 *sì:* four
白 *bái:* white

Alternate Name

Grain Gate   穀門   *gŭ mén*

Classical Location: Three fen below Tear Container (ST-1), in the hollow of the cheekbone, level with the pupil. *(Golden Mirror)*

Explanation of Point Name

The four white areas of the eye, located above, below and to either side of the iris, are the "four whites." ST-2 is used to treat such ailments in these areas as painful redness, nearsightedness, and eye screen.

Another interpretation claims that the "four whites" are the four white areas (above, below, and to either side) around the mouth. These areas are diagnostic indicators of the body's earth qi; therefore the point name may be considered as a reminder that this point belongs to the stomach (earth) channel. The alternate name Grain Gate is also a reference to the mouth, which is the gate to the stomach.

A locational association may be seen in its position in an area of white flesh, where it helps the eye see in the four directions.

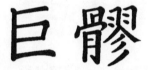

Great Bone-Hole

ST-3 (jù liáo)
巨 jù: great, big, giant
髎 liáo: bone-hole

Classical Location: Eight fen lateral to the nostril, directly below the pupil, level with Water Trough (GV-26).
(Great Compendium)

Point Associations: Intersection-jiaohui point of the hand yang ming large intestine and foot yang ming stomach channels and the yang motility vessel.

Explanation of Point Name
The Great Bone-Hole is so named because it is found in the largest bone-hole in the cheek.

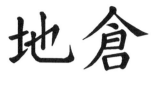

Earth Granary

ST-4 *(dì cāng)*

地 *dì:* earth
倉 *cāng:* granary, storehouse

Alternate Names

Stomach Link	胃維	*wèi wéi*
Linking Confluence	會維	*huì wéi*
Ghost Bed	鬼床	*guǐ chuǎng*

Classical Location: Below Great Bone-Hole (ST-3), a little more than four fen out from the corner of the mouth. A pulsating vessel can be faintly felt close below.
(Golden Mirror)

Point Associations: Intersection-jiaohui point of the foot yang ming stomach and hand yang ming large intestine channels and the conception and yang motility vessels.

Explanation of Point Name

The face is divided into three sections: the area above the nose corresponds to heaven, the nose to man, and the area below the nose to earth. This point is located next to the mouth and is thus called Earth Granary. ST-4 is called a "granary" because it is similar to a granary in that both receive the five grains, food, the material manifestations of earthly qi (地氣 *dì qi*). The character for granary, 倉 *cāng*, resembles a mouth (especially in its older form) and is formed from the character for food (食 *shí*) and the character for mouth (口 *kǒu*).

The stomach is associated with earth in five-phase theory, and although the five-phase character for earth is 土 *tǔ* and not 地 *dì*, the connection is not lost. The point may be named Earth Granary because it is located on the stomach channel (earth), the "granary organ," the organ that receives food.

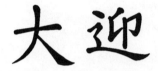

Great Reception

ST-5 *(dà yíng)*
大 *dà:* great, large
迎 *yíng:* to receive, to welcome

Alternate Name

Marrow Hole   髓孔   *suǐ kǒng*

Classical Location: One inch and two fen from the angle of the mandible, in the depression in the bone, in which a pulsation can be felt. [If the head is turned], the point is located where the shoulder touches the jawbone.
(Great Compendium)

Explanation of Point Name

ST-5 may be called Great Reception because it is proximal to the intersection of the large intestine and stomach channels, and is also a branching point of the stomach channel. It can be thought of as a point where the stomach channel receives or welcomes the large intestine channel and as an internal branch of its own channel.

Its name might also be derived from its proximity to the lower jawbone, 大迎骨 *dà yíng gǔ,* which is called great reception bone.

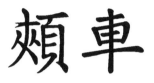

Jawbone

ST-6 *(jiá chē)*
頰 *jiá:* jaw
車 *chē:* vehicle, chariot, car

Alternate Names

Hinge	機關	*jī guān*
Tooth Bend	曲牙	*qū yá*
Ghost Bed	鬼床	*guǐ chuǎng*
Ghost Forest	鬼林	*guǐ lín*

Classical Location: Eight fen below the ear, in the depression just in front of the angle of the mandible. The point is found in lateral recumbent posture, in the hollow that appears when the mouth is opened. *(Great Compendium)*

Point Associations: The 7th of the thirteen ghost points.

Explanation of Point Name

The character combination 頰車 *jiá chē* is an ancient name for the jawbone. The location of the point near the angle of the mandible accounts for its appellation (and explains the alternate names Hinge and Tooth Bend as well). The name of both this point and the jawbone, 頰車, can be translated literally as "Jaw Vehicle," a perhaps more poetic yet less obvious rendering. The explanation that the jawbone is a "vehicle" that carries teeth becomes clearer when the name is compared with its synonym 牙車 *yá chē*, which means literally "tooth vehicle."

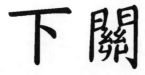

Below the Joint

ST-7 *(xià guān)*
下 *xià:* below, lower
關 *guān:* joint, hinge; barrier; to shut, to close

Classical Location: Below Guest-Host (an alternate name for GB-3), on the lower aspect of the pulsating vessel in front of the ear. A hollow felt when the mouth is closed disappears when the mouth is opened. The point is found in lateral recumbent posture with the mouth closed.
(Great Compendium)

Point Associations: Intersection-jiaohui point of the foot yang ming stomach and foot shao yang gallbladder channels.

Explanation of Point Name

ST-7 may derive its name from its location below the joint of the mandible. Also, it is located just below the zygomatic arch, an area that reminded the ancient Chinese of the door bolt (關 *guān*). Thus the point name may be considered a reference to the point's location below that arch. See also GB-3 (Above the Joint).

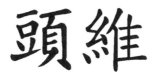

Head Corner

ST-8 *(tóu wéi)*
頭 *tóu:* head
維 *wéi:* to bind, to tie together (originally, a net for catching birds), corner

Alternate Name

Forehead Large   顙大   *sǎng dà*

Classical Location: At the corners of the forehead within the hairline, one inch and five fen to the side of Root Spirit (GB-13), four inches, five fen from Spirit Court (GV-24). *(Great Compendium)*

Point Associations: Intersection-jiaohui point of the foot yang ming stomach and foot shao yang gallbladder channels.

Explanation of Point Name

From its original meaning of net, the *wéi* character (維) came to mean to "bind or tie." If 維 is taken in this sense then the point name may be a reference to the point's location at the place where a crown or other headwear would be bound to the head.

However, the character 維 *wéi* often carries the meaning of corner. For example, the expression 四維 *(sì wéi)* refers to the four corners of a net, and by extension, the four cardinal points and the four limbs. ST-8 is located at the corner of the forehead and is therefore called Head Corner.

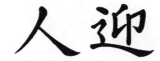

Man's Prognosis

ST-9 *(rén yíng)*

人 *rén:* man, person
迎 *yíng:* to predict, to calculate; to welcome, to receive;
　　　to face

Alternate Names

Fivefold Confluence	五會	*wǔ huì*
Celestial Fivefold Confluence	天五會	*tiān wǔ huì*

Classical Location: At the major pulsating vessel of the neck, one inch and five fen to the side of the Adam's apple. The point is found in supine posture. *(Great Compendium)*

Point Associations: Intersection-jiaohui point of foot yang ming stomach and foot shao yang gallbladder channels.

Explanation of Point Name

The name stresses the point's function of receiving the qi of the five viscera (氣所迎會 *qì suǒ yíng huì*).

Another association comes from the expression: 迎日推策 *yíng rì tuī cè,* which literally translates as "to receive the days and predict events," and is used to describe a type of astrological prediction. The use of the character 迎 *yíng* in this point name may therefore imply that palpation of ST-9 can aid in establishing a patient's prognosis. In other words, by "receiving" (迎 *yíng*) the pulse one can predict the patient's (人 *rén*) outcome.

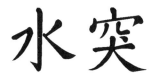

Water Prominence

ST-10 *(shuǐ tú)*

水 *shuǐ:* water
突 *tú:* prominence, to protrude; sudden, abrupt; splash

Alternate Name

Water Gate	水門	*shuǐ mén*
Water Heaven	水天	*shuǐ tiān*

Classical Location: In front of the major sinew of the neck, directly below Man's Prognosis (ST-9) and above Qi Abode (ST-11). *(Great Compendium)*

Explanation of Point Name

The pulsation of the carotid artery at this point resembles the gentle splash of water. The point name may thus reflect the feel of the point when palpated. When liquids are swallowed this point protrudes; thus a rendering as Water Protrusion is also possible.

The name may also be indicative of a function of the point in the treatment of phlegm-rheum counterflow qi ascent. The use of the character 水 *shuǐ* in the name of this point may be considered as a representation of phlegm-rheum, while 突 *tú* can be taken to refer to counterflow qi.

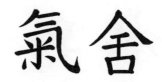

Qi Abode

ST-11 *(qì shè)*

氣 *qì:* qi, breath
舍 *shè:* residence, to reside; to bestow, to give away
something

Classical Location: Directly below Man's Prognosis (ST-9) on the neck, in the depression to the side of Celestial Chimney (CV-22). *(Great Compendium)*

Explanation of Point Name

The breath (氣 *qì*) passes by the area of ST-11. The rendering of the name Qi Abode brings to mind the point's location beside the trachea.

Therapeutically, ST-11 is employed in treating qi ascent cough. This may be viewed as if the stomach were giving its qi to aid the lung, because in Chinese medical theory it is the stomach that provides qi for the lung (earth engenders metal). In this sense Qi Bestowal might be an appropriate rendering of the point name.

As a further note, it should be pointed out that the functions of stomach channel points 11 through 16 and 18 are primarily associated with their location in relation to the chest and lung. The point names reflect these associations through the metaphor of the chest as a house. The house has a window, roof, door and storeroom, while ST-11 represents the abode itself.

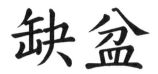

Empty Basin

ST-12 *(quē pén)*

缺 *què:* empty, vacant; imperfect, defective
盆 *pén:* basin, bowl

Alternate Names

| Celestial Cover | 天蓋 | *tiān gài* |
| Cubit Cover | 尺蓋 | *chǐ gài* |

Classical Location: Below Qi Abode (ST-11), in the depression at the horizontal bone [i.e., the clavicle].
(Golden Mirror)

Explanation of Point Name

Traditionally, the clavicle was called 盆骨 *pén gǔ,* a term which translates literally as "basin bone." The supraclavicular fossa was referred to as *què pén* (缺盆), because its shape is reminiscent of an "empty basin." The name of this point is an obvious reference to its location above the clavicle.

Because the clavicle resembles the broken rim of a basin, the location of ST-12 at the edge of that bone allows an additional rendering of the point name as Broken Basin.

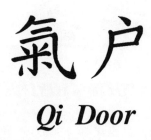

Qi Door

ST-13 (qì hù)
氣 qì: qi, breath
戶 hù: door, gate

Classical Location: Below the clavicle, in the depression two inches to the side of Shu Mansion (KI-27), four inches either side of the midline. The point is found in supine posture. *(Great Compendium)*

Explanation of Point Name

ST-13 is located at the upper portion of the lung. Celestial qi (and the breath) must pass down through this point in order to reach the lung; it is as if this region were a door through which qi passes. Additionally, ST-13 is used to treat asthma, bronchitis and other respiratory disorders, lending a functional interpretation to the point name.

庫房

Storeroom

ST-14 *(kù fáng)*

庫 *kù:* storehouse
房 *fáng:* house, room

Classical Location: In the depression, one inch and six fen below Qi Door (ST-13), four inches either side of the midline. *(Great Compendium)*

Explanation of Point Name

The chest can be seen to have the shape of a room and to store the heart and lung. This image is illustrative of the point's location on the chest.

Clinically, ST-14 is used in the treatment of qi ascent cough, difficult breathing and spitting of bloody, turbid, foamy spittle and pus. A functional perception is lent to the point name when we consider its relationship to the lung, the storeroom of the qi.

A third perspective comes from the Chinese word for breast, 乳房 *rǔ fáng*, rendered literally as milk room. Both the point name and the word for breast contain the character 房, and thus evoke the concept of breast. Chinese medical theory states that after giving birth women retain blood (manifested by the cessation of menstrual flow) and transform it into milk, which is stored in the breast. ST-14 is located above the breast and is used in the treatment of disorders of the breast such as mammary yong. The name Storeroom, if considered a reference to the breast, is then indicative of both the function and location of the point in regard to the breast.

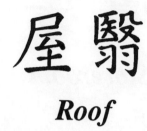

Roof

ST-15 *(wū yì)*
屋 *wū:* house, room
翳 *yì:* a shade, canopy; feather screen

Classical Location: In the depression one inch and six fen below Storeroom (ST-14), four inches from the midline. The point is found in supine posture. *(Great Compendium)*

Explanation of Point Name

This point is employed in treating counterflow cough qi ascent, phlegm rheum, spitting of blood or pus and other lung disorders. The position of the lung as the uppermost of the five viscera likens it to a roof; the name of the point is thus illustrative of its relationship to the lung in both location and function. The female breast rises at this point like the slanting roof of a house, providing further justification for the naming of this point as Roof.

膺窗

Breast Window

ST-16 *(yīng chuāng)*

膺 *yīng:* breast, chest
窗 *chuāng:* window

Classical Location: In the depression one inch and six fen below Roof (ST-15), four inches either side of the midline. *(Great Compendium)*

Explanation of Point Name

Qi and breast milk pass into the breast through this point as air and light pass through a window; hence the appellation Breast Window.

乳中

Breast Center

ST-17 *(rǔ zhōng)*

乳 *rǔ:* breast
中 *zhōng:* center

Alternate Name

On the Nipple 當乳 *dāng rǔ*

Classical Location: Center of the nipple. *(Great Compendium)*

Explanation of Point Name

This point derives its name from its location at the center of the nipple.

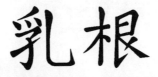

Breast Root

ST-18 *(rǔ gēn)*

乳 *rǔ:* breast
根 *gēn:* root

Alternate Name

Hemp Breathing 薛息 *bì xí*

Classical Location: In the depression one inch and six fen below Breast Center (ST-17), four inches either side of the midline. The point is found in supine posture.
(Great Compendium)

Explanation of Point Name

ST-18 is located at the root of the breast; hence the name.

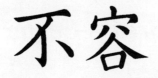

Not Contained

ST-19 *(bù róng)*

不 *bù:* not, negative
容 *róng:* to contain, to hold; to allow

Classical Location: One and a half inches lateral to Dark Gate (KI-21), two inches either side of the midline. *(Great Compendium)*

Explanation of Point Name

While the names of the stomach channel points on the rib cage relate primarily to the chest and lung, once the channel runs into the abdomen the names reflect the points' locations near the stomach and their functions in relation to that organ. ST-19 is the first point on the stomach channel after it leaves the thorax. It is "not contained" by the rib cage. Further, if the stomach is filled to this point it cannot receive any more food. The name 不容 *bù róng* in this sense carries a meaning of "cannot contain."

ST-19 is employed in the treatment of disorders such as vomiting, lack of appetite, and inability to ingest food and drink. These symptoms all result from the stomach not containing food. In addition, this point "does not allow" turbid qi to upflow.

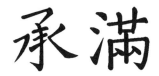

Assuming Fullness

ST-20 *(chéng măn)*
承 *chéng:* to take responsibility for; to receive, to support
滿 *măn:* full, fullness

Classical Location: One inch below Not Contained (ST-19), two inches either side of the midline. *(Great Compendium)*

Explanation of Point Name

This point is located just below the stomach, as if it were assuming a position of support for the ample fullness of the stomach. When the stomach is full it extends to this point. ST-20 can be employed to treat this fullness, and to treat fullness in the abdomen and ribs. Given this, it can be said that the point assumes responsibility for fullness. In this respect the name is a reminder of both the location and function of the point.

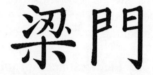

Beam Gate

ST-21 *(liáng mén)*
梁 *liáng:* crossbeam, beam
門 *mén:* gate, door

Classical Location: One inch below Assuming Fullness (ST-20), two inches either side of the midline. *(Golden Mirror)*

Explanation of Point Name

ST-21 may have acquired its name from one of the five accumulations (五積 *wŭ jĭ*) mentioned in the *Classic of Difficult Issues.* Known as 伏梁 *fú liáng,* "deep-lying beam," this condition is described as a condition in which a palpable mass the size of an arm located in the upper abdomen causes irritability and insomnia. Since ST-21 may be used in the treatment of this condition it is a gateway to the beam or, in other words, the Beam Gate.

The character 粱 *liáng* may be a misrepresentation of 粱 *liáng,* which is a kind of millet. If this is the case then the name may be considered as a reference to the location of this point, which is at approximately the level at which grain enters the stomach. Furthermore, since "sea of grain" is an epithet of the stomach, the point name can be indicative of the use of ST-21 in the treatment of disorders of that organ such as lack of appetite, untransformed digesta and diarrhea.

Additionally, 粱門 *liáng mén* is a place name.

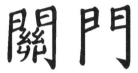

Pass Gate

ST-22 *(guān mén)*
關 *guān:* gate, barrier; to shut, to close
門 *mén:* gate, door

Classical Location: One inch below Beam Gate (ST-21), two inches either side of the midline. *(Golden Mirror)*

Explanation of Point Name

The "lower gate of the stomach" is located three inches above the navel as is ST-22. Digesta passes through this area on its way to the intestines, therefore this point is called Pass Gate.

ST-22 treats diarrhea, closing the lower gate and stopping the flow. A rendering of Shutting the Gate would clearly express this interpretation of the point name.

However, this point name could also be rendered simply as Gate since both 關 *guān* and 門 *mén* can have that meaning. The rendering Pass Gate is preferable because it shows the point's connection to the area three inches above the umbilicus, which is referred to as 關 *guān* (pass), and also draws attention to the point's proximity to Stone Pass (KI-18).

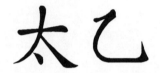

Supreme Unity

ST-23 *(tài yǐ)*

太 *tài* - supreme, most, excessive
乙 *yǐ* - one; the intestines of a fish; second of the ten
　　　heavenly stems

Alternate Name

　　　Supreme Unity　　太才　　*tài yī*

Classical Location: One inch below Pass Gate (ST-22), two inches either side of the midline.
(Golden Mirror)

Explanation of Point Name

The original meaning of 乙 *yǐ* was the intestines of a fish. The shape of the character represents the intestines, and in this point name it relates to the location and function of the point in regard to that bowel.

The term 太乙 *tài yǐ* is also the name of the supreme unity. Because, as Lao Tzu says in the *Tao Te Ching*, "the ten thousand things spring from one," the point name

Supreme Unity is a metaphor for the stomach (or the central burner), which is the source of post-natal qi. This appellation serves as a reminder that the point belongs to the stomach channel and treats disorders of the central burner. As the one thing (i.e., the supreme unity) splits to become heaven and earth, so the turbid and the clear are divided at ST-23. The name of this point further reflects its ability to aid the separation of the clear and the turbid. ST-23 possesses this function because it is located at the beginning of the small intestine, from which the clear ascends and the turbid descends.

That the term 太乙 *tài yǐ* is the name of a star that is related to the abdomen in Chinese astrological theory is also worthy of note.

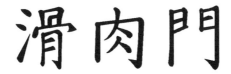

Slippery Flesh Gate

ST-24 (*huá ròu mén*)
滑 *huá:* slippery, glossy
肉 *ròu:* flesh, meat, muscle
門 *mén:* gate, door

Alternate Names

Slippery Dark Gate	滑幽門	*huá yōu mén*
Slippery Flesh	滑肉	*huá ròu*
Celestial Manager	司天	*sī tiān*

Classical Location: One inch below Supreme Unity (ST-23), two inches either side of the midline. *(Golden Mirror)*

Explanation of Point Name

The point is located near the opening of the small intestine (the pylorus), which is a "gate of slippery flesh." An alternate name for ST-24 is 滑幽門 *huá yōu mén,* which is the Chinese name for the pylorus (literally, "slippery dark gate"). It is possible that this name was the original name and that the now standard name is a mistranscription.

The characters 滑肉 *huá ròu* may be taken as a reference to the intestines, which are indeed "slippery flesh." Again, 門 *mén* is often simply a way of describing an acupuncture point.

Functionally, the spleen engenders flesh, and, as *Essential Questions* records, "The yang ming rules the flesh." This point treats both the spleen and the stomach and the point name reflects this. The word slippery (or glossy) could refer to the nature of the flesh at the part of the abdomen where the point is located.

Clinically, ST-24 treats tongue disorders such as swallowing of the tongue and thus is a way (a gate) to treat such "slippery flesh."

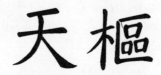

Celestial Pivot

ST-25 *(tiān shū)*
天 *tiān:* celestial, of the heavens; sky; Nature; heaven
樞 *shū:* pivot, axis

Alternate Names

Long Grain	長穀	*cháng gǔ*
Long Ravine	長谿	*cháng xī*
Long Chicken	長雞	*cháng jī*
Long Link	長維	*cháng wéi*
Valley Gate	谷門	*gǔ mén*
Cycle Border	循際	*xún jì*
Origin Supplementer	補元	*bǔ yu*

Classical Location: One inch below Slippery Flesh Gate (ST-24), in the depression two inches lateral to the center of the navel. *(Golden Mirror)*

Point Associations: Alarm-mu point of the large intestine.

Explanation of Point Name

Essential Questions states: "[The area] above the celestial pivot is ruled by celestial qi; [the area] below the celestial pivot is ruled by the earthly qi. The place where these qi intersect is the origin of man's qi and the ten thousand things." This quotation shows that the junction of celestial and earthly qi in the body is the Celestial Pivot. The point name refers to the point's location in the center of the body and to its relative importance as a juncture of celestial and earthly qi.

天樞 *tiān shū* is the ancient name of the central star in the Northern Dipper; the other six stars in that constellation rotate around it. The *Essential Questions* states that "the upper body has three qi's, this is the celestial part, and is ruled by celestial qi; the lower body has three qi's and is ruled by earthly qi." The three stars above and below the Celestial Pivot are representative of the three qi's above and below ST-25.

The numerous alternate names for ST-25 provide a good sample for the study of the effects of mistranscription on acupuncture point names.

外 陵

Outer Mound

ST-26 *(wài líng)*
外 *wài:* outside, outer
陵 *líng:* tomb, burial mound

Classical Location: One inch below Celestial Pivot (ST-25), two inches either side of the midline. *(Golden Mirror)*

Explanation of Point Name

The Chinese traditionally buried their dead in mounds. These mounds, called 陵 *líng,* are often seen on hillsides and other geomantically propitious locations in China. The bulges of the rectus abdominus muscle resemble mounds, and as ST-26 is located on the outer sides of these mounds it is called Outer Mound.

Piles of earth are called mounds or hills. The spleen and stomach channels have many "hill" and "mound" points because these two channels belong to the earth phase of the five phases.

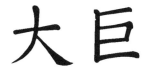

Great Gigantic

ST-27 *(dà jù)*

大 *dà:* big, great
巨 *jù:* large, big, great

Alternate Names

Humor Gate	液門	*yè mén*
Armpit Gate	掖門	*yè mén*
At the Spring	在泉	*zài quán*

Classical Location: One inch below Outer Mound (ST-26), two inches either side of the midline. *(Golden Mirror)*

Explanation of Point Name

The *Great Compendium* lists ST-27 as being appropriate for treatment of distention and swelling in the small intestine and for treatment of *kui shan*.   From this it can be seen that the point name may indicate the location of the point at the largest part of the lower abdomen. The point's function of freeing the intestines can be affirmed in translating the character 大 *dà* as "to free" or "unblock."
(康熙字典 *Kang-Xi Dictionary*).

One alternate name for ST-27, 液門 *yè mén,* is rendered here as Humor Gate. The point may have acquired this appellation because it can be used to treat vexation thirst, which arises when humor is depleted. It is more likely however, that 液門 is a mistranscription of the alternate name 腋門 *yè mén,* which is rendered here as Armpit Gate. 腋門 is the name for ST-22 found in the oldest extant acupuncture book, the *Systematized Canon of Acupuncture and Moxibustion.* The difference between 液 and 腋 is only that the former has a water radical on its left (three dots), while the latter has the radical 月 (*rù*), flesh, on its left. In addition, the two characters are homophones and could have been easily confused. TB-2 also has these two point names but in that case the name 液門 is older and 腋門 is probably a mistranscription.

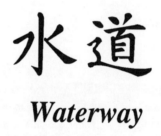

Waterway

ST-28 *(shuǐ dào)*
水 *shuǐ:* water
道 *dào:* path

Classical Location: Three inches below Great Gigantic (ST-27), two inches either side of the midline.
(Great Compendium)

Explanation of Point Name

The three organs most intimately connected with water metabolism are the bladder, kidney and triple burner. ST-28 clears damp-heat from the lower burner, disinhibits the lower burner, and clears triple burner heat bind. It may also be employed in treating urinary inhibition and cold bladder *(Great Compendium).* Because of its ability to affect the body's water metabolism (i.e., free the waterways), ST-28 is called Waterway.

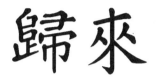

Return

ST-29 *(guī lái)*

歸 *guī:* to return; to restore
來 *lái:* to come, to arrive

Alternate Names

Ravine Hole	谿穴	*xī xuè*
Ravine Valley	谿谷	*xī gǔ*

Classical Location: Two inches below Waterway (ST-28), two inches either side of the midline. *(Great Compendium)*

Explanation of Point Name

A branch of the stomach channel that diverges from the main channel at ST-12 passes downward through the stomach, and then rejoins the main channel at ST-30. ST-29 is called Return because it is located just one body inch up from ST-30, the point where the divergent channel returns. In addition, ST-29 is used to treat many problems related to both male and female reproductive organs. ST-29 may also be called Return because it treats menstrual block and thus aids the return of the menstrual cycle.

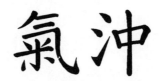

Surging Qi

ST-30 *(qì chōng)*

氣 *qì:* qi
沖 *chōng:* to flush, surge; a thoroughfare; important place;
to rush against

Alternate Name

Qi Thoroughfare	氣街	*qì jiē*
Sheep's Droppings	羊屎	*yáng shǐ*

Classical Location: One inch below Return (ST-29), two inches either side of the midline, in the depression where a pulsating vessel can be felt, at the starting point of the penetrating vessel. *(Great Compendium)*

Explanation of Point Name

The name Surging Qi reflects this point's location at the beginning of the penetrating vessel and its ability to treat disorders related to that vessel. In the term "penetrating vessel" (沖脈 *chōng mài*), the word 沖 is rendered as "penetrating" because of the function and pathway of the vessel. If this term is translated more literally as "surging vessel," its relationship to the name of this point becomes obvious. The penetrating vessel is employed in treating surging counterflow. ST-30 also treats disorders characterized by surging qi, such as running piglet and upward surge of qi attacking the heart.

An alternate name for ST-30 is Qi Thoroughfare, possibly a reference to the point's location on one of the body's four qi thoroughfares. This thoroughfare begins in the abdomen; the other three are in the head, chest and back. The other alternate name listed, Sheep's Droppings, may be taken as a reference to the lumps in the inguinal region formed by tendons and lymph nodes.

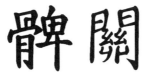

Thigh Joint

ST-31 (bì guān)

髀 bì: thigh; the lateral aspect of the groin
關 guān: gate; joint, hinge; pass

Classical Location: In the crease behind the crouching rabbit [i.e., the rise of flesh in the center of the thigh]. *(Great Compendium)*

Explanation of Point Name

In older Chinese texts 髀關 is an anatomical term referring to either the lateroanterior aspect of the thigh or the outer aspect of the inguinal region. The character 髀 bì, translated as thigh, renders the point name as Thigh Joint, referring to its location near the joint (關) of the thigh.

Another translation of 髀 bì, taken to mean the lateral aspect of the groin, again locationally defines ST-31. A 關 guān is a border pass; in this sense a reference to the place where the stomach channel enters the lower abdomen. In similar fashion, the character 髀 bì translated as inferior, combined with 關 guān, translated as hip joint, illustrates the point's location below the hip or its location near the hip and in the inferior (lower) part of the body.

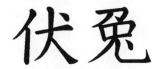

Crouching Rabbit

ST-32 *(fú tù)*

伏 *fú:* to bend over; lie prostrate; to hide
兔 *tù:* rabbit

Alternate Names

Outer Hill	外丘	*wài qiū*
Outer Hook	外勾	*wài gōu*

Classical Location: At the prominence of the flesh, six inches above the knee. *(Systematized Canon)*

Explanation of Point Name

This point derives its name from its location in the prominence of the thigh muscle, which is said to resemble a crouching rabbit. The alternate rendering, Hidden Rabbit, is justified because when the knee is bent the rise in the muscle at this point disappears like a rabbit in hiding.

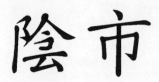

Yin Market

ST-33 *(yīn shì)*

陰 *yīn:* yin, the complement of yang
市 *shì:* city, market

Alternate Name

Yin Tripod 陰鼎 *yīn dǐng*

Classical Location: Three inches above the knee, in the depression below the crouching rabbit. The point is found in kneeling posture. *(Great Compendium)*

Explanation of Point Name

Although the stomach channel is a yang channel, it traverses the front of the body, which is considered yin. ST-33 is a point where qi and blood are gathered and dispersed, like goods at a marketplace; hence the meaning, Yin Market. In addition, the word market may be taken as a reference to the stomach, which receives and distributes the five grains.

The character 市 *shì* is a mistranscription of 市 *fú*. This latter character is an ancient word for a pad that was used to protect the knee when the wearer was kneeling in prayer. The lower body is yin, thus the point name reminds the practitioner of the location of the point in the lower body, just above the knee.

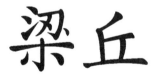

Beam Hill

ST-34 *(liáng qiū)*
梁 *liáng:* crossbeam, ridge
丘 *qiū:* mound, hill

Alternate Names

Hip Bone	骻骨	kuà gǔ
Chicken Top	雞頂	jī dǐng
Crane Top	鶴頂	hè dǐng

Classical Location: One inch below Yin Market (ST-33), in the depression between the two sinews. *(Golden Mirror)*

Point Associations: The cleft-xi point of the stomach channel.

Explanation of Point Name

ST-34 is located two body inches above the laterosuperior border of the patella. There is a rise in the muscle at this point that resembles a small mound. The name Beam Hill may stem from ST-34's ability to treat 伏梁 *fú liáng*, deeply-lying beam (see ST-21).

Optionally, this point name could be rendered as Hill Ridge because it is located on the ridge of the hill of flesh above the knee. The leg must be straightened and the muscle flexed in order to see the hill of flesh.

ST-34 is notably the cleft-xi point of the stomach channel. Cleft-xi points are where channel qi gathers. The name of this point reveals that this point is a gathering of earth qi, i.e., a hill. Were the character 梁 *liáng* taken as a mistranscription of 粱 *liáng*, as occurred in the point name in Beam Gate (ST-21), the point name would then become Grain Hill, a fitting epithet for the stomach.

梁丘 is also a place name from the Spring and Autumn Period of Chinese History.

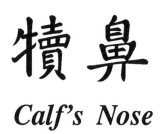

Calf's Nose

ST-35 (*dú bí*)

犢 *dú:* calf
鼻 *bí:* nose

Classical Location: Below the kneecap, above the lower leg bone, in the depression lateral to the large sinew that looks like an ox's nose, hence the name. *(Great Compendium)*

Explanation of Point Name

The diagram 坤 *kūn* is associated in the *Book of Changes (Yì Jīng)* with the earth phase and thus the stomach. The animal associated with 坤 is the ox. The kneecap and the tendon just below the kneecap resemble a calf's nose when viewed from the front. The point position corresponds to the lateral nostril; thus the name. A further expansion of this image is found in the name for the two points on either side of the tendon in front of the knee, these are called: 膝眼 *xī yǎn,* Knee Eyes.

足三里

Leg Three Li

ST-36 (zú sān lǐ)
足 zú: foot
三 sān: three
里 lǐ: measurement of distance (equal to approximately one third of an English mile)

Alternate Names

Lower Hollow Three Li	下虛三里	xià xū sān lǐ
Ghost Evil	鬼邪	guǐ xié
Lower Mound	下陵	xià líng
Lower Sea of Qi	下氣海	xià qì hǎi
Three Li	三里	sān lǐ
Lower Mound Three Li	下陵三里	xià líng sān lǐ
Lower Three Li	下三里	xià sān lǐ

Classical Location: Three body inches below the knee, on the outer side of the shinbone and in the inner side of the big sinew. Located with the leg raised, the point is where the flesh divides between two sinews; when extreme pressure is applied at the point, the pulse at Ravine Divide (ST-41) ceases. *(Great Compendium)*

Point Associations: Uniting-he (earth) point; one of the nine needles for returning yang; the command point of the abdomen.

Explanation of Point Name
As a reminder of its location, *Essential Questions* states, "...the spot called Three Li is three inches below the knee" (...所謂三里者,下膝三寸也).

In classical Chinese, the character 里 *lǐ* was used commonly to mean 理 *lǐ,* to regulate or rectify. Given this, the point name can be taken to mean that the point can regulate three things, which some books specify as being the spleen, stomach and kidney, and others as the upper, central and lower burners.

An oral tradition has it that in ancient times, when the primary means of travel was on foot, stimulation of ST-36 was thought to relieve fatigue sufficient to allow one to journey another three *lǐ.*

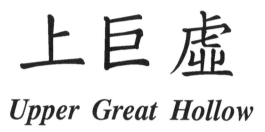

Upper Great Hollow

ST-37 (shàng jù xū)
上 *shàng:* upper
巨 *jù:* great, large
虚 *xū:* vacuous, empty; hollow

Alternate Names

Upper Ridge of Great Hollow	巨虚上廉	*jù xū shàng lián*
Upper Ridge	上廉	*shàng lián*
Upper Ridge of the Leg	足之上廉	*zú zhī shàng lián*
Great Hollow	巨虚	*jù xū*

Classical Location: Three inches below Three Li (ST-36), in the depression between the sinew and bone. The point is found with the leg raised. *(Great Compendium)*

Point Associations: Lower uniting-he point of the large intestine.

Explanation of Point Name

This name refers to the point's location in a hollow of the shin. It is called Upper Great Hollow because it is in the upper part of the hollow, in contrast to Lower Great Hollow (ST-39), which is in the lower part of the hollow.

Anecdotally, there was a type of wild horse in ancient China called 巨虛 *jù xū*. This type of horse was particularly quick and could roam far and wide. The point name, if taken to be derived from the name of the horse, is a reference to the point's effectiveness in treating leg disorders, and is also a reference to the traveling nature of qi here. As ST-37 is the lower uniting-he point of the large intestine, qi travels from here up to the large intestine.

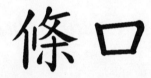

Ribbon Opening

ST-38 *(tiáo kǒu)*
條 *tiáo:* a long and narrow item, ribbon
口 *kǒu:* mouth, opening

Classical Location: Two inches below Upper Great Hollow (ST-37), located with the foot raised. *(Golden Mirror)*

Explanation of Point Name

One way to interpret the meaning of the point name is to visualize the qi flowing from the Upper Great Hollow (ST-37) to the Lower Great Hollow (ST-39). It must go through a narrow passage at ST-38; hence the name Ribbon Opening.

We can also imagine the large intestine and small intestine like ribbons in shape. ST-38 is located between the lower uniting-he points of the large and small intestines and is therefore like an opening between the two long, narrow bowels.

According to the *Great Compendium* this point may be used to treat wind qi, and thus is an opening to treat wind. The rendering Wind Opening is based on a translation of the character 條 *tiáo* as describing a wind from the northeast. Though not a literal translation, it would reflect this function of the point.

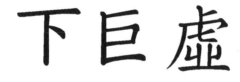

Lower Great Hollow

ST-39 *(xià jù xū)*
下 *xià:* lower
巨 *jù:* great, large
虚 *xū:* hollow, deficiency, vacancy

Alternate Names

Lower Ridge	下廉	*xià lián*
Lower Ridge of Great Hollow	巨虚下廉	*jù xū xià lián*

Classical Location: One inch below Ribbon Opening (ST-38), in the depression between the sinew and bone. *(Golden Mirror)*

Point Associations: Lower uniting-he point of the small intestine.

Explanation of Point Name

The explanation for this point name is the same as for Upper Great Hollow (see ST-37 above). The only differences are that this point is in the lower corner of the hollow as opposed to the upper corner, and that ST-39 is the lower uniting-he point of the small, and not the large, intestine.

豐隆

Bountiful Bulge

ST-40 *(fēng lóng)*
豐 *fēng:* abundant, great, bountiful
隆 *lóng:* prosperous; swell, bulge

Classical Location: Bountiful Bulge (ST-40) lies upward and outward from Lower Great Hollow (ST-39), eight inches above the outer anklebone, in a depression on the outer face of the lower leg bone. *(Golden Mirror)*

Point Associations: Connecting-luo point of the foot yang ming stomach channel, connecting to the foot tai yin spleen channel.

Explanation of Point Name

ST-40 is located at the belly of the calf muscle, the Bountiful Bulge. As the connecting-luo point of the stomach channel, ST-40 is also endowed with an abundance of earth qi. These elements give the name Bountiful Bulge a double meaning where the word bountiful can refer to both the abundance of earth qi at the connecting-luo point and the largeness of the bulge of muscle. Thus the name at once reminds us where the point is located and that it is the connecting-luo point of the channel.

This point name is also the name of a cloud spirit and an expression describing the sound of thunder.

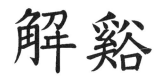

Ravine Divide

ST-41 *(jiě xī)*

解 *jiě:* separate, divide, untie, undo
谿 *xī:* brook, stream, gorge, ravine

Alternate Name

> Shoelace   鞋帶   *xié dài*

Classical Location: One and a half inches back from Surging Yang (ST-42), in the depression at the center of the ankle. Follow the depression between the large toe and the second toe straight up to locate the point.
(Great Compendium).

Point Associations: River-jing (fire) point.

Explanation of Point Name

ST-41 is located in a small cleft in the center of the ankle. The point name reminds us that the point is located in a gorge or ravine that "divides" the lateral and medial aspects of the ankle and separates the shinbone from the foot.

Pathogens collect in clefts such as the one in which this point is located. Needling this point can release (untie) the area, just as the shoelaces are untied at this point. An alternate name for this point is Shoelace since both qi and shoelaces can be bound here.

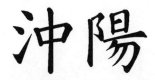

Surging Yang

ST-42 *(chōng yáng)*

沖 *chōng:* to flush, rinse, dash; thoroughfare
陽 *yáng:* yang, the complement of yin

Alternate Names

Meeting Bones	會骨	*huì gǔ*
Meeting Bend	會屈	*huì qū*
Meeting Gush	會湧	*huì yǒng*
Meeting Source	會原	*huì yuán*
Unrestrained Yang	跌陽	*dié yáng*

Classical Location: Going down from Ravine Divide (ST-41), [the point is] at a depression on the high point of the instep, where a pulse can be felt. *(Golden Mirror)*

Point Associations: Source-yuan point of the stomach channel.

Explanation of Point Name

The character 陽 *yáng* as used in this point name is a reference to the point's location on the top (back) of the foot (at the rise in the instep). It is called 沖 *chōng* as a reminder of the pulse at this point that dashes against the hand when palpated.

沖 (or 衝) *chōng,* hub or thoroughfare, is used to indicate an important point, and as the source point of the stomach channel, ST-42 is an important point in this part of the foot. A rendering as Yang Hub might best express this point name interpretation.

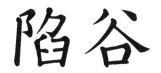

Sunken Valley

ST-43 *(xiàn gǔ)*
陷 *xiàn:* to sink
谷 *gǔ:* a valley

Classical Location: In the outer aspect of the space between the large and second toe, in the depression behind the base joint, two inches up from Inner Court (ST-44).
(Great Compendium)

Point Associations: Stream-shu (water) point.

Explanation of Point Name

The name refers to the concavity in which the point is located. It also hints at the effectiveness of ST-43 in the treatment of water swelling because a valley in the earth (stomach belongs to the earth phase) can contain and therefore regulate water.

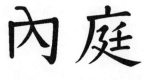

Inner Court

ST-44 *(nèi tíng)*

内 *nèi:* inside, inner
庭 *tíng:* courtyard, court

Classical Location: Below Sunken Valley (ST-43), on the outer side of the second toe, in the depression in front of the base joint. *(Golden Mirror)*

Point Associations: Spring-ying (water) point.

Explanation of Point Name

ST-44 lies between the toes, just as a courtyard lies between the rooms of a house. The point can be said to be inside the courtyard, or to be the inner courtyard itself. The fact that the character 内 *nèi* resembles the space between the toes supports this explanation.

The pictograph 内 *nèi* is a representation of a person 人 *rén* within an enclosure. It recalls a clinical association with the point name, for ST-44 may be used to treat loathing to hear human voices, which is a condition in which the patient shuts himself away, as in a room or court.

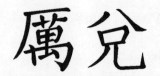

Severe Mouth

ST-45 *(lì duì)*

厲 *lì:* harsh, severe, fierce; to oppress; quick, rapid
兑 *duì:* exchange, convert; mouth, a hole

Classical Location: On the outer side of the end of the toe next to the great toe, the breadth of a Chinese leek leaf from the corner of the nail. *(Great Compendium)*

Point Associations: Well-jing (metal) point.

Explanation of Point Name

According to the *Book of Changes,* the character 兌 *duì* is equivalent to 口 *kǒu,* mouth. The point name may be considered as a reference to the effectiveness of ST-45 in treating serious disorders of the mouth such as wry mouth, tooth decay in the upper teeth and clenched jaw. Rendering the point name as Severe Mouth conveys this interpretation. In the same translational context, the point name may be connected to the fact that ST-45 is the point from which channel qi flows into the spleen channel (SP-1) and the opening of the spleen is the mouth.

厲 *lì* can also mean quick or rapid. ST-45 is located on a part of the foot that is instrumental in rapid ambulation. If 兌 *duì* were taken to mean acupuncture point, the name could justifiably be rendered as Running Point.

Some scholars believe that the character 厲 *lì* may have been mistranscribed from the homophone 癘, epidemic disease. ST-45 can be used to treat this type of disorder. In this instance the character 兌 *duì* would mean simply hole or acupuncture point, and a rendering of the name as Epidemic Point would be fitting.

Further association of point name with function can be made in rendering the character 厲 *lì* as descriptive of a serious wind pathogen (厲風). The point name could thus be taken as a reference to the point's effectiveness in treating wind-related disorders.

Spleen Channel
(Foot Tai Yin)

足太陰脾經

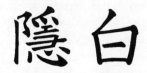

Hidden White

SP-1 *(yǐn bái)*
隱 *yǐn*: hidden, obscure
白 *bái*: white

Alternate Names

Yin White	陰白	*yīn bái*
Ghost Pile	鬼壘	*guǐ lěi*
Ghost Eye	鬼眼	*guǐ yǎn*

Classical Location: On the inner side of the big toe, the width of a Chinese leek leaf from the corner of the nail. *(Great Compendium)*

Point Associations: Well-jing (wood) point; the 3rd of the thirteen ghost points.

Explanation of Point Name

SP-1 is the first point on the earth channel. Earth engenders metal and thus the beginnings of metal exist subtly in earth and doubly so at the beginning of the earth channel. Because white is the color associated with metal, this point is called Hidden White.

Additionally, the character 隱 *yǐn*, which is similar to but not to be confused with 陰 *yín*, the opposite of 陽 *yáng*, may point to the fact that the spleen belongs to the tai yin channel, which is referred to as "the yin within yin." Because 陰 means shadow, cloudy, dark, etc., the yin within the yin is doubly obscure; thus 隱. The character 白 *bái*, white, can be taken as a reference to the location of the point on the border of the white flesh of the toe.

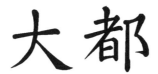

Great Metropolis

SP-2 *(dà dū)*
大 *dà*: great, big
都 *dū*: unit of government organization, a capital city;
    a pool (廣雅: 都, 池也.)

Classical Location: On the inner side of the big toe, on the border of the red and white flesh, in the depression formed by the cleft of the bone behind the base joint.
(Great Compendium)

Point Associations: Spring-ying (fire) point.

Explanation of Point Name

In ancient China, 都 *dū* was a name used for large or important municipal district. The character 大 *dà*, large or great, may be a reference to the fleshy part of the large toe where the point is located, or simply an adjective amplifying the importance implied by 都 . The point name reflects both this point's significance (which is due, in part, to its being the fire [mother] point of the earth channel) and its location on the great (大 *dà*) toe.

This point might also be rendered as Great Pool, for it stores earth qi just as a pool stores water.

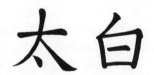

Supreme White

SP-3 *(tài bái)*
太 *tài*: very, extreme, supreme
白 *bái*: white

Classical Location: Back along the inside of the toe from Great Metropolis (SP-2), in the depression under the ball bone. *(Golden Mirror)*

Point Associations: Stream-shu (earth) and source-yuan point.

Explanation of Point Name

This point name has several associative interpretations. First, the flesh at this point is especially white: Supreme White. Also, the planet Venus is called 太白 *tài bái* in Chinese. Venus is in the western sky; west is related to metal and the color white. As the earth point of the spleen channel, SP-3 can fortify earth to engender metal. The point name, if rendered as Venus, is indicative of this function.

Additionally, there is a mountain in China called 太白 . The point name is a reminder that the point is located next to the "mountain" of the ball of the foot.

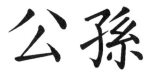

Yellow Emperor

SP-4 *(gōng sūn)*

公 *gōng*: grandfather; public; a surname
孫 *sūn*: grandson; a surname

Classical Location: One inch behind the base joint of the great toe. *(Systematized Canon)*

Point Associations: Connecting-luo point joining the stomach channel and a confluence-jiaohui point of the eight extraordinary channels (related to the penetrating vessel).

Explanation of Point Name

The Chinese divide their ancient history into epochs, associating each with one of the five phases. During the earth phase, from 2697 to 2597 B.C., China was ruled by the Yellow Emperor 黃帝 *huáng dì*, yellow being the color associated with earth. The Yellow Emperor's family name was 公孫 *gōng sūn*. SP-4 is the connecting-luo point between the two earth organs (spleen and stomach); as such it is as important to the earth phase in the body as the Yellow Emperor 黃帝 (公孫) was to the earth phase of history.

Additionally, if 公 *gōng* is thought of as the "grandfather" (home channel), then its offshoot could be thought of as 孫 *sūn*, the "grandson" (connecting vessel). The point name is hence a reminder that this is the connecting-luo point of the spleen channel.

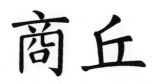

Shang Hill

SP-5 *(shāng qiū)*

商 *shāng*: one of five sounds of the musical scale; market
丘 *qiū*: hill

Alternate Name

Shang Hill   商坵   *shāng qiū*

Classical Location: In the slight depression under the inside anklebone, between Mound Center (LV-4) in front and Shining Sea (KI-6) behind. *(Great Compendium)*

Point Associations: River-jing (metal) point.

Explanation of Point Name

SP-5 is the river-jing (metal) point of the spleen channel; the sound associated with metal is 商 *shāng*. The character 丘 *qiū*, meaning hill, refers to the bone that bulges out beside the hollow in which this point lies. As SP-5 is the metal point of the earth channel, the name implies a high point of earth (hill) where the ore that makes metal (*shāng*) is mined.

This point name is also a place name and a surname.

三陰交

Three Yin Intersection

SP-6 *(sān yīn jiāo)*

三 *sān*: three
陰 *yīn*: yin, the complement of yang
交 *jiāo*: to intersect, join, meet, cross

Alternate Names

Great Yin	大陰	*dà yīn*
Tai Yin	太陰	*tài yīn*
Life Support	承命	*chéng mìng*
Lower Three Li	下三里	*xià sān lǐ*

Classical Location: In the depression beneath the bone, three inches above the tip of the [inner] anklebone. *(Great Compendium)*

Point Associations: Intersection-jiaohui point of the foot tai yin spleen, foot jue yin liver and foot shao yin kidney channels; one of the nine needles for returning yang.

Explanation of Point Name

SP-6 is the point of intersection of the three leg yin channels (liver, spleen and kidney). For this reason, the point is called Three Yin Intersection.

漏谷

Leaking Valley

SP-7 *(lòu gǔ)*

漏 *lòu*: to leak, to drip
谷 *gǔ*: valley

Alternate Names

Yin Channel	陰經	*yīn jīng*
Tai Yin Connection	太陰絡	*tài yīn luò*

Classical Location: In the depression under the leg bone, six inches above the inner anklebone. *(Great Compendium)*

Explanation of Point Name

The character 谷 *gǔ* means valley, but is a common substitute for the homophone 穀 *gǔ,* which means grain. If the spleen qi is not properly controlled, the 谷氣 (grain qi) essence can drain out, resulting in emaciation and fatigue. SP-7 treats this type of disorder, so its Chinese name could be rendered as Leaking Grain.

The point is located in the longitudinal gully formed by the calf muscle, whose resemblance to a valley justifies a literal translation of the point name as Leaking Valley. Thus, we see that this point's function of percolating damp from the spleen, combined with its location in a groove, provides association for its name. As is often the case, the Chinese point name has a double meaning that gets lost in translation.

In *The Systematized Canon of Acupuncture and Moxibustion* 太陰絡 *tài yīn luò* is used; many believe this indicates that SP-7 is a connecting-luo point. If this were the case, the fact that connecting-luo points leak qi and blood to the related channel could be a further reason that this point is called Leaking Valley. Yet, wording in the *Systematized Canon* is insufficiently clear to determine with certainty whether its author was positing the existence of a connecting vessel at this point. No mention of SP-7 being a connecting-luo point is to be found in any other classic.

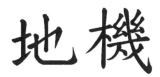

Earth's Crux

SP-8 *(dì jī)*
地 *dì*: earth
機 *jī*: crucial point; to cure; machine

Alternate Names

Earth Winnower	地箕	*dì jī*
Spleen Abode	脾舍	*pí shè*

Classical Location: In the depression by the bone five inches above Leaking Valley (SP-7) and five inches below the knee on the inner side. The point is found with the leg outstretched. *(Great Compendium)*

Explanation of Point Name

As the *Ode to Elucidate Mysteries* says: "Man consists of top, middle and bottom. The major points for these three areas are Great Embracement (SP-21), Celestial Pivot

(ST-25), and Earth's Crux (SP-8) [respectively].'' To the Chinese it is obvious that ''top, middle and bottom'' are parallel with the concepts of heaven, man and earth. It can thus be seen that SP-8 is an essential point for treatment of diseases of the earth portion of the body. It is also an important point in the treatment of splenogastric (earth) disorders, and is furthermore the cleft-xi point of the earth channel (where earth qi gathers). SP-8 is therefore the Earth's Crux.

The character 機 *jī* can mean to cure. (淮南:精神: 機, 喻疾也.) SP-8 can treat disorders of the earth phase (spleenstomach) such as lack of appetite and thin stool diarrhea; therefore the name 地機 *dì jī* could also be rendered as Earth's Cure.

The alternate name 地箕 *dì jī* is homophonic with 地機 . This is a good example of how the primarily oral transmission of acupuncture through the ages led to alternate names.

陰陵泉

Yin Mound Spring

SP-9 *(yīn líng quán)*

陰 *yīn*: yin, the complement of yang
陵 *líng*: mound, hill, tomb
泉 *quán*: a spring

Alternate Name

Yin's Mound Spring   陰之陵泉 *yīn zhī líng quán*

Classical Location: Below the knee and above Earth's Crux

(SP-8), at the depression at the end of the crease when the knee is flexed. *(Golden Mirror)*

Point Associations: Uniting-he (water) point.

Explanation of Point Name

In the landscape of the body, the knee can be said to resemble a hill or mound. Since SP-9 is located near the knee and is the water point of the spleen channel, it can be thought of as a spring beside a mound. The "mound spring" on the yin aspect of the leg is called Yin Mound Spring. (See also GB-34, Yang Mound Spring.)

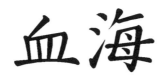

Sea of Blood

SP-10 *(xuè hǎi)*
血 *xuè*: blood
海 *hǎi*: sea

Alternate Names

Blood Cleft	血郄	*xuè xī*
Hundred Worm Burrow	百蟲窠	*bǎi chóng kē*

Classical Location: Two and a half inches above the kneecap, on the border of the white flesh on the inner side. *(Great Compendium)*

Explanation of Point Name

SP-10 is called Sea of Blood because it treats menstrual irregularity, fulminant uterine bleeding and other blood and circulatory disorders.

箕門

Winnower Gate

SP-11 *(jī mén)*

箕 *jī*: winnowing basket; dustpan
門 *mén*: door, gate

Alternate Name

Tai Yin Inner Market 太陰內市 *tài yīn nèi shì*

Classical Location: Moving up from Sea of Blood (SP-10), on to the fish's belly and between the two sinews, a pulse can be felt at the point. *(Great Compendium)*

Explanation of Point Name

The pictograph 箕 *jī* translates as winnowing basket. A classical Chinese term for squatting with the legs spread open, exposing the inner thighs, is 箕坐 *jī zuò* (literally, "winnow-sit," the position taken while winnowing). The point can be located in this position and so the name is a reminder of the site of the point. As is often the case, 門 *mén*, gate or door, is a reference to an acupuncture point: a place where the qi enters and leaves.

As a further locational reminder, the space between the two sinews of the inner thigh can be seen as wide at the front and narrowing as it approaches the groin, a configuration that resembles a dustpan. The point name, if rendered as "Dustpan Gate," serves to remind the practitioner that the point lies within the border of the two sinews.

It is also worth noting that in ancient Chinese astronomy one of the 28 constellations was a dustpan-shaped one called 箕 *jī*.

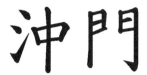

Surging Gate

SP-12 *(chōng mén)*

沖 *(衝)* *chong*: surge, dash, flush, rinse; thoroughfare, hub
門 *mén*: gate, door

Alternate Names

Palace of Charity	慈宮	*cí gōng*
Upper Palace of Charity	上慈宮	*shàng cí gōng*
Front Camphorwood Gate	前章門	*qián zhāng mén*

Classical Location: One inch below Bowel Abode (SP-13) at the pulsating vessel in the crease at the extremity of the pubic bone, four and a half inches from the midline of the abdomen. *(Great Compendium)*

Explanation of Point Name

The character 沖 or 衝 *chōng* may refer to the surging nature of the pulse at the point, or to the fact that the point treats upsurging qi (as in surge of fetal qi to the heart in pregnant women). The character 門 *mén*, gate, has the same meaning here as in Winnower Gate (SP-11) i.e., an acupuncture point.

SP-12 is also the intersection-jiaohui point of the spleen and liver channels, and as such represents a major thoroughfare in the qi network. A rendering as Thoroughfare Gate is therefore justified.

府舍

Bowel Abode

SP-13 *(fǔ shè)*

府 *fǔ*: mansion, residence; (ancient: 腑 *fǔ, bowel*)
舍 *shè*: house, abode

Classical Location: Three inches below Abdominal Bind (SP-14), four and a half inches lateral to the midline of the abdomen. *(Great Compendium)*

Point Associations: Intersection-jiaohui point of the foot tai yin spleen and foot jue yin liver channels and the yin linking vessel.

Explanation of Point Name

府 *fǔ*, meaning residence, was used metaphorically in ancient books to represent the bowels, which are now depicted by 腑 *fǔ*, where the radical 肉 *rù* (simplified to 月) is added to the original character 府. SP-13 is located in the area of the large and small intestines, and is thus called the Bowel Abode. Retaining the original analogy of 府 , the name could be simply Residence.

腹結

Abdominal Bind

SP-14 *(fù jié)*

腹 *fù*: abdomen
結 *jié*: a knot; to tie, weave, congeal

Alternate Names

Intestinal Bind	腸結	*cháng jié*
Abdominal Hole	腹窟	*fù kū*
Abdominal Bend	腹屈	*fù qū*
Abdominal Exit	腹出	*fù chū*

Classical Location: One inch and three fen below Great Horizontal (SP-15), four and a half inches from the midline of the abdomen. *(Great Compendium)* The *Golden Mirror* locates the spleen channel abdominal points three and a half inches from the midline.

Explanation of Point Name

The name Abdominal Bind and the alternate name Intestinal Bind both refer to the effectiveness of this point in treating pain and stagnation in the abdomen presenting as constipation, hernia or abdominal pain.

By itself, the character 結 *jié* can mean a curve or a bend. (廣雅:釋詁: 結, 曲也.) The point name may therefore refer to the turn in the intestine beneath this point. The alternate name Abdominal Bend supports this interpretation.

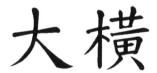

Great Horizontal

SP-15 *(dà héng)*
大 *dà*: great, big
橫 *héng*: horizontal, crosswise

Alternate Names

| Human's Horizontal | 人橫 | *rén héng* |
| Kidney Qi | 腎氣 | *shèn qì* |

Classical Location: Three inches and five fen below Abdominal Lament (SP-16), four and a half inches from the midline of the abdomen. *(Great Compendium)*

Point Associations: Intersection-jiaohui point of the foot tai yin spleen channel and the yin linking vessel.

Explanation of Point Name

The characters 大 *dà* (large) and 横 *héng* (horizontal) refer to the large intestine (大腸 *dà cháng*), which lies beneath this point, and its alarm-mu point (ST-25), to which SP-15 is horizontal. The point name may also be considered a reference to the large horizontal crease on which the point is located.

腹哀

Abdominal Lament

SP-16 (*fù āi*)
腹 *fù*: abdomen
哀 *āi*: to lament, to sympathize with, to pity; sorrow, grief

Alternate Names

Intestinal Bend	腸屈	*cháng qū*
Intestinal Lament	腸哀	*cháng āi*

Classical Location: One inch and five fen below Sun and Moon (GB-24), four and a half inches from the midline. *(Great Compendium)*

Point Associations: Intersection-jiaohui point of the foot tai yin spleen channel and the yin linking vessel.

Explanation of Point Name

A distressed abdomen makes a sound that resembles wailing. In Chinese, this is expressed as 哀鳴 *āi míng*, to lament. SP-16 treats abdominal disorders such as indigestion, center cold, pus and blood in the stool, and abdominal pain, and thus eases Abdominal Lament.

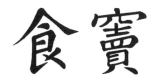

Food Hole

SP-17 *(shí dòu)*

食 *shí*: food

竇 *dòu*: a hole, a drain

Alternate Name

| Life Pass | 命關 | *mìng guān* |

Classical Location: One inch and six fen below Celestial Ravine (SP-18), and six inches from the midline of the chest. *(Great Compendium)*

Explanation of Point Name

The spleen's function of ruling digestion and providing the body with nourishment is reflected by a character meaning food: 食 *shí* . The character 竇 *dòu* is another word for hole. We may visualize the essence of grain qi rising to the lung and passing through the diaphragm at this point, the Food Hole.

The name Food Hole may also be taken as a reference to the nipple. Thus we may associate the point name with the location of the point near the breast.

天 谿

Celestial Ravine

SP-18 *(tiān xī)*

天 *tiān*: celestial, of the heavens; sky; Nature; heaven
谿 *xī*: ravine

Classical Location: In a depression one inch and six fen below Chest Village (SP-19), six inches from the midline of the chest. The point is located in supine posture.
(Great Compendium)

Explanation of Point Name

The area above the diaphragm is often referred to as "heaven," 天 *tiān*, (see SP-8). The ideograph 谿 *xī* refers to the cleft formed by the ribs and sinews that contain this point. The point name is a reminder of the point's location in a cleft of the upper body.

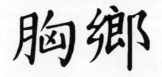

胸 鄉

Chest Village

SP-19 *(xiōng xiāng)*

胸 *xiōng*: chest
鄉 *xiāng*: countryside, village (district under 50,000)

Classical Location: One inch and six fen below All-Round Fluorishing (SP-20), six inches from the midline of the chest. The point is found in supine posture. *(Golden Mirror)*

Explanation of Point Name

The character 鄉 *xiāng*, village, was chosen for reasons similar to those that account for points being named 都 *dū*, metropolis (SP-2, LV-6, KI-19), and 里 *lǐ* (LI-13). Conjuring the image of a rural backwater, "village" reflects the relative unimportance of SP-19. The character 鄉 may also have been picked because of its similarity in form and pronunciation to 響 *xiāng,* meaning sound, since the beat of the heart can be heard at this point. In either case, the appellation Chest Village is basically locational in nature.

The character 鄉 *xiāng* can also mean the space between stairs. If that interpretation of the word is applied then the point name may be construed as a reference to the location of the point between the ribs.

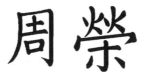

All-Round Flourishing

SP-20 *(zhōu róng)*
周 *zhōu*: all, whole, circumference
榮 *róng*: flourish; honor, glory; to nourish

Alternate Name

All-Round Construction　　　周營　　*zhōu yíng*

Classical Location: One inch and six fen below Celestial Treasury (LU-1), six inches from the midline. The point is found in supine posture. *(Great Compendium)*

Explanation of Point Name

The spleen manages the blood and disperses essence, thus nourishing the body. The lung distributes this nourishment in the form of the qi and fluids through the body. SP-20 is located just below LU-1; because of its location it can influence both the lung and the spleen and contribute to the nourishment of the whole body. Rendering this point name as Complete Nourishment or All-Round Flourishing expresses this meaning.

周营 *zhōu yíng*, All-Round Construction, is an alternate name for this point. This name more directly relates the nourishing nature of the point because 营 is the character that represents the nourishing aspect of qi-blood (i.e., 营氣) *yíng qì*, construction qi (the theoreticl complement of 衛氣 *wèi qì*, defense qi).

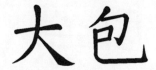

Great Embracement

SP-21 *(dà bāo)*

大 *dà*: great, big
包 *bāo*: to wrap, to contain, to include, to embrace; bag, sack

Alternate Name

      Great Bladder   大胞   *dà bāo*

Classical Location: Downward and outward from All Round Fluorishing (SP-20), crossing the shao yang gallbladder channel, three inches below Armpit Abyss (GB-22), a little over six inches below the armpit. *(Golden Mirror)*

Point Associations: Great connecting-luo point of the spleen. This connecting vessel presides over yin and yang, and via the spleen, irrigates the five viscera.

Explanation of Point Name

SP-21 is the connecting-luo point of the great connecting channel of the spleen (脾之大絡). The character 大 *dà* is a reference to this connecting channel, which disperses over the chest, thus "embracing" (包 *bāo*) the body in a net.

In another sense, we see the spleen as the central viscus, bordered by the lung and heart above and the liver and kidney below. In this view it is contained by the other four viscera. The name Great Embracement is illustrative of this arrangement.

The alternate name 大胞 *dà bāo*, Great Bladder, is most likely a mistranscription of the more common name, 大包 *dà bāo*. The rendering of the former as Great Bladder is not meant to imply the urinary bladder, but is simply a way of indicating a flesh (月) bag (包).

Heart Channel
(Hand Shao Yin)

手少陰心經

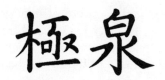

Highest Spring

HT-1 *(jí quán)*
極 *jí*: extreme, most venerable, best
泉 *quán*: spring, fountain

Classical Location: Amid the sinews of the armpit, on the inner side of the arm, where the pulsating vessel enters the chest. *(Great Compendium)*

Explanation of Point Name

The qi of the heart channel issues at this point and flows down the channel toward the hand. This is analogous to water bubbling forth from a spring and flowing toward the sea. The heart is the sovereign organ because of its crucial role in the body, therefore the epithet "highest" or "most venerable" is applied to the first point on this channel. Note that the rendering Highest Spring is not meant to imply that this spring is the highest one in the body, but the most respected one. Ridge Spring (CV-22) is above Highest Spring in physical position.

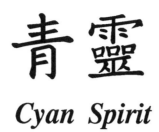

Cyan Spirit

HT-2 *(qīng líng)*
青 *qīng*: cyan, blue-green, purple
靈 *líng*: spirit; divine; efficacious

Alternate Name

Cyan Spirit Spring   青靈泉   *qīng líng quán*

Classical Location: Three inches above the elbow, as located when the arm is raised and the elbow stretched out. *(Great Compendium)*

Explanation of Point Name

The epithet spirit is a reference to the heart's function of storing the spirit. The character 神 *shén* is usually used for the spirit that the heart stores. In this case, 靈 *líng*, the yin aspect of spirit, is used to represent that spirit.

The character 青 *qīng* is most commonly used to represent the colors green and blue (cyan). In older texts it is also used to indicate black or purple. In this point name, 青 may refer to green as the color associated with wood (plant life), which engenders fire (the heart), or as the color of life, exemplified by the sprouting of green leaves in springtime (the heart rules life and death). It may be further construed as a reference to the deep red color of the blood in the vessels, which are ruled by the heart, or the color purple, which is associated with royalty (the heart being the sovereign viscus).

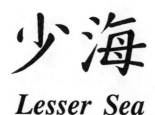

Lesser Sea

HT-3 *(shào hǎi)*
少 *shào*: less, few
海 *hǎi*: sea

Alternate Name
      Bending Joint   曲節   *qū jié*

Classical Location: On the inner side of the elbow, behind the joint, off the big bone [i.e., the medial epicondyle of the humerus], five fen from the tip of the elbow when the arm is flexed toward the head. *(Great Compendium)*

Point Associations: Uniting-he (water) point.

Explanation of Point Name

HT-3 is the uniting-he point of the heart channel as well as the water point. Where the waters unite is the sea; because this is the shao yin (lesser yin) channel, this point is called Lesser Sea. The quality of the qi at uniting-he points is described as a river uniting with the sea. Thus the name recalls the nature of the qi at the point.

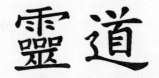

Spirit Pathway

HT-4 *(líng dào)*
靈 *líng*: spirit
道 *dào*: pathway

Classical Location: One inch and five fen behind the palm. *(Great Compendium)*

Point Associations: Jing-river (metal) point.

Explanation of Point Name

HT-4 is the river-jing (metal) point of the heart channel. The qi at river-jing points moves as a mighty river moves along its broad path. Because this particular point is related to the heart, which stores the spirit, it is called Spirit Pathway. Spirit is a reference to the heart and pathway is a reference to the channel. The point name thus reveals that HT-4 is a point on the heart channel and is a point that is itself a pathway for treatment of the spirit.

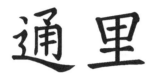

Connecting Li

HT-5 *(tōng lǐ)*
通 *tōng*: to go through, unblock; connect
里 *lǐ*: unit of measurement; ward (neighborhood), village

Alternate Name

Connecting Grain	通理	*tōng lǐ*

Classical Location: In the depression one inch behind the palm. *(Great Compendium)*

Point Associations: Connecting-luo point of the heart channel joining to the small intestine channel.

Explanation of Point Name

If 里 *lǐ* is taken to mean a place, i.e., a village or ward, then the point name indicates a connecting place, a crossroads village. The rendering of the point name as Connecting Li conveys the fact that HT-5 is the connecting-luo point of the heart channel. The phrase 通里, *tōng lǐ,* can furthermore connote a return to one's home village (里), highlighting HT-5 as the place where qi returns to the home channel.

In ancient China, the character 里 *lǐ* was often employed to express the meaning associated with 裡 *lǐ,* a homophone meaning inner or interior. Since 通 *tōng* means to connect, rendering the point name Inward Connection also serves to illustrate that this is the connecting-luo point of the channel. We see this also in the alternate name Connecting Grain, where the character 理 implies a streak or vein like the grain in wood. The word grain is used to indicate the fiber-like structure of wood and, by extension, the connecting vessel at HT-5.

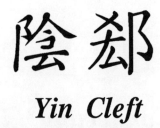

Yin Cleft

HT-6 *(yīn xī)*
陰 *yīn*: yin, the complement of yang
郄 *xī*: cleft

Alternate Names

Shao Yin Bone-Hole	少陰郄	*shào yīn xī*
Stone Palace	石宮	*shí gōng*
Shao Yin Cleft-Xi	少陰郄	*shào yīn xī*

Classical Location: In the vessel behind the palm, five fen from the wrist. *(Great Compendium)*

Point Associations: Cleft-xi point of the heart channel.

Explanation of Point Name

HT-6 is the cleft-xi point of the shao yin heart channel and is therefore called Yin Cleft.

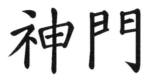

Spirit Gate

HT-7 *(shén mén)*

神 *shén*: spirit
門 *mén*: gate, door

Alternate Names

Protuberant Bone	兌骨	*duì gǔ*
Protuberant Hub	兌衝	*duì chōng*
Protuberance	兌中	*duì zhōng*
Edge	鋭中	*ruì zhōng*
Central Metropolis	中都	*zhōng dū*

Classical Location: Behind the palm, in the depression at the end of the protuberant bone [i.e., at the head of the ulna]. *(Great Compendium)*

Point Associations: Stream-shu (earth) and source-yuan point.

Explanation of Point Name

HT-7 is especially effective in treating disorders of the spirit such as vexation, mania, poor memory and insomnia. The character 神 *shén*, spirit, thus brings to mind this point's ability to treat spirit disorders as well as the heart's function of storing the spirit. The pictograph 門 *mén*, meaning gate, can be thought of as a reference to acupuncture points in general, or as a way of likening this point to a gateway for treatment of the spirit.

少府

Lesser Mansion

HT-8 *(shào fǔ)*

少 *shào*: lesser, minor; few, little
府 *fǔ*: residence, storehouse, mansion

Alternate Name

Protuberant Bone   兌骨   *duì gǔ*

Classical Location: Behind the base joint of the little finger, in the gap between the bones, level with Palace of Toil (PC-8). *(Great Compendium)*

Point Associations: Spring-ying (fire) point.

Explanation of Point Name

HT-8 is the fire point of the heart channel. The heart itself is associated with fire, so the fire point is its home or residence (府 *fǔ*). The character 少 *shào*, meaning lesser, refers to the fact that this is the hand shao yin (lesser yin) channel.

Historically, 少府 *shào fǔ* was the title of an ancient Chinese official equivalent to a modern-day Secretary of Agriculture. The point name may thus refer to the heart's responsibility of storing the spirit, just as the 少府 ruled over the storage of grain. The 少府 was furthermore in charge of distributing produce among the people in much the same way that the heart commands the blood and thus distributes nourishment throughout the body.

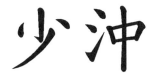

Lesser Surge

HT-9 *(shào chōng)*

少 *shào*: lesser, minor
沖 *chōng*: thoroughfare, a hub; to surge, clash

Alternate Name

Lesser Thoroughfare	少衝	*shào chōng*
Channel Start	經始	*jīng shǐ*

Classical Location: On the inner side of the little finger, the width of a Chinese leek leaf from the corner of the nail. *(Great Compendium)*

Point Associations: Well-jing (wood) point.

Explanation of Point Name

The *Systematized Canon of Acupuncture* describes HT-9 as the point where the hand shao yin heart channel surges forth. The point name is illustrative of the idea that this point is the surging (沖 *chōng*) point of the hand shao yin (lesser yin) channel.

HT-9 is the last point on the heart channel; from here qi travels to the small intestine channel. The point serves as a thoroughfare for the qi of the shao yin (lesser yin) channel, a function substantiating the alternate rendering as Lesser Thoroughfare.

Small Intestine Channel
(Hand Tai Yang)

手太陽小腸經

少澤

Lesser Marsh

SI-1 *(shào zé)*
少 *shào*: lesser, minor; few, little
澤 *zé*: marsh, damp place

Alternate Name

Small Propitiousness　　　小吉　　*xiǎo jí*

Classical Location: On the outer side of the little finger, in the depression one fen from the corner of the nail. *(Great Compendium)*

Point Associations: Well-jing (metal) point.

Explanation of Point Name

The character 澤 *zé* (marsh) refers to a low place where water collects, much like a well. SI-1, which is located in a small depression, is the well-jing point of the small intestine channel. The character 澤 *zé* is a reminder of both the location and the transporting-shu association of this point. The character 少 *shào* is a reference to the hand shao (lesser) yin channel of the heart. This point is related to the heart channel because it is the first point after the heart channel in the qi cycle, and because it is used in treating disorders of that channel.

The name Lesser Marsh may also relate to the point function in moistening heart fire. In this interpretation lesser refers to the heart channel (*shao yin*, lesser yin), while marsh is a reference to the moistening nature of the point. SI-1 treats dry mouth and vexation, both of which are symptoms of insufficient yin humor.

The pictograph 少 *shào* can also mean little (少 , 小也), a reminder that the point is on the little finger.

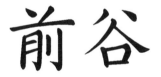

Front Valley

SI-2 *(qián gǔ)*
前 *qián*: in front of, before
谷 *gǔ*: valley

Alternate Name

      Hand Tai Yang   手太陽   *shǒu tài yáng*

Classical Location: On the outer side of the little finger, in the depression in front of the base joint.
(Great Compendium)

Point Associations: Spring-ying (water) point.

Explanation of Point Name

The character 谷 *gǔ* (valley) refers to the depression in which this point is located, while 前 *qián* (front) refers to the position of that depression just distal to the metacarpophalangeal joint of the little finger. Hence the name Front Valley.

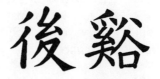

Back Ravine

SI-3 (*hòu xī*)
後 *hòu*: back, behind
谿 *xī*: ravine, creek

Classical Location: On the outer side of the little finger, in the depression behind the base joint, located by making a fist. *(Great Compendium)*

Point Associations: Stream-shu (wood) point.

Explanation of Point Name

SI-3 is called Back Ravine in reference to its location in a narrow depression proximal to the metacarpophalangeal joint. The character 谿 *xī* refers not only to the depression in which the point is located, but also to the quality of the qi at this point. SI-3 is the stream-shu point of this channel, and the qi at stream-shu points is said to flow rapidly like a stream flowing through a ravine.

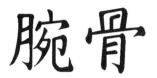

Wrist Bone

SI-4 *(wàn gǔ)*
腕 *wǎn*: wrist
骨 *gǔ*: bone

Classical Location: On the outer side of the hand, in the depression by the prominent bone in front of the wrist. *(Great Compendium)*

Point Associations: Source-yuan point.

Explanation of Point Name

The point name is a reference to the point's location distal to the prominent bone of the wrist.

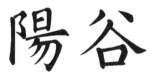

Yang Valley

SI-5 *(yáng gǔ)*
陽 *yáng*: yang, the complement of yin
谷 *gǔ*: valley

Classical Location: At the wrist, in the depression at protuberant bone [i.e., the distal extremity of the ulna]. *(Great Compendium)*

Point Associations: River-jing (fire) point.

Explanation of Point Name

The three points across the yang side of the wrist are Yang Ravine (LI-5), Yang Pool (TB-4), and Yang Valley (SI-5). SI-5 is located in a hollow that is less deep than a ravine and less wide than a pool; thus it is given the appellation Yang Valley.

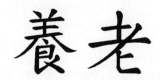

Nursing the Aged

SI-6 (yǎng lǎo)

養 *yǎng*: to support, nourish; to raise (children);
to nurse (the elderly)
老 *lǎo*: aged, old

Classical Location: In a hole on the protuberant bone of the wrist; in a depression one inch behind the wrist.
(Systematized Canon)

Point Associations: Cleft-xi point of the small intestine channel.

Explanation of Point Name

In one's later years the wrist joints are often afflicted with stiffness and pain. SI-6 can be used to prevent or cure this ailment and a variety of other problems associated with old age such as lower back pain, shoulder pain, poor eyesight and deafness; for this reason it is called Nursing the Aged.

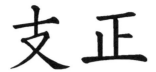

Branch to the Correct

SI-7 (zhī zhèng)

支 *zhī*: a branch; to support
正 *zhèng*: correct; to put right; true; to regulate

Classical Location: Five inches behind the wrist.
(Great Compendium)

Point Associations: Connecting-luo point of the small intestine channel connecting to the heart channel.

Explanation of Point Name

The word used for a channel branch is 支 *zhī*. Here, because the heart is the ruling organ it is called "the correct" (正 *zhèng*); therefore SI-7 is the Branch to the Correct. If the character 正 *zhèng* is taken to indicate the true (regular) channel and 支 *zhī* is taken to represent the connecting vessel, then the name Branch from the True is also justified.

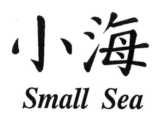

Small Sea

SI-8 (xiǎo hǎi)

小 *xiǎo*: small
海 *hǎi*: sea

Classical Location: On the outer side of the elbow on the outer side of the big bone, in the depression five fen from the tip of the elbow. The point is found by flexing the arm toward the head. *(Great Compendium)*

Point Associations: Uniting-he (earth) point.

Explanation of Point Name

The character 小 *xiǎo*, small, is a reference to the small intestine. SI-8 is the uniting-he point of the small intestine channel, where the qi flows deep and enters the small intestine much like a river flowing into the sea; thus the point is called Small Sea. Note that this point is directly opposite Lesser Sea (HT-3), and that both are uniting-he points.

Because it is the earth point of the small intestine channel, SI-8 is related to the earth bowel, the stomach, which is the "sea of grain." It nourishes the five organs, which in turn are the "sea of the channels and connecting vessels." The name Small Sea brings to mind the sea of grain and the sea of the channels and thus highlights SI-8's association with earth among the five phases.

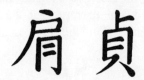

True Shoulder

SI-9 (jiān zhēn)
肩 *jiān*: shoulder
貞 *zhēn*: true, correct; upright; central; divination

Classical Location: Between the two bones below the curve of the shoulder blade, in the depression behind Shoulder Bone (LI-15). *(Great Compendium)*

Explanation of Point Name

The character 貞 *zhēn* can be equivalent to 正 *zhèng* in the sense that they both carry a meaning of true, accurate, central or essential. SI-9 is located "right on" the shoulder and is an important point in the region; hence the rendering True Shoulder. Shoulder Divination is fitting in view of the usefulness of SI-9 for palpatory diagnosis of shoulder problems. Correct Shoulder calls to mind the usefulness of SI-9 in correcting shoulder problems.

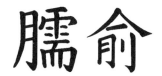

Upper Arm Shu

SI-10 *(nào shū)*

臑 *nào*: upper arm; shoulder bone, outer arm bone
俞 *shū*: acupuncture point

Classical Location: Behind Shoulder Bone-Hole (TB-14), below the large bone, in the depression above the shoulder blade. The point is found with the arm raised.
(Great Compendium)

Point Associations: Intersection-jiaohui point of the hand tai yang small intestine channel and the yang linking and yang motility vessels.

Explanation of Point Name

The character 臑 *nào* is the ancient Chinese word for the upper arm. As might be expected, SI-10 is a major point for treating shoulder and arm problems.

天宗

Celestial Gathering

SI-11 *(tiān zōng)*

天 *tiān*: celestial, of the heavens; sky; Nature; heaven
宗 *zōng*: to gather; ancestor; religion, to believe in

Classical Location: Behind Grasping the Wind (SI-12), in the depression of the shoulder blade. *(Great Compendium)*

Explanation of Point Name

SI-11 is closely tied to the heart because the small intestine and heart have an internal-external relationship, and because the point is located next to Heart Shu (BL-15). The heavens are supreme, and the heart is called the sovereign viscus. Since both are charged with the function of ruling, the point name bears the epithet "celestial." The character 宗 *zōng* may be considered either as a reference to ancestral (宗) qi (disorders of which can be treated through this point), or as a reference to SI-11 as a gathering point of qi.

The name given to this point is also a star name.

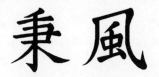

Grasping the Wind

SI-12 *(bǐng fēng)*

秉 *bǐng*: grasp, control
風 *fēng*: wind

Classical Location: Outward from Celestial Bone-Hole (TB-15), on the shoulder behind the small protuberance of the shoulder blade [i.e., the coracoid process]. A hole appears when the arm is raised. *(Great Compendium)*

Explanation of Point Name

A deep depression is found at this spot when the arm is raised. An invasion of external wind can get caught in this depression and cause shoulder disorders. In a manner of speaking, the point catches or "grasps" the wind. SI-12 is treated to relieve this type of shoulder pain accompanied by inability to raise the arm. It can literally "grasp the wind" and relieve the pain.

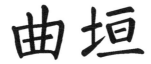

Crooked Wall

SI-13 *(qū yuán)*
曲 *qū*: crooked, curved
垣 *yuán*: a wall; an ancient Chinese astronomical division

Classical Location: In the center of the shoulder, in the depression in the bend of the blade. The point hurts when pressed. *(Great Compendium)*

Explanation of Point Name

This name is a reference to the point location above the curved wall of the scapula. The character 垣 *yuán* may also have been chosen for its astronomical connotations. In ancient China, heavenly bodies were organized in three 垣 *yuán* and twenty-eight constellations. In this part of the body, the microcosmic equivalent of the heavens, the names of many points coincide with those of heavenly bodies or contain the character 天 *tiān*, celestial.

肩外俞

Outer Shoulder Shu

SI-14 *(jiān wài shū)*
肩 *jiān*: shoulder
外 *wài*: outside, exterior
俞 *shū*: acupuncture point

Classical Location: Above Crooked Wall (SI-13) on the upper face of the shoulder, in the depression three inches from the spinal column. *(Golden Mirror)*

Explanation of Point Name

The point is called Outer Shoulder Shu because it is located on the outer shoulder and is used primarily to treat pain in the scapula, shoulder and back.

肩中俞

Central Shoulder Shu

SI-15 *(jiān zhōng shū)*
肩 *jiān*: shoulder
中 *zhōng*: center
俞 *shū*: acupuncture point

Classical Location: At the inner side of the corner of the shoulder blade, two inches from the spinal column. *(Great Compendium)*

Explanation of Point Name

This point is named for its location in the middle of the shoulder. It should be noted that modern sources place this point at the center of an imaginary line drawn between Shoulder Well (GB-21) and Great Hammer (GV-14).

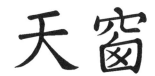

Celestial Window

SI-16 *(tiān chuāng)*

天 *tiān*: celestial, of the heavens; sky; Nature; heaven
窗 *chuāng*: window, shutter

Alternate Names

Lofty Window	窗聳	*chuāng sǒng*
Window Basket	窗籠	*chuāng lóng*
Window Dragon	窗龍	*chuāng lóng*

Classical Location: In the cleft in the major sinew of the neck, below the corner of the jaw, and behind Protuberance Assistant (LI-18), in the depression where a pulsating vessel can be felt. *(Great Compendium)*

Explanation of Point Name

In this point name 天 *tiān*, celestial, is a reference to the location of the point in the upper body. Just as a window allows movement of air (qi), the character 窗 *chuāng* may be construed as a reference to the point's ability to move qi. SI-16 is employed in treating qi blockage disorders such as throat bi, shoulder and neck pain, and pain and swelling of the cheeks.

As a further analogy, we can picture the eyes and ears as the "windows" of the head. 窗 *chuāng* may be taken as a reference to the use of this point in the treatment of ear disorders such as deafness and tinnitus.

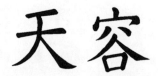

Celestial Countenance

SI-17 *(tiān róng)*
天 *tiān*: celestial, of the heavens; sky; Nature; heaven
容 *róng*: contain, receive; a hood

Classical Location: Below the ear, behind the corner of the jaw. *(Great Compendium)*

Explanation of Point Name

The name for SI-17, Celestial Countenance, refers to its location in the upper body (天 *tiān*) just below the head. From here the channel qi flows to the face.

Translated as hood (容 *róng*), it conjures the image of protection from the wind. This point is treated to relieve wind disorders such as wind bi and sore throat.

顴髎

Cheek Bone-Hole

SI-18 *(quán liáo)*
顴 *quán*: cheekbone
髎 *liáo*: bone hole

Alternate Names

Mouth Bone	兌骨	*duì gǔ*
Influential Bone-Hole	權髎	*quán liáo*
Hammer Bone-Hole	椎髎	*zhuī liáo*

Classical Location: In the depression below the protuberance of the cheek bone. *(Great Compendium)*

Explanation of Point Name

This point is named for its location in a crevice just below the cheekbone. The alternate names, Influential Bone-Hole and Hammer Bone-Hole, are good examples of mistranscription from oral and written sources respectively.

聽宮

Auditory Palace

SI-19 *(tīng gōng)*

聽 *tīng*: to hear
宮 *gōng*: palace

Alternate Names

Heard	所聞	*suǒ wén*
More Heard	多所聞	*duō suǒ wén*

Classical Location: At the pearl of the ear, which is the size of an adzuki bean. *(Great Compendium)*

Explanation of Point Name

SI-19 is located just in front of the ear and is employed to treat many kinds of ear disorders such as purulent ear discharge, deafness and tinnitus. Its importance in treating these disorders is underlined by the epithet "palace."

Bladder Channel

(Foot Tai Yang)

足太陽膀胱經

睛明

Bright Eyes

BL-1 *(jīng míng)*

睛 *jīng*: eye, pupil
明 *míng*: to brighten, bright

Alternate Names

Bright Essence	精明	*jīng míng*
Inner Canthus	目內眥	*mù nèi zì*
Outside the Inner Canthus	內眥外	*nèi zì wài*
Tear Hole	淚孔	*lèi kǒng*

Classical Location: In the depression one fen outward from the inner canthus. *(Golden Mirror)*

Point Associations: Intersection-jiaohui point of the hand tai yang small intestine, foot tai yang bladder, and foot yang ming stomach channels and the yin motility and yang motility vessels.

Explanation of Point Name

BL-1 is called Bright Eyes because it treats a variety of eye problems and improves the eyesight. The point name brings to mind both the function and location of the point. The character 明 *míng* is particularly appropriate for representing the eyes because it is composed of 日 *rì*, sun, and 月 *yuè*, moon, and the sun and moon are called "the two eyes of heaven and earth." Furthermore, it is said that when the five viscera flourish, the eyes shine like the sun and moon.

The alternate name, Bright Essence, if not due to mistranscription of the character 睛 *jīng* into 精 *jīng*, is a reference to the theory that essence manifests in the eyes. As the *Spiritual Axis* (靈樞:脈度篇) states, "The essential qi of the five viscera and six bowels flows up into the eyes to manifest as essence." (五臟六腑之精氣，皆上注於目而爲之精.)

攢竹

Bamboo Gathering

BL-2 *(zǎn zhú)*
攢 *cuàn*: to gather, collect, bring together;
    zǎn: save, accumulate
竹 *zhú*: bamboo

Alternate Names

At the Eyebrow	眉中	*méi zhōng*
Eyebrow	眉頭	*méi tóu*
Root of the Eyebrow	眉本	*méi běn*
Origin Pillar	元柱	*yuán zhù*
Pillar Border	員柱	*yuán zhù*
Man Present	員在	*yuán zài*

Beginning of Light	始光	*shǐ guāng*
Bright Light	明光	*míng guāng*
Night Light	夜光	*yè guāng*
Tear Hole	淚空	*lèi kǒng*

Classical Location: In the depression on the eyebrow above Bright Eyes (BL-1). *(Golden Mirror)*

Explanation of Point Name

When bamboo is gathered and put in bunches, it can be seen to resemble a large eyebrow. The character 攢 *cuàn*, meaning to gather, has a hand radical, 手 *shǒu*. Because BL-2 is located at the inner extreme of the eyebrow, its position is analogous to the hand that gathers the bamboo.

BL-2 may be translated as Bamboo Gathering because the eyebrow resembles a bamboo leaf and the inner corner, where the point is located, is the spot where the brow (or leaf) gathers.

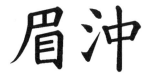

Eyebrow Ascension

BL-3 *(méi chōng)*
眉 *méi*: eyebrow
沖 *chōng*: to pour, rinse, flush; to change

Classical Location: Above the eyebrow, between Spirit Court (GV-24) and Deviating Turn (BL-4). *(Great Compendium)*

Explanation of Point Name

In this instance the ideograph 沖 may be taken to mean "to rise up," as in the phrase 沖天 *chōng tiān*, "to rise to heaven." BL-3 is located directly above the eyebrow, half an inch behind the hairline. The name Eyebrow Ascension depicts channel qi rising from the eyebrow to this point.

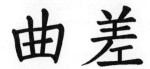

Deviating Turn

BL-4 *(qū chā)*

曲 *qū*: bent, crooked
差 *chā*: difference; chai: to send on an errand

Alternate Name

Nose Flush　　　鼻衝　　*bí chōng*

Classical Location: Above Eyebrow Ascension (BL-3) within the hairline, one inch and five fen each side of Spirit Court (GV-24). *(Golden Mirror)*

Explanation of Point Name

This point name is a reference to the point's location askew from the straight alignment of points on the bladder channel, that is, where the channel deviates from the course it is expected to take.

BL-4 is alternately named Nose Flush in reference to its ability to treat nasal congestion and other disorders of the nose.

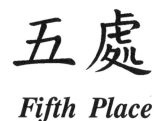

Fifth Place

BL-5 *(wǔ chù)*

五 *wǔ*: five
處 *chù*: a place

Alternate Name

Great Place　　　　巨處　　　*jù chù*

Classical Location: Five fen backward from Deviating Turn (BL-4), one inch and five fen each side of Upper Star on the governing vessel (GV-23). *(Golden Mirror)*

Explanation of Point Name

Fifth Place is an allusion to this point's position as the fifth point on the bladder channel.

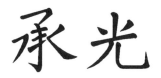

Light Guard

BL-6 *(chéng guāng)*

承 *chéng*: to undertake as one's responsibility;
　　　to carry, to receive, hold
光 *guāng*: light, to shine

Classical Location: One inch and five fen behind Fifth Place (BL-5). *(Great Compendium)*

Explanation of Point Name

The character 承 *chéng* can mean to take on responsibility for a task. The second character, 光 *guāng*, means light and may be taken as a representation of the eyesight. Because BL-6 protects the eyesight and treats related disorders, this point can be said to bear responsibility for or to be a guardian of the eyesight. The translation of this name as Light Guard conveys this meaning.

This point name might also be rendered as Receiving the Light, as 承 *chéng* can also mean to receive (the light in this instance being sunlight, or perhaps the glow of the head's yang qi). Thus translated, the name reminds us of the point's location on the top of the head.

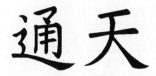

Celestial Connection

BL-7 (*tōng tiān*)

通 *tōng*: to free, unblock; to be freed, unblocked;
    to connect, communicate
天 *tiān*: celestial, of the heavens; sky; Nature; heaven

Alternate Names

Celestial Lord	天伯	*tiān bó*
Celestial White	·天白	*tiān bái*
Celestial Mortar	天臼	*tiān jiù*
Old as the Heavens	天舊	*tiān jiù*

Classical Location: One inch and five fen behind Light Guard (BL-6), one inch and five fen each side of Hundred Convergences on the governing vessel (GV-20).
(Golden Mirror)

Explanation of Point Name

The character 天 *tiān* can be considered as a reference to the vertex of the head, while the pictograph 通 *tōng* may be construed as indicating the connecting vessel that runs from BL-7 to Hundred Convergences (GV-20); hence the rendering Celestial Connection.

Rendered as Unblock Heaven, the name is a reflection of this point's function of clearing the nose. Heaven (天) here refers to the uppermost viscus, the lung, which opens at the nose.

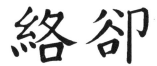

Declining Connection

BL-8 *(luò què)*

絡 *luò*: mesh, connect; connecting vessel
卻 *què*: to retreat; refuse

Alternate Names

Brain Cover	腦蓋	*nǎo gài*
Connecting Cleft	絡郤	*luò xī*
Strong Yang	強陽	*qiáng yáng*

Classical Location: One inch and five fen behind Celestial Connection (BL-7). *(Great Compendium)*

Explanation of Point Name

The path of the bladder channel begins its steep decline (卻) after crossing the vertex of the head and passing through BL-8. The ideogram 絡 *luò* may be a reference to the connecting vessels (絡脈 *luò mài*) located in the vicinity of this point (one vessel connects to the brain).

絡 *luò* are small red vessels in the eye. Needling this point causes these vessels to recede, thus the point name could also be rendered as Vessel Recession.

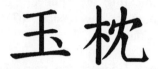

Jade Pillow

BL-9 *(yù zhěn)*
玉 *yù*: jade
枕 *zhěn*: pillow

Classical Location: One inch and five fen behind Declining Connection (BL-8), one inch and three fen to each side of Brain's Door (GV-17). *(Great Compendium)*

Explanation of Point Name

The occipital bone is called 枕骨 *zhěn gǔ*, literally "pillow bone," the name given to BL-9 in *Essential Questions*. An obsolete synonym was 玉枕骨 *yù zhěn gǔ*, "jade pillow bone," the word jade being added for aesthetic reasons or to emphasize the bone's importance. The name can be seen to derive from its location on the occipital protuberance.

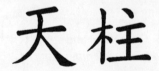

Celestial Pillar

BL-10 *(tiān zhù)*
天 *tiān*: celestial, of the heavens; sky; Nature; heaven
注 *zhù*: pillar

Classical Location: At the hairline on either side of the nape, in the depression on the outer face of the major sinew. *(Great Compendium)*

Explanation of Point Name

The two muscles at the nape of the neck (trapezius) appear like two pillars supporting the head (heaven). BL-10 may derive its appellation from its location on these pillars. The word pillar can also be interpreted as alluding to the cervical vertebrae, because in ancient times the vertebrae of the neck were collectively called 天柱骨 *tiān zhù gǔ*, the celestial pillar bone. As might be expected from the point's location, BL-10 treats disorders of the neck. The point name could also be considered to refer to the neck, which is yet another "pillar" supporting the head.

BL-10 is another of the many points that have star names: 天柱 *tiān zhù* is a star in the constellation Draco.

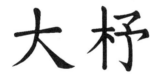

Great Shuttle

BL-11 *(dà zhù)*

大 *dà*: large
杼 *zhù*: a reed, a weaver's shuttle

Alternate Name

Back Shu 背俞 *bèi shū*

Classical Location: In the depression on the nape of the neck, one inch and five fen either side of the spine, below the first vertebra. The point is found in straight sitting posture. *(Great Compendium)*

Point Associations: The meeting-hui point of the bones; intersection-jiaohui point of the foot tai yang bladder, hand tai yang small intestine, foot shao yang gallbladder, and hand shao yang triple burner.

Explanation of Point Name

In ancient China the spinal vertebrae were referred to as 杼 骨 *zhù gǔ*, shuttle bones, because the vertebrae resembled a shuttle weaving in and out of the pattern formed by the posterior of the rib cage. The first vertebra, being the most prominent, is labeled with the epithet "great" (大椎: see Great Hammer - GV-14). This point is located just lateral to that bone; hence the appellation.

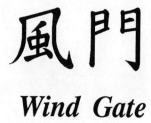

Wind Gate

BL-12 *(fēng mén)*
風 *fēng*: wind
門 *mén*: gate

Alternate Names

Heat Mansion	熱府	*rè fǔ*
Wind Mansion	風府	*fēng fǔ*

Classical Location: One inch and five fen either side of the spine, below the second vertebra. The point is found in straight sitting posture. *(Great Compendium)*

Point Associations: Intersection-jiaohui point of the governing vessel and the foot tai yang bladder channel.

Explanation of Point Name

BL-12 is called Wind Gate both because wind pathogens enter the body there, and because the point can be used to treat exterior wind patterns. The alternate names 風府 *fēng fǔ*, Wind Mansion, and 熱府 *rè fǔ*, Heat Mansion, also reflect this line of reasoning.

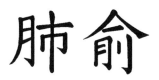

Lung Shu

BL-13 *(fèi shū)*
肺 *fèi*: lung
俞 *shū:* acupuncture point

Classical Location: One inch and five fen either side of the spine, below the third vertebra. *(Great Compendium)*

Point Associations: Associated-shu point of the lung.

Explanation of Point Name

On the bladder channel, each of the twelve organs has an associated-shu (俞 *shū*) point. These points are used in both the diagnosis and treatment of their associated organ, and are generally located at about the level of that organ. Since the lung is the highest organ in the body, the associated-shu point of the lung is the first in this series of points. (More is said about the character 俞 in the **Glossary of Single Characters** at the end of the book.)

厥陰俞

Jue Yin Shu

BL-14 *(jué yīn shū)*

厥 *jué*: faint, lose consciousness
陰 *yīn*: yin, the complement of yang
俞 *shū*: acupuncture point

Alternate Names

Jue Shu	厥俞	*jué shū*
Gate Tower Shu	闕俞	*què shū*

Classical Location: One inch and five fen either side of the spine, below the fourth vertebra. The point is found in straight sitting posture. *(Great Compendium)*

Point Associations: Associated-shu point of the pericardium (jue yin).

Explanation of Point Name

According to the *Great Compendium* this point is the associated-shu point of the pericardium connecting vessel. Since the pericardium belongs to the jue yin the point is called Jue Yin Shu. It is the pericardium connecting vessel that has an associated-shu point and not the viscus itself; at the time these points were named, the pericardium was not one of the eleven organs.

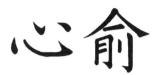

Heart Shu

BL-15 *(xīn shū)*

心 *xīn*: heart
俞 *shū*: acupuncture point

Alternate Names

Back Shu	背俞	*bèi shū*
Heart's Shu	心之俞	*xīn zhī shū*

Classical Location: One inch and five fen either side of the spine, below the fifth vertebra. The point is found in straight sitting posture. *(Great Compendium)*

Point Associations: Associated-shu point of the heart.

Explanation of Point Name

Associated-shu points are located near their associated organs. BL-15 is level with the heart.

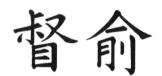

Governing Shu

BL-16 *(dū shū)*

督 *dū*: to govern
俞 *shū*: acupuncture point

Alternate Names

| High Boost | 高盇 | *gāo yì* |
| High Cover | 高蓋 | *gāo gài* |

Classical Location: One inch and five fen either side of the spine, below the sixth vertebra. The point is found in straight sitting posture. *(Great Compendium)*

Explanation of Point Name

Not only the organs, but other anatomical entities as well, have associated-shu points. BL-16 is the associated-shu point of the governing vessel.

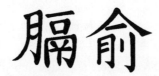

Diaphragm Shu

BL-17 *(gé shū)*
膈 *gé*: diaphragm
俞 *shū*: acupuncture point

Alternate Name

Within the Seventh Burner　　七焦之間 *qī jiāo zhī jian*

Classical Location: One inch and five fen either side of the spine, below the seventh vertebra. The point is found in straight sitting posture. *(Great Compendium)*

Point Associations: Meeting-hui point of the blood.

Explanation of Point Name

This point is located at the level of the diaphragm and is the diaphragm shu. The alternate name is likely a transcription error. 焦 *jiāo*, burner, was probably mistakenly substituted for 椎 *zhuī*, vertebra. The name should have been Within the Seventh Vertebra.

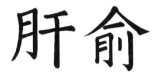

Liver Shu

BL-18 *(gān shū)*
肝 *gǎn*: liver
俞 *shū*: acupuncture point

Classical Location: One inch and five fen either side of the spine, below the ninth vertebra. The point is found in straight sitting posture. *(Great Compendium)*

Point Associations: Associated-shu point of the liver.

Explanation of Point Name
The point's association with the liver accounts for its name.

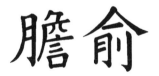

Gallbladder Shu

BL-19 *(dǎn shū)*
膽 *dǎn*: gallbladder
俞 *shū*: acupuncture point

Classical Location: One inch and five fen either side of the spine, below the tenth vertebra. The point is found in straight sitting posture. *(Great Compendium)*

Point Associations: Associated-shu point of the gallbladder.

Explanation of Point Name

Association with the gallbladder explains the name.

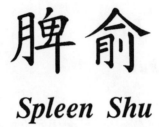

Spleen Shu

BL-20 *(pí shū)*
脾 *pí*: spleen
俞 *shū*: acupuncture point

Alternate Name

Within the Eleventh Burner
十今J之間   *shí yī jiāo zhī jian*

Classical Location: One inch and five fen either side of the spine, below the eleventh vertebra. This point is found in straight sitting posture. *(Great Compendium)*

Point Associations: Associated-shu point of the spleen.

Explanation of Point Name

The association with the spleen explains the name.

胃俞

Stomach Shu

BL-21 *(wèi shū)*
胃 *wèi*: stomach
俞 *shū*: acupuncture point

Classical Location: One inch and five fen either side of the spine, below the twelfth vertebra. The point is found in straight sitting posture. *(Great Compendium)*

Point Associations: Associated-shu point of the stomach.

Explanation of Point Name
The point's association with the stomach accounts for its name.

三焦俞

Triple Burner Shu

BL-22 *(sān jiāo shū)*
三 *sān*: three
焦 *jiāo*: burn, char
俞 *shū*: acupuncture point

Classical Location: One inch and five fen either side of the spine, below the thirteenth vertebra. The point is found in straight sitting posture. *(Great Compendium)*

Point Associations: Associated-shu point of the triple burner.

Explanation of Point Name

The point's association with the triple burner accounts for its name.

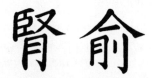

Kidney Shu

BL-23 *(shèn shū)*
腎 *shèn*: kidney
俞 *shū*: acupuncture point

Alternate Name

High Cover   高蓋   *gāo gài*

Classical Location: One inch and five fen either side of the spine, below the fourteenth vertebra, at the level of the navel. The point is found in straight sitting posture.
(Great Compendium)

Point Associations: Associated-shu point of the kidney.

Explanation of Point Name

The point's association with the kidney accounts for its name.

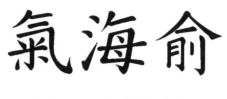

Sea-of-Qi Shu

BL-24 *(qì hǎi shū)*
氣 *qì*: qi
海 *hǎi*: sea
俞 *shū*: acupuncture point

Classical Location: One inch and five fen either side of the spine, below the fifteenth vertebra. The point is found in straight sitting posture. *(Great Compendium)*

Explanation of Point Name

BL-24 is located directly opposite Sea of Qi (CV-6), and is named Sea-of-Qi Shu because of its location and for reasons that are similar to those that account for CV-6 being named Sea of Qi (see CV-6).

大腸俞

Large Intestine Shu

BL-25 *(dà cháng shū)*
大 *dà*: large
腸 *cháng*: intestine
俞 *shū*: acupuncture point

Classical Location: One inch and five fen either side of the spine, below the sixteenth vertebra. The point is found in prostrate posture. *(Great Compendium)*

Point Associations: Associated-shu point of the large intestine.

Explanation of Point Name

The point's association with the large intestine accounts for its name.

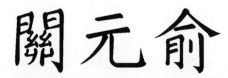

Origin Pass Shu

BL-26 *(guān yuán shū)*

關 *guān*: pass, gate
元 *yuán*: origin, source
俞 *shū*: acupuncture point

Classical Location: One inch and five fen either side of the spine, below the seventeenth vertebra. The point is found in prostrate posture. *(Great Compendium)*

Explanation of Point Name

BL-26 is anatomically opposite to Origin Pass (CV-4). It is called Origin Pass Shu because of its location and for reasons that are similar to those that account for CV-4 being named Origin Pass (see CV-4).

小腸俞

Small Intestine Shu

BL-27 *(xiǎo cháng shū)*

小 *xiǎo*: small
腸 *cháng*: intestine
俞 *shū*: acupuncture point

Classical Location: One inch and five fen either side of the spine, below the eighteenth vertebra. The point is found in prostrate posture. *(Great Compendium)*

Point Associations: Associated-shu point of the small intestine.

Explanation of Point Name

The point's association with the small intestine accounts for its name.

膀胱俞

Bladder Shu

BL-28 *(páng guāng shū)*

膀胱 *páng guāng*: urinary bladder
俞 *shū*: acupuncture point

Classical Location: One inch and five fen either side of the spine, below the nineteenth vertebra. The point is found in prostrate posture. *(Great Compendium)*

Point Associations: Associated-shu point of the bladder.

Explanation of Point Name

The association with the bladder explains the name.

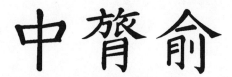

Central Backbone Shu

BL-29 *(zhōng lǚ shū)*
中 *zhōng*: center, middle
膂 *lǚ*: backbone; muscles parallel to the backbone
俞 *shū*: acupuncture point

Alternate Names

Central Backbone Inner Shu	中膂内俞	*zhōng lǚ nèi shū*
Central Backbone	中膂	*zhōng lǚ*
Spine Inner Shu	脊内俞	*jí nèi shū*
Return Shu	旋俞	*xuán shū*

Classical Location: One inch and five fen either side of the spine, below the twentieth vertebra. The point is found in prostrate posture. *(Great Compendium)*

Explanation of Point Name

Deriving the name Central Backbone Shu from its location at the center of the body, amongst the muscles that run parallel to the spine, this point functions in treating disorders of the back and spine. In addition, BL-29 is located lateral to BL-33, Central Bone-Hole. The parallel in name and location are a useful mnemonic and may be part of the reason BL-29 is called Central Backbone Shu as opposed to just Backbone Shu.

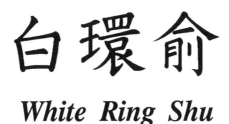

White Ring Shu

BL-30 *(bái huán shū)*

白 *bái*: white
環 *huán*: a ring, a bracelet; to encircle
俞 *shū*: acupuncture point

Alternate Names

Jade Ring Shu	玉環俞	*yù huán shū*
Jade House Shu	玉房俞	*yù fáng shū*

Classical Location: One inch and five fen either side of the spine, below the twenty-first vertebra. The point is found in prostrate posture. *(Great Compendium)*

Explanation of Point Name

"White ring" in Taoist metaphysics refers to the area of the body where essence is stored. The point name implies that BL-30 connects with this area. This interpretation is confirmed by the description of the term jade ring (an alternate term for white ring) provided by Zhang Zi-Yang (張紫陽):

"The heart above, the kidney below, the spleen to the left, liver to the right, life's door [i.e., genitals] to the front, the secret door [i.e., anus] to the rear, it connects like a ring, white like silk one inch in diameter. It wraps the body's essence

and is called the jade ring; this area is directly behind the navel and is the root of man's lifeline.''

The alternate names reinforce this explanation in their use of the word jade.

The bladder channel circles back up to Upper Bone-Hole (BL-31) after passing through this point. Clinically, BL-30 treats disorders that are described with the word white such as white vaginal discharge and white turbidity (urethral discharge).

上髎

Upper Bone-Hole

BL-31 (shàng liáo)

上 *shàng*: up, upper, upward; to rise
髎 *liáo*: bone-hole

Classical Location: In the first opening one inch below the lumbar bone, in the depression either side of the spine. *(Systematized Canon)*

Point Associations: According to the *Great Compendium of Acupuncture and Moxibustion,* Upper Bone-Hole is the site of a connecting vessel communicating with the kidney and gallbladder channels.

Explanation of Point Name

The BL-31 points are the top two of the Eight Bone-Holes (八 髎), which also include BL-32, BL-33, and BL-34.
  The point names for the Eight Bone-Holes derive from their location in the sacral foramina.

次髎

Second Bone-Hole

BL-32 *(cì liáo)*

次 *cì*: second; next in a sequence
髎 *liáo*: bone-hole

Classical Location: In the second opening, in the depression either side of the spine. *(Great Compendium)*

Explanation of Point Name

BL-32 is located at the second sacral foramen.

中髎

Central Bone-Hole

BL-33 *(zhōng liáo)*

中 *zhōng*: center, middle
髎 *liáo*: bone-hole

Alternate Name

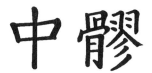

Central Hole   中空   *zhōng kōng*

Classical Location: In the third opening, in the depression on either side of the spine. *(Great Compendium)*

Point Associations: According to the *Great Compendium of Acupuncture and Moxibustion,* BL-33 is a meeting point of the bladder, liver, and gallbladder channels.

Explanation of Point Name

Located between the Upper Bone-Hole (BL-30) and the Lower Bone-Hole (BL-34), BL-33 is the Central Bone-Hole.

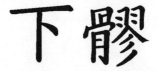

Lower Bone-Hole

BL-34 *(xià liáo)*
下 *xià*: lower, below
髎 *liáo*: bone-hole

Classical Location: In the fourth opening, in the depression on either side of the spine. *(Great Compendium)*

Explanation of Point Name

The point is named for its location in the lowest part of the sacral foramen.

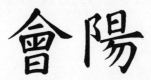

Meeting of Yang

BL-35 *(huì yáng)*
會 *huì*: to meet
陽 *yáng*: yang, the complement of yin

Alternate Names

Hub Disinhibitor	利機	*lì jī*
Leg Bone-Hole	足窌	*zú liáo*

Classical Location: On either side of the tailbone. *(Systematized Canon)*

Explanation of Point Name

Qi from the bladder and governing channels, the two most yang channels of the body, are present at BL-35, and explain its choice of name, Meeting of Yang. Fittingly, the Meeting of Yin (CV-1) is located on the yin complement to the governing vessel - the conception vessel.

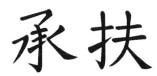

Support

BL-36 *(chéng fú)*

承 *chéng*: to hold, to carry; to receive;
    to bear responsibility
扶 *fú*: support, aid, assist

Alternate Names

Skin Region Support	承扶皮部	*chéng fú pí bù*
Flesh Cleft	肉郄	*ròu xī*
Skin Cleft	皮郄	*pí xī*
Skin Region	皮部	*pí bù*
Yin Joint	陰關	*yīn guān*

Classical Location: In the crease below the buttock and above the inner face of the thigh. *(Great Compendium)*

Explanation of Point Name

Located at the junction of the legs and the trunk of the body, BL-36 derives its name, Support, because it bears the weight of and supports the upper body.

The character 扶 *fú* was a term used in antiquity to describe a wind that carried disease (淮南： 扶風，疾風也). The point name may be considered a reflection of the point's function in treating wind disorders.

殷門

Gate of Abundance

BL-37 *(yīn mén)*
殷 *yīn*: abundant, great, many; center, exactly
門 *mén*: door, gate

Classical Location: Six inches below Support (BL-36).
(Great Compendium)

Explanation of Point Name

BL-37 is located in the abundant (殷 *yīn*) flesh on the back of the upper leg. Again, the character 門 *mén* carries the meaning of acupuncture point. Since BL-37 is in approximately the center of the back face of the upper leg, the meaning of 殷 *yīn* as "center" is also applicable.

浮郄

Superficial Cleft

BL-38 *(fú xī)*

浮 *fú*: superficial, unsubstantial; to float
郄 *xī*: cleft, crevice

Classical Location: One inch above Bend Yang (BL-39). The point is found with the knee flexed.
(Great Compendium)

Explanation of Point Name

This point name is a reference to the point's location in a cleft, and to the superficial needling depth recommended for the point (0.5 inches).

The word superficial in the point name may also be a reference to the shallowness of the flesh at this point.

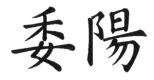

Bend Yang

BL-39 *(wěi yáng)*

委 *wěi*: crooked, bent; to bow under a burden
陽 *yáng*: yang, the complement of yin

Classical Location: Six inches below BL-36. The point is in front of the foot tai yang and behind the shao yang, between the two sinews on the outer end of the popliteal fossa. *(Great Compendium)*

Point Associations: Lower uniting-he point of the triple burner channel.

Explanation of Point Name

This point's name is explained by its location on the yang side of the bend of the knee, i.e., the popliteal crease.

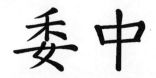

Bend Middle

BL-40 *(wěi zhōng)*
委 *wěi*: crooked, bent; to bow under a burden
中 *zhōng*: center, middle

Alternate Names

Blood Cleft	血郄	*xuè xī*
Central Cleft	中郄	*zhōng xī*
Cleft Center	郄中	*xī zhōng*

Classical Location: At the pulsating vessel in the center of the popliteal crease. *(Systematized Canon)*

Point Associations: Uniting-he (earth) point; command point of the back.

Explanation of Point Name

This point is at the center of the crease at the bend of the knee and is thus named Bend Middle.

The functions of BL-40 to clear the blood, drain heat, and treat acute back sprain are best activated by drawing blood from the small veins surrounding the point. Thus, it is sometimes referred to by the alternate name Blood Cleft.

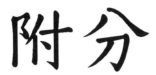

Attached Branch

BL-41 (fù fēn)
附 fù: attach, append
分 fēn: to part, a part

Classical Location: Below the second vertebra, on the inner border of the shoulder blade, three inches either side of the spine. *(Systematized Canon)*

Point Associations: Intersection-jiaohui point of the foot tai yang bladder and hand tai yang small intestine channels.

Explanation of Point Name

This is the first point on the second line of the bladder channel. It is as if an extra branch has been added to the channel, affirming the name, Attached Branch.

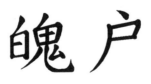

Po Door

BL-42 (pò hù)
魄 pò: soul, spirit
戸 hù: door

Classical Location: Below Attached Branch (BL-41), three inches either side of the spine, below the third vertebra. The point is found in straight sitting posture.
(Great Compendium)

Explanation of Point Name

According to *Essential Questions* the *pò* (soul) is stored in the lung. BL-42 is located lateral to Lung Shu (BL-13) and is called Po Door. 戶 *hù*, door, gives us the image of a place where qi enters and exits.

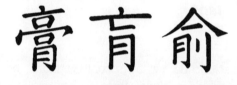

Gao Huang Shu

BL-43 (*gāo huāng shū*)
膏 *gāo*: area below the heart
肓 *huāng*: membrane just above the diaphragm
俞 *shū*: acupuncture point

Classical Location: Three inches either side of the spine, below the fourth vertebra and just above the fifth.
(Glorious Anthology)

Explanation of Point Name

The area labeled 膏肓 *gāo huāng* is just below the heart. In ancient texts it is said to contain vital organs and to defy all cure if affected by disease. "The Four Books of Acupuncture" states that diseases located above *huāng* and below *gāo* can be treated by neither herbs nor acupuncture, although moxa on BL-43 can bring results. For this reason the point is called Gao Huang Shu.

神堂

Spirit Hall

BL-44 *(shén táng)*

神 *shén*: spirit

堂 *táng*: hall, main room of a house; temple, memorial

Classical Location: In the depression three inches either side of the spine, below the fifth vertebra. The point is found in straight sitting posture. *(Great Compendium)*

Explanation of Point Name

The heart stores the spirit. BL-44 is lateral to Heart Shu (BL-15), and is therefore called Spirit Hall. The frequent usage of 堂 *táng*, hall, in acupuncture point names may be simply poetic, or perhaps has some abstruse meaning. In this case, it is more concretely appropriate because in ancient times 堂 was a word for temple, which is a place where a spirit resides.

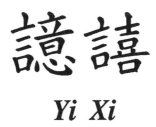

Yi Xi

BL-45 *(yì xī)*

譩 *yì*: a sighing, laughing sound

譆 *xī*: a sighing, laughing sound

Classical Location: On the inner side of the shoulder, three inches either side of the spine, below the sixth vertebra. The point is found in straight sitting posture. When firm pressure is applied, the patient cries "ee shee" indicating that the point has been found. *(Golden Mirror)*

Explanation of Point Name

Numerous texts state that when BL-45 is palpated firmly the patient will put forth an "yi xi" sound. This is the reason for the point name.

膈 關

Diaphragm Pass

BL-46 *(gé guān)*

膈 *gé*: diaphragm
關 *guān*: pass, gate

Classical Location: In the depression three inches either side of the spine, below the seventh vertebra. The point is found in straight sitting posture with shoulders spread. *(Great Compendium)*

Explanation of Point Name

This point is located 1.5 inches lateral to Diaphragm Shu (BL-17), and is thus called Diaphragm Pass. The ancients may have chosen the 關 *guān* (pass) appellation because the diaphragm represents a type of border separating the upper burner from the middle burner, In those times, roads had passes, called 關 *guān*, at political borders. Pass could also, as is often the case, be simply a way of indicating a place of entry and exit of qi.

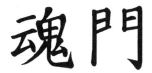

Hun Gate

BL-47 *(hún mén)*
魂 *hún*: soul, spirit
門 *mén*: gate, door

Classical Location: In the depression three inches either side of the spine, below the ninth vertebra. The point is found in straight sitting posture. *(Great Compendium)*

Explanation of Point Name

The 魂 *hún* (spirit stored in the liver) is said to enter and leave the body through this point. This may be an extrapolation of the fact that BL-47 is located lateral to the Liver Shu (BL-18), or that, like BL-18, this point is located at about the level of the liver.

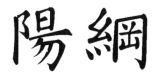

Yang Headrope

BL-48 *(yáng gāng)*
陽 *yáng*: yang, the complement of yin
綱 *gāng*: headrope of a fishing net; a key link;
　　principle, essence

Classical Location: In the depression three inches either side of the spine, below the tenth vertebra. The point is found in straight sitting posture with shoulders spread. *(Great Compendium)*

Explanation of Point Name

Generally speaking, a given point on the outer branch of the bladder channel shares to some extent the functions of the point located medially to it on the inner branch. Since Gallbladder Shu (BL-19) is located 1.5 inches medial to BL-48, we can say that BL-48 is also related to the gallbladder. Thus seen, this pair of points is the uppermost representation of a bowel (腑 *fǔ*, as opposed to 臟 *zàng*, viscus) on the bladder channel. As the viscera are considered to be yin in nature while the bowels are yang, these points therefore resemble the headrope of the yang-associated points on the channel. Since the gallbladder is the yang manifestation of wood-spring, and spring is the head season of the yang, this might be a further reason for naming BL-48 Yang Headrope.

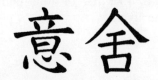

Reflection Abode

BL-49 *(yì shè)*
意 *yì*: idea, wish, meaning
舍 *shè*: a house, a shed; to reside

Classical Location: Three inches either side of the spine, below the eleventh vertebra. The point is found in straight sitting posture. *(Great Compendium)*

Explanation of Point Name

BL-49 is located 1.5 inches lateral to Spleen Shu (BL-20). Spleen qi resides at these points and since the spleen stores the faculty of reflection (for example, in *Essential Questions* 脾藏意), BL-49 is called Reflection Abode.

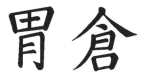

Stomach Granary

BL-50 *(wèi cāng)*
胃 *wèi*: stomach
倉 *cāng*: granary, storehouse, warehouse,

Classical Location: Three inches either side of the spine, below the twelfth vertebra. The point is found in straight sitting posture. *(Great Compendium)*

Explanation of Point Name

The stomach is termed "the granary organ" in classical texts. BL-50 is located 1.5 inches lateral to Stomach Shu (BL-21), and can be thought of as a place where stomach qi is stored, the Stomach Granary.

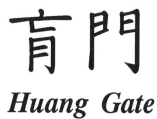

Huang Gate

BL-51 *(huāng mén)*
肓 *huāng*: membrane just superior to the diaphragm
門 *mén*: gate, door

Classical Location: In the depression either side of the spine, below the thirteenth vertebra. The point is located in straight sitting posture. *(Great Compendium)*

Explanation of Point Name

BL-51 most probably derives its name from the fact that it is used to treat tightness and pain in the region below the heart, the 肓 *huāng* area.

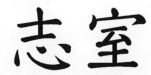

Will Chamber

BL-52 *(zhì shì)*
志 *zhì*: will, ambition
室 *shì*: room, chamber

Alternate Name

Palace of Essence   精宮   *jīng gōng*

Classical Location: In the depression three inches either side of the spine, below the fourteenth vertebra. The point is found in straight sitting posture. *(Great Compendium)*

Explanation of Point Name

The kidney stores the will. Since BL-52 is located 1.5 inches lateral to the kidney associated-shu point, it is intimately connected with that viscus. The appellation Will Chamber reveals this relationship.

胞肓

Bladder Huang

BL-53 *(bāo huāng)*

胞 *bāo*: bladder; womb, uterus; afterbirth
肓 *huāng*: the membrane located above the diaphragm

Classical Location: In the depression three inches either side of the spine, below the nineteenth vertebra. The point is located in prostrate posture. *(Great Compendium)*

Explanation of Point Name

The character 胞 *bāo* is composed of a flesh radical (月) and 包 *bāo*, meaning to wrap. It is used in older texts to refer to bladders in general or the womb in particular. Since *Essential Questions* states that "the huang originates below the navel," the name is probably a reference to the womb or the urinary bladder. BL-53 is closely related to the urinary bladder because it is a bladder channel point, it is located lateral to Bladder Shu, and it is used to treat urinary system disorders such as strangury and urinary block. In theory, BL-53 is also related to the womb because the bladder and kidney are a yin-yang pair and the womb is dependent on kidney qi. However, Bladder Huang was chosen because the point is not used to treat female reproductive disorders.

秩邊
Sequential Limit

BL-54 *(zhì biān)*

秩 *zhì*: sequence, order
邊 *biān*: side; border, limit, edge; close by

Classical Location: In the depression three inches either side of the spine, below the twentieth vertebra. The point is found in prostrate posture. *(Great Compendium)*

Explanation of Point Name

BL-54 is the last outer branch point before the channel path runs down the back of the leg. It is therefore the lower limit (邊 *biān*) of that sequence (秩 *zhì*) and is appropriately named Sequential Limit. Although 秩 *zhì*, sequence, is certainly a reference to the outer branch, 邊 *biān*, if it is taken to mean "side", may be a way of indicating that BL-54 treats diseases affecting the side of the body. This is a clinically relevant idea because BL-54 is important in the treatment of sciatic pain and sciatica often involves the lateral aspect of the legs.

合陽
Yang Union

BL-55 *(hé yáng)*

合 *hé*: to unite, to meet
陽 *yáng*: yang, the complement of yin

Classical Location: Three inches below the crease of the knee. *(Great Compendium)*

Explanation of Point Name

This point is located just below the uniting-he point of the bladder channel. It is furthermore situated just below the area of the popliteal crease where an internal branch of the bladder channel unites with the main channel. The character 合 *hé*, meaning union, reflects both these facts, while 陽 *yáng* can be taken as a representation of the bladder, which is a yang organ.

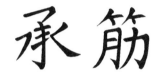

Sinew Support

BL-56 *(chéng jīn)*

承 *chéng*: to support; to receive
筋 *jīn*: sinew, muscle, tendon

Alternate Names

Calf Intestine	腨腸	*chuài cháng*
Rectum	直腸	*zhí cháng*

Classical Location: Below Yang Union (BL-55), in the depression at the center of the calf, seven inches above the heel. *(Golden Mirror)*

Explanation of Point Name

Located in the upper gastrocnemius muscle and useful in treating spasm of that muscle and other similar ailments in the local area, BL-56 truly provides Sinew Support. As it is located below the two sinews at the back of the knee, the point name may also refer specifically to those sinews.

In the *Systematized Canon of Acupuncture and Moxibustion* there are references to the area at the top of the back of the lower leg as "calf intestine." The alternate point name, Calf Intestine, probably derives from this reference.

The alternate name Rectum may refer to the fact that a branch of the bladder channel departs from the main channel at the popliteal fossa and rises to the rectal region. Additionally, many points in the calf area treat rectal disorders.

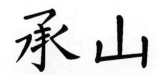

Mountain Support

BL-57 (chéng shān)
承 chéng: to support, to receive
山 shān: mountain

Alternate Names

Intestine Mountain	腸山	cháng shān
Damage Mountain	傷山	shāng shān
Fish Belly	魚腹	yú fù
Fish's Lumbus	魚腰	yú yāo
Fleshy Cinnamon	肉桂	ròu guì

Classical Location: Below Sinew Support (BL-56), in the parting of the flesh at the lower tip of the belly of the calf. *(Golden Mirror)*

Explanation of Point Name

The gastrocnemius muscle can be seen to resemble a mountain. This point is located in a position that supports the weight of that "mountain." Additionally, the gastrocnemius muscle divides at this point, creating an indentation that resembles the character 人 *rén*, which means man. The point may therefore be called Mountain Support because the area resembles a man bearing the weight of a mountain.

The alternate name Fish Belly refers to the calf muscle's resemblance to the belly of a fish.

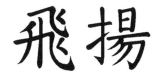

Taking Flight

BL-58 *(fēi yáng)*

飛 *fēi*: to fly, hover; swift
揚 *yáng*: to raise (e.g., the head);
    to throw upward and scatter; to spread

Alternate Names

Flying Yang	飛陽	*fēi yáng*
Jue Yang	厥陽	*jué yáng*
Jue Poplar	厥楊	*jué yáng*

Classical Location: Moving obliquely [i.e.,outward and downward] from Mountain Support (BL-57), in the depression seven inches above the outer anklebone.
(Golden Mirror)

Point Associations: Connecting-luo point of the bladder channel connecting to the kidney channel.

Explanation of Point Name

BL-58 is the connecting-luo point that connects the tai yang bladder channel to the shao yin kidney channel. The qi "leaps" from the yang to the yin side of the leg, "taking flight." After this point is needled patients who were suffering from leg pain are able to run freely, or "take flight."

In the alternate name Flying Yang, 陽 *yáng*, the complement of yin, is used instead of 揚 *yáng*. The use here of the character 陽 is either a mistranscription or a reference to the point's location on the foot tai yang channel. Since the name Jue Yang 厥陽 dates back as far as the *Systematized Canon*, it is also possible that it is the character 揚 that is a mistranscription.

跗陽

Instep Yang

BL-59 (*fū yáng*)
跗 *fū*: the instep, the metatarsus
陽 *yáng*: yang, the complement of yin

Alternate Names

Give Yang	付陽	*fù yáng*
Yang Attachment	附陽	*fù yáng*
Yang Correction	陽矯	*yáng jiǎo*

Classical Location: Below Taking Flight (BL-58), between the sinew and bone, three inches above the outer anklebone. *(Golden Mirror)*

Point Associations: Cleft-xi point of the yang motility vessel; intersection-jiaohui point of the foot tai yang bladder channel and the yang motility vessel.

Explanation of Point Name

The point's location above the yang aspect of the instep is one way of accounting for its name.

趺 *(fū, instep)* is similar to 扶 *fú* , which means to assist. This would imply that because the three leg yang channels run close together at this point, they work to assist each other. The similarity of the two characters gives the point name a double meaning.

BL-59 is also known by the appellations of 付陽 Give Yang and 附陽 Yang Attachment. Both these characters are pronounced *fù yáng*. This pronunciation differs only in tone and has resulted in considerable confusion as to which is original. The character 付 *fù* means "to give," thus the name 付陽 is probably a reference to the point's location adjacent to the connecting-luo point, where the yang qi of the bladder channel is "given" to the kidney channel. The character 附 *fù* can mean "to be near" or "to be attached." If it is considered to mean "to be near," then the name 附陽 implies the point's location near the other two yang channels of the leg. If, on the other hand, 附 is taken to mean "to be attached," then the name is either a reference to the point being the cleft-xi point of the yang motility vessel or to its proximity to the connecting-luo point of the channel (BL-58). This would render the name as either Nearby Yang or Yang Attachment.

昆侖

Kunlun Mountains

BL-60 *(kūn lún)*

昆 *kūn*: first half of the name of a mountain range
侖 *lún*: second half of the name of a mountain range

Alternate Name

Lower Kunlun Mountains　下崑崙　*xià kūn lún*

Classical Location: Below Instep Yang (BL-59), five fen behind the outer anklebone, in the depression above the heel bone, where a fine pulsating vessel can be felt.
(Golden Mirror)

Point Associations: River-jing (water) point.

Explanation of Point Name

The resemblance of the exterior (lateral) malleolus to a mountain suggested this name for the point to the ancient Chinese. The point itself is located just below the "mountain," and possibly for this reason it is also referred to as 下崑崙 *xià kūn lún*, Lower Kun Lun Mountains. This name may also be a way of distinguishing this point from Origin Pass (CV-4), which bears the alternate name of Kunlun Mountains.

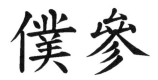

Subservient Visitor

BL-61 *(pú cān)*

僕 *pú*: subservient; servant, slave
參 *cān*: to visit a superior; shen:
      root, as in ginseng, 人參, rén sh*ēn*

Alternate Name

      Quieting of Evil   安邪   *ān xié*

Classical Location: In the depression below the heel bone. The point is found with the foot arched.
(Great Compendium)

Point Associations: Intersection-jiaohui point of the foot tai yang bladder channel and the yang motility vessel.

Explanation of Point Name

The character 僕 *pú* means a servant or person of inferior rank. BL-61 is an intersection-jiaohui point of the yang motility vessel and the bladder channel. The yang motility vessel can therefore be likened to a visitor of inferior rank at the bladder channel, a Subservient Visitor. When a visitor of inferior rank arrives he kneels down in front of the host. The visitor's hands fall to where the point is located. One must get down on hands and knees to locate the point on oneself, thus assuming the position of a Subservient Visitor.

The character 參 *cān* is equivalent to 驂 *cān*. This latter character originally represented the outer two horses in a team of four, and by extension has come to mean "outer." Since the character 僕 *pú* means subservient, or "lower," the point name can also be taken as a reminder of the point's location on the outer and lower aspect of the foot.

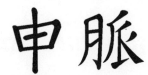

Extending Vessel

BL-62 *(shēn mài)*

申 *shēn*: to extend; the ninth of the 12 earthly branches
脈 *mài*: vessel; pulse

Alternate Names

Yang Motility	陽蹺	*yáng qiāo*
Yang Motility	陽蹻	*yáng qiāo*
Ghost Road	鬼路	*guǐ lù*

Classical Location: In the depression five fen below the outer anklebone between the two sinews.
(Great Compendium)

Point Associations: Confluence-jiaohui point of the eight extraordinary vessels (yang motility vessel); intersection-jiaohui point of the foot tai yang bladder channel and the yang motility vessel. The fifth of the thirteen ghost points.

Explanation of Point Name

The yang motility vessel extends upward from this point; hence the rendering Extending Vessel. Supporting this interpretation is the fact that an alternate name for BL-62 is 陽蹺 *yáng qiāo*, Yang Motility.

申 *shēn* brings to mind 伸 *shēn*, which is similar in form and identical in pronunciation. This latter character means to stretch out, and suggests that BL-62 can treat disorders that prevent the patient from straightening the leg.

When the character 申 *shēn* is used to denote the ninth of the twelve earthly branches (EB-9), it may be interpreted as referring to 申時 *shēn shí* , the ninth watch of the day (3:00 to 5:00 p.m.), which is a time associated with the bladder channel. The point name could therefore be rendered as Shen Vessel, or EB-9 Vessel.

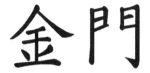

Metal Gate

BL-63 (*jīn mén*)
金 *jīn*: metal, gold
門 *mén*: gate, door

Alternate Names

| Gate Beam | 關梁 | *guān liáng* |
| Beam Gate | 梁關 | *liáng guān* |

Classical Location: Slightly behind the outer anklebone, behind Hill Ruins (GB-40), in front of Extending Vessel (BL-62). *(Great Compendium)*

Point Associations: Cleft-xi point of the bladder channel; intersection-jiaohui point of the foot tai yang bladder channel and the yang linking vessel.

Explanation of Point Name

Metal is the element of the five phases that is associated with 申, the ninth watch (申時 *shēn shí* : EB-9 watch, 3:00 to 5:00 p.m.), with which the bladder channel is associated. Bladder channel qi and blood flows through this point during that period; hence the name Metal Gate.

BL-63 is also the intersection-jiaohui point of the bladder channel and the yang linking vessel, and may thus be likened to a gate between the two. As the yang linking vessel is associated with yang metal, the point is named Metal Gate.

This point has the function of treating liver wind spasms. Although BL-63 is not directly associated with metal, the name is a reminder that the point's function is similar to the restraint of wood (liver) by metal in the restraining cycle of the five phases.

This point name is also a place name.

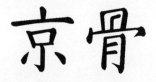

Capital Bone

BL-64 (*jīng gǔ*)
京 *jīng*: capital; large, big; source, origin
骨 *gǔ*: bone

Alternate Name

Large Bone   大骨   *dà gǔ*

Classical Location: On the outer side of the foot, below the large bone, in the depression at the border of the red and white flesh. *(Systematized Canon)*

Point Associations: Source-yuan point.

Explanation of Point Name

The pictograph 京 *jīng* carries the meaning of great or big (capital). The metatarsal bone was in ancient times called 京骨 *jīng gǔ*, "capital bone." The point name thus reveals the point's location below that bone. The alternate name 大骨 *dà gǔ*, Large Bone, confirms this interpretation. Because the character 京 also had, in the past, a meaning of 原 *yuan*, source or origin, the name is also an indication that BL-64 is the source-yuan point of the bladder channel.

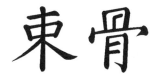

Bundle Bone

BL-65 *(shù gǔ)*
束 *shù*: a bundle; to bind, tie, restrain
骨 *gǔ*: bone

Classical Location: On the outer side of the small toe, in the depression behind the base joint. *(Systematized Canon)*

Point Associations: Stream-shu (wood) point.

Explanation of Point Name

The joint at the base of the small toe was at one time called the 束骨 *shù gǔ*, meaning "bundle bone," probably because it appears to be the place where the foot bones are bundled together. This point, located just proximal to that joint, derives its name from the location.

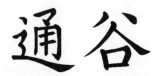

Valley Passage

BL-66 *(tōng gǔ)*

通 *tōng*: to pass through, to unblock;
to conduct i.e., a substance
谷 *gǔ*: valley

Alternate Name

Foot Valley Passage 足通谷 *zú tōng gǔ*

Classical Location: On the outer side of the small toe, in the depression in front of the base joint.
(Great Compendium)

Point Associations: Spring-ying (water) point.

Explanation of Point Name

This point is near the end of the bladder channel and the beginning of the kidney channel. After qi passes through BL-67 and KI-1 it arrives at Blazing Valley (KI-2). BL-66 is a passage to that valley, or a Valley Passage. As well, BL-66 is the spring-ying (water) point of the bladder channel. The point is like a Valley Passage that conducts the qi onward to the stream-shu, river-jing, and uniting-he points.

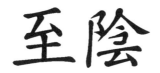

Reaching Yin

BL-67 *(zhì yīn)*

至 *zhì*: to arrive at, to reach; extremely, most
陰 *yīn*: yin, the complement of yang

Alternate Name

Digit Well 指井 *zhǐ jǐng*

Classical Location: On the outer side of the small toe, the width of a Chinese leek leaf away from the corner of the nail. *(Great Compendium)*

Point Associations: Well-jing (metal) point.

Explanation of Point Name

The pictograph 至 *zhì* can mean to arrive at or to reach. BL-67 is the last point of the bladder (yang) channel, from which the qi then passes to the kidney (yin) channel. Therefore BL-67 is said to be Reaching Yin. Alternately, we may recall that the kidney is referred to in *Essential Questions* as "extreme yin" (腎者至陰也). If the character 至 *zhì* is interpreted as meaning extreme, then the point name is indicative of the point's connection to the kidney. A rendering of this point's name as Extremity of Yin is also valid if we consider the tenet that the extreme of yin or yang engenders its complement. Thus we are reminded that the very end of the yang channel contains the beginnings of the yin channel and vice versa.

Kidney Channel

(Foot Shao Yin)

足少陰腎經

湧泉

Gushing Spring

KI-1 (yǒng quán)

湧 yōng: to gush, well up, surge
泉 quán: a spring; ancient term for coin

Alternate Names

Earth Surge	地沖	dì chōng
Earth Thoroughfare	地衝	dì chōng
Yin Valley	陰谷	yīn gǔ
Stumbling Heart	蹶心	jué xīn
Foot Shao Yin Union	足少陰合	zú shào yīn hé
Vessel in the Center of the Sole		
足下中央之脈	zú xià zhōng yāng zhī mài	

Classical Location: In the depression in the heart of the sole, as felt when the leg is stretched, the foot bent and the toes curled. *(Golden Mirror)*

Point Associations: Well-jing (wood) point; one of the nine needles for returning yang.

Explanation of Point Name

The sole of the foot is the lowest part of the body, analogous to the earth of the Chinese cosmology. A place where water gushes forth from the earth is, obviously, a spring. Because KI-1 is located at this "earth" position, and because it is the beginning point of the water (kidney) channel, it is the "gushing spring" of the body.

KI-1 is the well-jing point of the kidney channel. The qi at the well-jing points is said to "come forth," and anyone who has felt the needle sensation at this point will understand the use of the word "gushing." The origin of the kidney channel is thus fittingly called the Gushing Spring.

The alternate name Earth Surge is explained by combining the explanations above. In the alternate name Yin Valley, "yin" refers to both the shao yin kidney channel and the bottom of the foot, while "valley" is a reference to the depression in which the point is found.

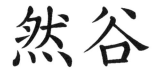

Blazing Valley

KI-2 *(rán gǔ)*

然 *rán*: so, however; suddenly; same as 燃, *rán*, burn
谷 *gǔ*: valley

Alternate Names

Blazing Bone	然骨	*rán gǔ*
Dragon in the Abyss	龍淵	*lóng yuān*
Dragon in the Spring	龍泉	*lóng quán*
Grain Connection	通穀	*tōng gǔ*

Classical Location: In the depression below the large bone that lies in front of the inner ankle. *(Great Compendium)*

Point Associations: Spring-ying (fire) point; also, a branch departs from the channel here and connects to Earth's Crux (SP-8) *(Great Compendium)*.

Explanation of Point Name

The ideogram 然 *rán* originally meant the same as its homophone 燃, to burn, which differs only by having a 火 *huǒ*, fire radical, on the left (the four dots at the bottom of these characters also represent fire). KI-2 is the fire point of the kidney channel and is located in a depression, or "valley," on the medial aspect of the foot. The point is therefore aptly named Blazing Valley.

The alternate name, Dragon in the Abyss, is a reminder that KI-2 is the fire point of the water channel. The dragon stands for the fire nature of the point while the character 淵 *yuān*, abyss, which has a water radical, represents a deep source of water, i.e., the kidney. The derivation of the alternate name Dragon in the Spring follows the same rationale.

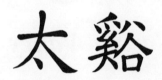

Great Ravine

KI-3 *(tài xī)*
太 *tài*: great, big, the most
谿 *xī*: a mountain stream, ravine

Alternate Names

Small Lu	呂細	*lǔ xì*
Lu Palace	呂宮	*lǔ gōng*

Classical Location: Five fen behind the inner anklebone, in the depression above the heel bone where a pulsating vessel can be felt. *(Great Compendium)*

Point Associations: Stream-shu (earth) and source-yuan point; one of the nine needles for returning yang.

Explanation of Point Name

KI-3 is the source point of the channel, and palpation of the pulse here can reveal the condition of the kidney qi. The use of 太 *tài*, meaning great, is an indication of the importance of this point in these respects. The narrow depression in which the point is located, along with the fact that this is the water channel, make "ravine" (谿 *xī*) an appropriate appellation.

The character 呂 *lǔ* that is used in the alternate name for this point represents the fifth note of the Chinese musical scale. 呂 is a yin sound and is associated with the kidney. The alternate name Small Lu is the yin (small) aspect of the yin sound and represents yin within yin, just as the kidney is yin within yin, lowest of the yin organs and associated with shao yin (lesser yin).

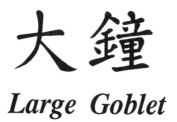

大鐘

Large Goblet

KI-4 (*dà zhōng*)

大 *dà*: large, great
鐘 *zhōng*: a handleless cup; a bell; to gather

Alternate Name
Great Goblet   太鐘   *tài zhōng*

Classical Location: At the back of the heel, between the two sinews above the large bone. *(Great Compendium)*

Point Associations: Connecting-luo point of the kidney channel connecting to the bladder channel.

Explanation of Point Name

The kidney is said to store essence, and its related organ, the bladder, holds fluids until they are released from the body. KI-4 is the connecting-luo point of the kidney channel, which connects to the bladder channel. The point name helps recall this connection by invoking the image of a Large Goblet, which serves to represent the storing functions of both the kidney and bladder.

In classical Chinese the homophones 鐘 and 鍾 (both pronounced *zhōng*) were often used interchangeably, referring to either a liquor goblet or a bell. The character 踵, which means heel, is quite similar to 鍾 in appearance, differing only in respect to the radicals on the left, which in the former character is foot, 足 *zú*, and in the latter is metal, 金 *jīn*. It is likely that the bell or goblet-like shape of the heel bone resulted in the formation of the character 踵. Thus the name Large Goblet may further serve to remind the practitioner of the location of the point at the heel.

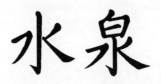

Water Spring

KI-5 *(shuǐ quán)*
水 *shuǐ*: water
泉 *quán*: spring

Classical Location: One inch below Great Ravine (KI-3), below the inner anklebone. *(Great Compendium)*

Point Associations: Cleft-xi point of the kidney channel.

Explanation of Point Name

KI-5 is the cleft-xi point of the kidney channel, and as such, is located in a cleft where kidney (water) qi collects. A spring is a deep place where water collects; hence the name.

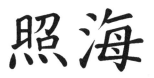

Shining Sea

KI-6 *(zhào hǎi)*
照 *zhào*: to shine, to reflect
海 *hǎi*: sea

Alternate Names

Leaky Yin	漏陰	*lòu yīn*
Yin Motility	陰蹺	*yīn qiǎo*
Yin Motility	陰蹻	*yīn qiǎo*

Classical Location: Four fen below the inner anklebone, in the depression bordered by sinews in front and behind, the anklebone above, and the soft bone below.
(Great Compendium)

Point Associations: A confluence-jiaohui point of the eight extraordinary vessels (yin motility vessel); intersection-jiaohui point of the foot shao yin kidney channel and the yin motility vessel.

Explanation of Point Name

KI-6 is located next to Blazing Valley (KI-2), the fire point of the kidney channel. The brightness of fire (see KI-2) shining on water (i.e., the kidney channel) gives KI-6 its name.

The character 海 *hǎi*, sea, may be a reference to the point's location at the beginning of the yin motility vessel, and recognition of the fact that kidney qi serves as the source (i.e., the sea) for that vessel. For this reason, KI-6 is also known by the alternate name of 陰蹻 *yīn qiǎo*, yin motility.

復溜

Recover Flow

KI-7 *(fù liū)*

復 *fù*: to recover; to turn around
溜 *liū*: to slide, glide, flow; smooth; a swift current

Alternate Names

Deep-Lying White	伏白	*fú bái*
Deep-Lying Mortar	伏臼	*fú jiù*
Returning White	復白	*fù bái*
Glorious Yang	昌陽	*chāng yáng*
Outer Life	外命	*wài mìng*

Classical Location: In the depression two inches above the inner anklebone. *(Systematized Canon)*

Point Associations: River-jing (metal) point.

Explanation of Point Name

KI-7 is an important point for inducing perspiration to aid a patient's recovery (復 *fù*) from exterior patterns by promoting the flow (流 *liú*) of sweat. The point is therefore called Recover Flow. KI-7 is also an instrumental point for stopping perspiration, thereby helping the patient to recover from the flow of sweat. Further, kidney qi leaves the channel at KI-6 to flow into the yin motility vessel. The flow then returns to the kidney channel at KI-7, so that the channel "recovers" the "flow" that it lost at KI-6.

The points below KI-7 on the kidney channel (KI-3 to KI-6) make a circular path behind the inner malleolus. After KI-7 the qi resumes a straight path up the leg; the point name could thus be rendered as Returning Flow.

In modern usage the characters 留 *liǔ*, meaning to remain or stay, and 溜 *liū*, meaning to flow, are clearly distinguished from one another, but they were not so in classical usage. With both the above meanings in mind the point name can serve as a reminder of the two main diseases that KI-7 treats, i.e., water swelling (in which water remains at some location) and spontaneous perspiration (where there is repeated flow of sweat).

KI-7 is alternately called Deep-Lying White because it is the metal point on the kidney (water) channel, and is thus metal (i.e., white) within water. The alternate names Deep-Lying Mortar and Returning White are presumably mistranscriptions of Deep-Lying White due to the similarity of either the characters themselves or their pronunciation.

交信

Intersection Reach

KI-8 (*jiāo xìn*)

交 *jiāo*: to connect, intersect; to deliver
信 *xìn*: faith, trust, evidence; true

Classical Location: Two inches above the inner anklebone, between the bone and sinew. *(Systematized Canon)*

Point Associations: Cleft-xi point of the yin motility vessel; intersection-jiaohui point of the foot shao yin kidney channel and the yin motility vessel.

Explanation of Point Name

The Chinese character 信 *xìn* implies reaching out, in much the same way as does the English word "faith." Since after KI-8 the kidney channel proceeds to intersect with the liver and spleen channels at Three Yin Intersection (SP-6), it could be said that from this point the channel is reaching toward that intersection. The rendering of the point name as Intersection Reach seeks to express this idea.

Faith, 信 *xìn*, is the virtue related to the earth phase; this character can therefore be construed as a representation of spleen-earth, giving the point name the implied meaning of an intersection with earth (i.e., at SP-6). Rendering the point name as Faith Intersection conveys, albeit abstrusely, the meaning inherent in the Chinese.

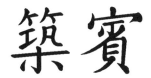

Guest House

KI-9 *(zhú bīn)*

築 *zhú*: to build, to construct; to pound, to attack
賓 *bīn*: guest; to submit

Alternate Names

Calf Intestine	腨腸	*chuài cháng*
Leg Belly	腿肚	*tuǐ dù*

Classical Location: To locate the point move upward and outward from Intersection Reach (KI-8), passing Three Yin Intersection (SP-6), up into the belly of the calf.
(Great Compendium)

Point Associations: Cleft-xi point of the yin linking vessel; intersection-jiaohui point of the foot shao yin kidney channel and the yin linking vessel.

Explanation of Point Name

The kidney channel hosts the yang motility vessel at this point and is said to have constructed (築 *zhú*) a dwelling or house for the guest (賓 *bīn*). In ancient times the character 賓 *bīn* was sometimes used as an equivalent of 擯 , to expel. Considered in this light, if 築 *zhú* is taken to mean "attack," the point name takes on the meaning of "to expel attack," and can be interpreted as referring to the point's ability to expel pathogenic qi that attacks the kidney. Rendering the name as Attack Expulsion would convey this meaning.

The alternate names, Calf Intestine and Leg Belly, refer to the location on the calf. Compare these names to Sinew Support (BL-56) and Mountain Support (BL-57).

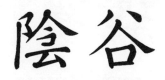

Yin Valley

KI-10 (yīn gǔ)
陰 yīn: yin, the complement of yang
谷 gǔ: valley

Classical Location: Below the knee, behind the inner leg bone, below the large sinew and above the small sinew. *(Systematized Canon)*

Point Associations: Uniting-he (water) point.

Explanation of Point Name

KI-10 is located between two tendons on the yin (inner) side of the knee. The depression between the tendons can be seen to resemble a valley; hence the name. The character 陰 yīn may furthermore be taken as a reference to the shao yin kidney channel.

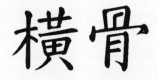

Pubic Bone

KI-11 (héng gǔ)
橫 héng: horizontal, crosswise
谷 gǔ: bone

Alternate Names

Lower Extreme	下極	*xià jí*
Curved Bone	曲骨	*qū gǔ*
Crooked Bone	屈骨	*qū gǔ*
Curved Bone's End	曲骨端	*qū gǔ duān*
Crooked Bone's End	曲骨端	*qū gǔ duān*

Classical Location: One inch below Great Manifestation (KI-12), on the bone, one inch either side of the center line of the abdomen, in the depression shaped like an upturned moon. *(Great Compendium)*

Point Associations: Intersection-jiaohui point of the foot shao yin kidney channel and the penetrating vessel.

Explanation of Point Name

The character combination 橫骨 *héng gǔ* was the ancient Chinese name for the pubic bone. As this point is positioned just above that bone, its name is obviously derived from its location.

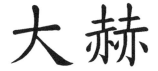

Great Manifestation

KI-12 *(dà hè)*

大 *dà*: large, big, great
赫 *hè*: bright, luminous or awe-inspiring (manifestation)

Alternate Names

Yin Gate	陰關	*yīn guān*
Yin Link	陰維	*yīn wéi*

Classical Location: One inch below Qi Hole (KI-13), one inch either side of the midline. *(Great Compendium)*

Point Associations: Intersection-jiaohui point of the foot shao yin kidney channel and the penetrating vessel.

Explanation of Point Name

KI-12 shares the exuberant yin qi of the penetrating vessel, which intersects the kidney channel at this point, and in females is close to the womb, where essence gathers. Great Manifestation somewhat exaggeratedly reflects this abundance of yin enjoyed by the point.

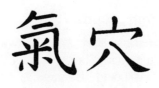

Qi Hole

KI-13 *(qì xuè)*
氣 *qì*: qi
穴 *xuè*: acupuncture point; cave, hole

Alternate Names

Infant's Door	子戸	*zǐ hù*
Uterine Gate	胞門	*bāo mén*

Classical Location: One inch below Fourfold Fullness (KI-14), one inch either side of the midline.
(Great Compendium)

Point Associations: Intersection-jiaohui point of the foot shao yin kidney channel and the penetrating vessel.

Explanation of Point Name

This point is cited in *A Treatise on Cold Damage* as the location of the manifestation of kidney qi. Furthermore, the kidney rules qi absorption and KI-13 is located close to where that absorption takes place. For these reasons it is named Qi Hole.

The alternate names for KI-13 differ for each side of the body. Infant's Door, 子户 *zǐ hù* is the point on the right. Uterine Gate, 胞門 *bāo mén* is the name given to the point on the left.

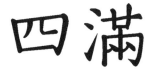

Fourfold Fullness

KI-14 *(sì mǎn)*
四 *sì*: four
滿 *mǎn*: full, complete

Alternate Names

Marrow Mansion	髓府	*suí fǔ*
Marrow Center	髓中	*suí zhōng*

Classical Location: One inch below Central Flow (KI-15), one inch either side of the midline. *(Great Compendium)*

Point Associations: Intersection-jiaohui point of the foot shao yin kidney channel and the penetrating vessel.

Explanation of Point Name

This point treats distention and fullness of the abdomen due to accumulation of any of four things: blood, qi, digesta, or water-damp. Thus the name can be thought of as indicating that the point treats Fourfold Fullness.

Fourfold Fullness also refers to the fullness in the lower abdomen that distends in the four directions, a condition relieved by treating KI-14. The word four in this instance is meant to emphasize the completeness of the distention and is not to be taken literally.

In the Chinese calendar, 小滿 *xiǎo mǎn*, meaning "brief fullness," is the eighth solar term, which occurs between May 21 and June 4. During this time a constellation of four (四 *sì*) stars is prominent in the night sky. KI-14 may be named Fourfold Fullness in reference to this period because the eighth solar term (小滿) is a time of flourishing on the earth, and KI-14 is located near the Cinnabar Field 丹田 *dān tián*, which is the place on the body where qi thrives.

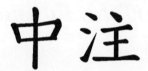

Central Flow

KI-15 *(zhōng zhù)*
中 *zhōng*: center, middle
注 *zhù*: to flow, to pour; to fix on

Classical Location: One inch below Huang Shu (KI-16), one inch each side of the midline. *(Great Compendium)*

Point Associations: Intersection-jiaohui point of the foot shao yin kidney channel and the penetrating vessel.

Explanation of Point Name

The name Central Flow can be thought of as a reminder that the point is located in the center of the body at a place where the kidney qi flows into the penetrating vessel. Alternatively, it is also where water qi flows down into the bladder. This point is located in the area from which the essential qi that is extracted from digesta flows from the central burner out to the five viscera; the name Central Flow conveys this meaning. Consider too, that the ministerial fire flows down from this point into the Cinnabar Field (丹田 *dān tián*). Thus the name Central Flow marks a flowing into the place of central importance.

Viewing 中 *zhōng* as representing 中衣 *zhōng yī*, an old name for underwear, introduces another interpretation. The point marks the site of the border of underwear and in this case 注 *zhù* means to attach. The point name could be interpreted as meaning the point where the underwear hangs on the body.

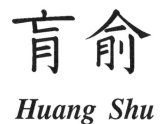

Huang Shu

KI-16 *(huāng shū)*
肓 *huāng*: the area just below the diaphragm
俞 *shū*: acupuncture point

Classical Location: One inch below Shang Bend (KI-17), one inch either side of the midline. *(Great Compendium)*

Point Associations: Intersection-jiaohui point of the foot shao yin kidney channel and the penetrating vessel.

Explanation of Point Name
The kidney channel passes through the abdomen and then proceeds up to the *huāng* area. Because of this and the

point's effectiveness in treating disorders of the *huāng* area, it is called Huang Shu. The character 肓 *huāng* can refer to either the bladder or the region below the heart. In either case it is related to the kidney because the bladder and kidney stand in interior-exterior relationship and because the kidney channel passes through the *huāng* region. It is not surprising that all the point names that contain the character 肓 *huāng* are found on the kidney and bladder channels.

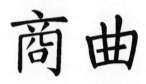

Shang Bend

KI-17 *(shāng qū)*
商 *shāng*: the musical tone associated with metal
曲 *qū*: bent, curved

Alternate Names

Shang Abode	商舍	*shāng shè*
High Bend	高曲	*gāo qū*

Classical Location: One inch below Stone Pass (KI-18),one and a half inches either side of the midline.
(Great Compendium)

Point Associations: Intersection-jiaohui point of the foot shao yin kidney channel with the penetrating vessel.

Explanation of Point Name

KI-17 is found at a place on the abdomen beneath which there is a bend in the large intestine. Shang is the fifth note in the Chinese musical scale and is associated with the metal phase and, by extension, the large intestine. The point name reveals that the point is located above the bend of the large intestine.

The character 高 *gǎo*, meaning high, is most likely a mistranscription of the character 商 *shāng* that produced the alternate name High Bend.

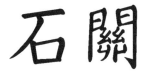

Stone Pass

KI-18 *(shí guān)*
石 *shí*: stone
關 *guān*: gate, passageway, pass

Alternate Names

Stone Gate Tower	石闕	*shí què*
Food Palace	食宮	*shí gōng*
Food Tube	食呂	*shí lǚ*
Stone Palace	石宮	*shí gōng*
Free Passage	通關	*tōng guān*

Classical Location: One inch below Yin Metropolis (KI-19), one and a half inches either side of the midline.
(Great Compendium)

Point Associations: Intersection-jiaohui point of the foot shao yin kidney channel and the penetrating vessel.

Explanation of Point Name

In this name 石 *shí* , meaning stone, may imply a blockage or a tightness and can thus be construed as a reference to KI-18's function of treating such disorders as difficult defecation, conglomerations, inhibited urination, and female infertility. In this connotation, pass would denote an acupuncture point.

Stone is fundamental to earth and can thus serve as a metaphor for digesta, which is fundamental to the earth phase in the body. Thus the point name may be a reference to the place through which food passes (i.e., the large intestine, which is situated beneath this point).

This point may be employed in treating stone water swelling (石水 *shí shuǐ*), which is a disorder characterized by hard, tight, water swelling in the lower abdomen. Stimulating KI-18 can open the pass (i.e., disinhibit the waterways) and thus disperse swelling. This provides another reason for naming the point Stone Pass.

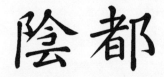

Yin Metropolis

KI-19 *(yīn dū)*
陰 *yīn*: yin, the complement of yang
都 *dū*: metropolis, capital

Classical Location: One inch below Open Valley (KI-20), one and a half inches either side of the midline.
(Great Compendium)

Point Associations: Intersection-jiaohui point of the foot shao yin kidney channel and the penetrating vessel.

Explanation of Point Name

A metropolis is an important gathering place. KI-19 is located at a spot just lateral to CV-12, which is the alarm-mu point of the stomach. This area is regarded as the place where the qi of the earth phase gathers. The point is thus named Yin Metropolis because it is an important gathering place on the yin channel. Since the point is located on the abdomen, which is the anatomical yin within the yin, and because it is located on the kidney channel, which is also yin within yin, the adjective yin in this name is doubly fitting.

The alternate name Food Palace reinforces this point's relationship to earth (stomach) qi.

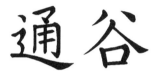

Open Valley

KI-20 *(tōng gǔ)*

通 *tōng*: to free, unblock; to pass through
谷 *gǔ*: valley; grain

Alternate Names

Freeing the Grain	通穀	*tōng gǔ*
Upper Gate	上門	*shàng mén*

Classical Location: One inch below Dark Gate (KI-21), one and a half inches from the midline. *(Great Compendium)*

Point Associations: Intersection-jiaohui point of the foot shao yin kidney channel and the penetrating vessel.

Explanation of Point Name

This point name refers to location, as is often the case. *Essential Questions* mentions that large areas of flesh are called valleys. This is why such points as LI-4 and KI-20, which are in fleshy areas, are called valleys (especially in contrast to ravines, such as KI-3 and SI-3, which are located where the flesh is much less abundant). KI-20 is in the valley formed by the muscles of the central abdomen. The qi of the kidney channel passes though this region as if it were traversing a mountain valley. Open Valley is a translation that highlights this interpretation of the point name.

The ideogram 谷 *gǔ*, in addition to its meaning of "valley," is frequently used as a substitute for the homophone 穀, meaning grain (which, perhaps coincidentally, is often grown in a valley). If taken in this way, the point name can be said to refer to the use of this point in aiding digestion, or to the fact that digesta passes through this area. In this case the alternate translation of Freeing the Grain might serve well.

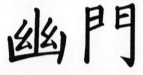

Dark Gate

KI-21 (*yōu mén*)

幽 *yōu*: dark, gloomy; secret, subtle, hidden
門 *mén*: gate, door

Alternate Name

Upper Gate   上門   *shàng mén*

Classical Location: In a depression one inch and five fen either side of Great Tower Gate (CV-14).
(Great Compendium)

Point Associations: Intersection-jiaohui point of the foot shao yin kidney channel and the penetrating vessel.

Explanation of Point Name

The meeting of the penetrating vessel (yin) with the kidney (yin) makes this point doubly yin. 幽 *yōu* conveys the aspect of yin that is dark and mysterious. The pictograph 門 *mén* refers either to the acupuncture point itself or to KI-21 being the exit point of the penetrating vessel, which, after passing through this point, disperses over the chest. For these reasons the point is called the Dark Gate.

The bottom opening of the stomach is also called 幽門, which in modern medicine the Chinese adopted as the equivalent of pylorus. KI-21 is nevertheless closer to the upper opening of the stomach (the cardia), as the alternate name Upper Gate suggests.

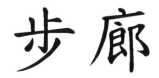

Corridor Walk

KI-22 *(bù láng)*

步 *bù*: a step; on foot
廊 *láng*: corridor, veranda, porch;
    an upward path (新華字典)

Alternate Name

    Walking Gentleman   步郎   *bù láng*

Classical Location: In the depression one inch and six fen above Dark Gate (KI-21), two inches either side of the midline. The point is found in supine posture. *(Golden Mirror)*

Explanation of Point Name

This point marks the advance of the kidney channel up to the rib cage. The character 步 *bù*, meaning to step, can be seen as a reference to the channel stepping up into the chest, or could be a reference to the nature of the channel in the region of the chest. The points proceed stepwise up the rib cage one rib at a time. The ideograph 廊 *láng* can mean either a path upward (toward a summit) or a corridor. The former interpretation simply describes the path of the kidney channel. As regards the latter interpretation, the left and right kidney channels, when charted on the chest, resemble a corridor.

Two translations of this name become possible in this light. Corridor Walk encompasses the idea of a corridor and the rib-by-rib, step-by-step nature of the channel, while Step Upward would include the idea of the channel advancing into the region of the chest and the notion of an upward path.

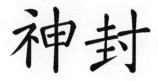

Spirit Seal

KI-23 *(shén fēng)*
神 *shén*: spirit
封 *fēng*: to seal; a border

Classical Location: One inch and six fen above Corridor Walk (KI-22), two inches either side of the midline. The point is found in supine posture. *(Golden Mirror)*

Explanation of Point Name

This point is located in the region of the heart. The heart stores the spirit. The heart yin directly, and the heart spirit indirectly, rely on kidney water for nourishment. This connection between the two organs accounts for the presence of the word "spirit" in the names of several kidney channel points in this area (神 *shén* or 靈 *líng*). The character 封 *fēng* can mean "to seal," and as such is a reference to kidney water containing or sealing in the yang nature of the spirit. 封 *fēng* may also mean "border," in which case it can be taken as a reference to the point's location on the edge of the cardiac region.

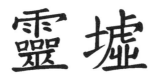

Spirit Ruins

KI-24 *(líng xū)*

靈 *líng*: spirit (similar, but more yin than 神 *shén*)
墟 *xū*: ruins; old burial grounds; residence 帝王布擭

Alternate Name

Spirit Wall 靈墙 *líng qiáng*

Classical Location: One inch and six fen above Spirit Seal (KI-23), two inches either side of the midline. The point is found in supine posture. *(Golden Mirror)*

Explanation of Point Name

Spirit Ruins represents the region where the spirit resides and thus reminds us that the point is near the heart. The character 墟 *xū* is associated with yin qualities, i.e., mysterious, hidden or obscure, and 靈 *líng* indicates the yin aspect of the spirit. The point name emphasizes the yin nature of the kidney as well as the point's location in the cardiac region.

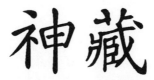

Spirit Storehouse

KI-25 (shén cáng)
神 *shén*: spirit
藏 *cáng*: to store; the viscera

Classical Location: One inch and six fen above Spirit Ruins (KI-24), two inches either side of the midline. The point is found in supine posture. *(Golden Mirror)*

Explanation of Point Name

The yin spirit (靈 *líng*) of the five viscera is transformed by heart fire into spirit (神 *shén*). This spirit is then stored in the heart. This point name refers to the point's location near the heart, which is the Spirit Storehouse.

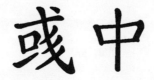

Lively Center

KI-26 (yù zhōng)
彧 *yù*: elegant, cultured; flourishing
中 *zhōng*: center, middle

Alternate Names

| Possible Center | 或中 | *huò zhōng* |
| Within Bounds | 域中 | *yù zhōng* |

Classical Location: One inch and six fen above Spirit Storehouse (KI-25), in the depression two inches either side of the midline. The point is found in supine posture. *(Golden Mirror)*

Explanation of Point Name

KI-26 is located where the heart fire flourishes and so is called Lively Center. In this point name 中 *zhōng*, meaning center, may be considered as a reference to the center of the chest, which is the seat of the emotions. The epithet Lively is attached because the point has the function of causing the qi in the chest to flow smoothly in the chest, thus lifting the spirits.

The character 或 *yù* originally meant "patterned." If understood in this sense it may be seen as a reference to the pattern of veins on the lung. The name thus becomes locational and could be rendered as Patterned Center. Possible Center and Within Bounds probably evolved from mistranscriptions of the character 或.

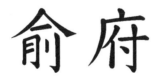

Shu Mansion

KI-27 (*shū fǔ*)

俞 *shū*: acupuncture point; to transport
府 *fǔ*: mansion; storehouse, treasury

Alternate Name

Transport Mansion   輸府   *shū fǔ*

Classical Location: Below the clavicle, in the depression two inches from Jade Pivot (CV-21). *(Systematized Canon)*

Explanation of Point Name

KI-27 is the last point on the kidney channel, and as such, is the point to which the kidney channel qi is transported (兪 *shū*) and at which it gathers (府 *fǔ*). Though commonly termed Shu Mansion, a rendering as Shu Storehouse or Shu Treasury is equally appropriate.

The character 府 *fǔ* can mean an important government building housing the highest political offices. The point may be likened to this type of building because it is the uppermost point on the kidney channel and is the highest point with the label *shū* (兪) on the body.

Another explanation describes the throat as a multi-story building (府 *fǔ*). Kidney qi is transported (兪 *shū*) to the throat through this point. A rendering of the point name as Mansion Transport reflects this idea. Because the character 輸 *shū*, which generally means transport, is often interchanged with the character 兪 *shū*, the alternate name for the point is also Transport Mansion.

Pericardium Channel

(Hand Jue Yin)

手厥陰心包經

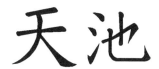

Celestial Pool

PC-1 *(tiān chí)*

天 *tiān*: celestial, of the heavens; sky; Nature; heaven
池 *chí*: pool, pond

Alternate Name

> Celestial Convergence   天會   *tiān huì*

Classical Location: Three inches below the armpit, one or two inches behind the nipple, between the protuberances of the ribs. *(Golden Mirror)*

Point Associations: Intersection-jiaohui point of the hand jue yin pericardium, foot jue yin liver and foot shao yang gallbladder channels.

Explanation of Point Name

This point is located in a type of depression which is often labeled a pool because qi may collect there, just as water collects in low-lying areas to form pools. At the same time, it may also be considered as a mountain pool from which water flows to the sea, an image that reflects the way in which qi flows down from PC-1 to PC-9. (PC-1 may well have been named after a mountain pool, since there are several in China named 天池 *tiān chí* .) The honorific "celestial" is a reference to the point's location high on the body or near the heart (which rules the body as heaven rules the earth).

It is interesting to note that the names for the first three points on the pericardium channel all relate to water, possibly in part because the channel originates in the often damp area of the armpit. Also, PC-1 is another point that shares its name with the name of a star.

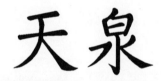

Celestial Spring

PC-2 *(tiān quán)*
天 *tiān*: celestial, of the heavens; sky; Nature; heaven
泉 *quán*: source, spring

Alternate Names

Celestial Warmth	天溫	*tiān wēn*
Celestial Damp	天濕	*tiān shī*

Classical Location: Two inches below the armpit fold. The point is located with the arm raised.
(Great Compendium)

Explanation of Point Name

The logic of this point name is much the same as that for Celestial Pool (PC-1 above). The epithet "celestial" owes its presence to the point's location in the upper part of the body, while "spring" is a metaphor for the downward flow of qi from this point, much like the flow of water from a mountain spring.

天泉 *tiān quán* is also a star name.

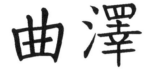

Marsh at the Bend

PC-3 *(qū zé)*
曲 *qū*: bend, curve, crook; bent
澤 *zé*: marsh

Classical Location: On the inner side of the elbow, where a pulsating vessel can be felt on the inside of the large sinew on the transverse crease. *(Great Compendium)*

Point Associations: Uniting-he (water) point.

Explanation of Point Name

In this point name the word marsh reflects the appellation of PC-3 as the water point of the pericardium channel. The location of the point at the crook of the elbow accounts for the name Marsh at the Bend. In addition, because marshes often exist at the mouths of rivers, the point name is a reminder that this is a uniting-he point, where the flow of qi is likened to the water of a river uniting with the sea.

郄門

Cleft-Xi Gate

PC-4 *(xī mén)*

郄 *xī*: cleft, crevice
門 *mén*: door, gate

Classical Location: Below Marsh at the Bend (PC-3), five inches behind the wrist. *(Golden Mirror)*

Point Associations: Cleft-xi point of the pericardium.

Explanation of Point Name

PC-4 is the cleft-xi point, and is by definition located in a cleft (郄 *xī*), the one formed by two ligaments. The word gate (門 *mén*) may be considered a reference to the entry and exit of qi at the point.

間使

Intermediary Courier

PC-5 *(jiān shǐ)*

間 *jiān*: among, between; to separate
使 *shǐ*: a messenger; to employ; to cause, to allow

Alternate Name

Ghost Road   鬼路   *guǐ lù*

Classical Location: In the depression between the two sinews, three inches from the wrist. *(Golden Mirror)*

Point Associations: River-jing (metal) point; the ninth of the thirteen ghost points.

Explanation of Point Name

In this point name, 間 *jiān*, meaning between, recalls the location of PC-5 between the two sinews. 使 *shǐ*, to employ, refers to the function of the pericardium to protect the heart, the sovereign viscus. If 間 is taken in the slightly different sense of "to come between," the point name can be seen to emphasize the pericardium's function of interceding for the heart, just as a minister "takes the heat" for the emperor.

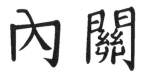

Inner Pass

PC-6 *(nèi guān)*
內 *nèi*: inner, inside
關 *guān*: gate, passage; to shut, to close

Classical Location: Between the sinews two inches behind the wrist, at the point opposite to Outer Pass (TB-5).
(Great Compendium)

Point Associations: Connecting-luo point of the pericardium channel connecting to the triple burner channel; confluence-jiaohui point of the eight extraordinary vessels (yin linking vessel).

Explanation of Point Name

In this instance 內 *nèi*, meaning inner, has a double connotation. The first is that of the inner surface of the arm, where the point is located; the second implies lying in between, describing the location of the pericardium channel between the other two hand yin channels (heart and lung). 關 *guān*, pass, refers to the connecting vessel that leads to the triple burner channel, reminding us that PC-6 is a connecting-luo point. For these reasons, the point is called Inner Pass. See also Outer Pass (外關 *wài guān*: TB-5).

The character combination 內關 *nèi guān* is an ancient disease name, which could be translated as "inner block." This disease is characterized by glomus and oppression in the chest. Since PC-6 can free the thoracic region, rendering the name of this point as Inner Block would reflect its ability to treat this disorder.

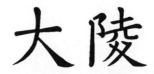

Great Mound

PC-7 *(dà líng)*
大 *dà*: great, large, big
陵 *líng*: mound, small hill

Alternate Names

Heart Governor	主心	*zhǔ xīn*
Ghost Heart	鬼心	*guǐ xīn*
Hand Heart Governor	手心主	*shǒu xīn zhǔ*

Classical Location: In the depression between the two sinews behind the hand. *(Systematized Canon)*

Point Associations: Stream-shu (earth) point; source-yuan point; the fourth of the thirteen ghost points; one of the nine needles for returning yang.

Explanation of Point Name

This point is located on the inner aspect of the arm just proximal to the wrist. The heel of the hand resembles two large mounds, thus giving PC-7 its name. In addition, a mound is a gathering of earth; therefore the name of this point further reflects its being the earth point of the pericardium channel.

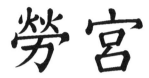

Palace of Toil

PC-8 *(láo gōng)*

勞 *láo*: toil, labor; taxation, weariness
宮 *gōng*: palace

Alternate Names

Construction Palace	營宮	*yíng gōng*
Center of the Palm	掌中	*zhǎng zhōng*
Five Li	五里	*wǔ lǐ*
Ghost Cave	鬼窟	*guǐ kū*
Ghost Road	鬼路	*guǐ lù*

Classical Location: At the pulsating vessel on the palm of the hand, located by bending the fourth finger.
(Great Compendium)

Point Associations: Spring-ying (water) point; one of the nine needles for returning yang.

Explanation of Point Name

PC-8 is located in the center of the palm. The point may be named Palace of Toil in reference to its location on the hand, which is the actual Palace of Toil because of all the work that the hands do.

The word "toil" (勞 *láo*) in this point name recalls the task that the pericardium performs in protecting the heart. Palace (宮 *gōng*) may be taken as a reminder of the close relationship of the pericardium and the heart, the emperor (the heart) residing within the palace (the pericardium).

PC-8 is used in the treatment of taxation fatigue, lending meaning to its translation as Taxation Palace.

中 衝

Central Hub

PC-9 (zhōng chōng)
中 zhōng: central, center, middle
衝 chōng: a hub, thoroughfare; (沖) to surge, to flush

Classical Location: At the tip of the middle finger, in the depression the width of a Chinese leek leaf away from the nail. *(Great Compendium)*

Point Associations: Well-jing (wood) point.

Explanation of Point Name

The location of PC-9 on the tip of the middle (central) finger makes it a centrally located, strategic point. The appellation Central Hub reflects this idea. Also, the pericardium channel traverses the center of the inner arm. Though the qi at well-jing points is usually described as small and still like water in a well, numerous sources say that the qi at PC-9 surges forth. (采艾編: 此其沖气也.) Therefore the point name could also be rendered as Central Surge.

Triple Burner Channel
(Hand Shao Yang)

手少陽三焦經

關 衝

Passage Hub

TB-1 *(guān chōng)*
關 *guān*: passage, gate, door
衝 *chōng*: hub, thoroughfare; 沖 surge, flush

Classical Location: On outer side of the finger next to the little finger, the width of a Chinese leek leaf away from the corner of the nail. (Great Compendium)

Point Associations: Well-jing (metal) point.

Explanation of Point Name

The word passage (關 *guān*) in the point name reflects the function of the triple burner as a conduit for the passage of qi from the upper to the lower body. Here, the character 衝 *chōng* may be considered as a reference to PC-1 as a point where the qi changes channels i.e., a hub.

This point is located on the tip of the ring finger. The names of the points on the tips of the middle and small fingers include the character 衝 (沖). The ring finger lies in between the other hubs, PC-9 and HT-9, resembling a passageway between them. The character 沖 *chōng* also may refer to the surging flow of qi at this point.

The qi at the well-jing points is usually described as small and still, like the water of a well. It is perhaps the nature of the reaction that these points evoke when they are needled that results in them also being described as places of surging qi. PC-9 and HT-9 are other well-jing points that have the character 沖 *chōng*, to surge, in their point names.

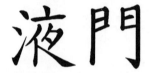

Humor Gate

TB-2 *(yè mén)*

液 *yè*: humor, water, fluid
門 *mén*: gate, door

Alternate Names

Armpit Gate	掖門	*yè mén*
Humor Gate	液門	*yè mén*

Classical Location: In the depression between the little finger and the one next to it. *(Systematized Canon)*

Point Associations: Spring-ying (water) point.

Explanation of Point Name

TB-2 is the spring-ying (water) point of the triple burner channel. Since the triple burner channel is responsible for water distribution in the three burners, its water point is especially important. The character 液 *yè* means humor, i.e., the thicker fluids in the body, and highlights the moistening function of this point. The ideograph 門 *mén* refers to the entry and exit of qi at this point; hence the appellation Humor Gate. The functions of this point of addressing vexation heat, increasing fluids and regulating the waterways are all reflected in its name.

In the earliest extant text devoted entirely to acupuncture, the *Systematized Canon of Acupuncture and Moxibustion*, this point is called Armpit Gate. Note the similarity of the characters 腋 *yè*, armpit, and 液 *yè*, humor. This earlier name may have referred to the effectiveness of this point in treating disorders of the upper arm. Formerly the word for armpit was sometimes written 掖 instead of 腋, i.e., with the hand (or arm) radical instead of the flesh radical, thus resulting in two alternate names of the same meaning.

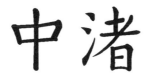

Central Islet

TB-3 *(zhōng zhǔ)*
中 *zhōng*: central, middle
渚 *zhǔ*: an islet

Alternate Name

    Lower Metropolis   下都   *xià dū*

Classical Location: In the depression behind the base joints of the little finger and the one next to it, one inch from Humor Gate (TB-2). *(Great Compendium)*

Point Associations: Stream-shu (wood) point.

Explanation of Point Name

This point is located between Humor Gate (TB-2) and Yang

Pool (TB-4). The name Central Islet can be seen to liken the point to a small island between two bodies of water.

The name of this point may be further considered as a reminder of triple burner functions. The character 中 *zhōng* (center) may be construed as a reference to source qi, which is sometimes called 中 and is moved by the triple burner, while 渚 *zhǔ* (islet) calls to mind the triple burner's governance of the waterways since an island can also dictate the flow of water.

This point is also the wood point of the triple burner channel. Wood can block the flow of water, causing water to flow around it just as if it were a small island.

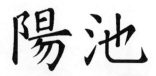

Yang Pool

TB-4 *(yáng chí)*
陽 *yáng*: yang, the complement of yin
池 *chí*: pool, pond

Alternate Name

> Divergent Yang　別陽　*bié yáng*

Classical Location: In a depression on the back of the wrist; feel straight along from the base joint of the fingers to the center of the wrist. *(Great Compendium)*

Point Associations: Source-yuan point of the triple burner.

Explanation of Point Name

In the landscape of the body the spot where TB-4 is located resembles a pond, i.e., a shallow depression where water (or in this case source qi, which collects at source-yuan points) can collect. This point is located on the yang aspect of the wrist and is thus called Yang Pool.

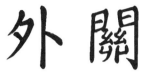

Outer Pass

TB-5 (wài guān)
外 wài: outer, outside
關 guān: pass, gate

Classical Location: Between the two bones two inches behind the wrist, opposite Inner Pass (PC-6).
(Great Compendium)

Point Associations: Connecting-luo point of the triple burner channel connecting to the pericardium channel; confluence-jiaohui point of the eight extraordinary channels (yang linking channel).

Explanation of Point Name

Located on the outer surface of the arm, this point marks the passage (i.e., connecting vessel) to the pericardium channel. See also Inner Passage (PC-6).

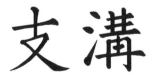

Branch Ditch

TB-6 (zhī gōu)
支 zhī: branch, limb; descendants
溝 gōu: ditch, water gully

Alternate Name

Flying Tiger 飛虎 *fēi hǔ*

Classical Location: On the outer face of the arm, three inches back from the wrist, in the depression between the two bones. *(Great Compendium)*

Point Associations: River-jing (wood) point.

Explanation of Point Name

This point is located on the upper limb (i.e., branch) and can be found in the gully-like depression between the sinews of the forearm. Because the triple burner helps to regulate water flow in the body, this depression can be likened to a water ditch. The name of this point therefore reminds the practitioner that just as water ditches are used to irrigate fields, the triple burner channel helps to irrigate the body. The point name also brings to mind TB-6's function of moistening the intestines.

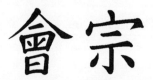

Convergence and Gathering

TB-7 *(huì zōng)*
會 *huì*: to converge, to gather, to meet
宗 *zōng*: a meeting of officials; a suzerain; ancestor; clan

Classical Location: In the space between the bones three inches behind the wrist. *(Great Compendium)*

Point Associations: Cleft-xi point of the triple burner.

Explanation of Point Name

Both 會 *huì* and 宗 *zōng* mean to meet or to gather. This point is the cleft-xi point of the triple burner channel, which is where triple burner qi collects.

Some sources invoke the meaning of suzerain for 宗 *zōng*. Just as a suzerainty is a part of a country yet rules from afar, this point is located off the direct line of the triple burner channel yet is still an important point.

The triple burner is associated with fire and, by extension, summer. The meeting (會 *huì*) of officials during the summer in ancient China was termed 宗 *zōng*. This point may be named after this summertime gathering because it is also a "gathering of fire," i.e., the cleft-xi point of the fire channel.

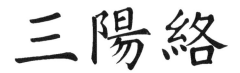

Three Yang Connection

TB-8 *(sān yáng luò)*

三 *sān*: three
陽 *yáng*: yang, the complement of yin
絡 *luò*: to connect, to mesh; to spin (into yarn); connecting vessel

Alternate Names

Connect Between	通間	*tōng jiān*
Connecting Gate	通門	*tōng mén*

Classical Location: Obliquely inward one inch up from Convergence and Gathering (TB-7). *(Golden Mirror)*

Explanation of Point Name

The three yang channels of the hand all pass near this point. In *The Systematized Canon of Acupuncture and Moxibustion* this is called the "great intersecting vessel." There is no connecting vessel at this point, so the word 絡 *luò* simply implies the connection of the three hand yang channels through physical proximity and functional similarity.

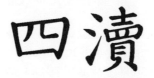

Four Rivers

TB-9 (sì dú)
四 *sì*: four
瀆 *dú*: a large river; to show contempt; ditch, drain

Classical Location: Five inches in front of the elbow, in the depression on the outer side. *(Great Compendium)*

Explanation of Point Name

In this point name the character 瀆 *dú*, meaning river, is drawn from the *Spiritual Axis,* where the triple burner is called 中瀆 *zhōng dú*, "the central river." The term "four rivers" is a reference to the four main rivers in China and, by extension, rivers and streams in general. It could be that the number four was chosen because it nicely follows Three Yang Connection (TB-8).

The spleen is intimately connected with the number four because four is the number of tai yin, with which the spleen is associated, and because the spleen governs the four limbs. The spleen is associated with damp and belongs to the earth phase. TB-9 is like a ditch joining to TB-10, which is the earth point of the triple burner channel.

In view of this and the triple burner's function in relationship to the water path, this point name could be rendered as Four Ditch, meaning a ditch to the earth phase, or to the spleen.

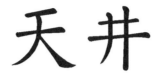

Celestial Well

TB-10 *(tiān jǐng)*

天 *tiān*: celestial, of the heavens, sky; Nature; heaven
井 *jǐng*: water well

Classical Location: Up one inch from the back of the tip of the large bone on the outer side of the elbow, in the depression between two sinews and the bone. The point is located with the arm bent over the chest. *(Golden Mirror)*

Point Associations: Uniting-he (earth) point.

Explanation of Point Name

The fact that the triple burner governs the waterways, combined with the location of this point in a depression, explains why the word "well" was chosen. Its location in the upper body led to the name Celestial Well. Also, the character combination 天井 *tiān jǐng* describes a small pond surrounded by high cliffs, i.e., a "celestial well." TB-10's location in a depression behind the elbow can be seen to resemble such an area.

Celestial Well is the name of an astrological constellation that resembles a well, and is further the name for the courtyard in certain styles of Chinese houses. It was thus a name quite familiar to the ancient Chinese.

清冷淵

Clear Cold Abyss

TB-11 *(qīng lěng yuān)*

清 *qīng*: clear
冷 *lěng*: cold, frigid
淵 *yuān*: a deep lake or abyss

Alternate Names

Clear Cold Spring	清冷泉	*qīng lěng quán*
Clear Sky	清昊	*qīng hào*
Clear Spirit	清靈	*qīng líng*

Classical Location: Two inches above the elbow. The point is found with the elbow stretched and the arm raised. *(Great Compendium)*

Explanation of Point Name

This phrase is found in ancient geography books in reference to various lakes. It implies the ability of this point to clear heat and drain fire.

消濼

Dispersing Riverbed

TB-12 *(xiāo luò)*

消 *xiāo*: to disperse, to eliminate
濼 *luò*: a riverbed

Alternate Name

Dispersing Brilliance　　消爍　　*xiāo shuò*

Classical Location: Up from Clear Cold Abyss (TB-11), on the outer aspect of the arm below the shoulder, in the depression at the parting of the flesh on the slanting line drawn from the end of the axillary crease to the elbow. *(Golden Mirror)*

Explanation of Point Name

The character 消 *xiāo* means to relieve or eliminate, while 濼 *luò* means riverbed, representing water (note the water radical on the left). The point name refers to the clear, cool nature of water (i.e., the waterways regulated by the triple burner) that can clear heat and relieve thirst. Also brought to mind by this point name is the dispersal of water over a riverbed as a metaphor for the triple burner function of dispersing water throughout the body.

The translation of this point name as Dispersed Riverbed gives us the image of a depression left in the earth after a river has dispersed, just as the point is located in a depression.

The character 濼 is also pronounced *pò*, and 淫濼 *yīn pò* is a name for either of two disease conditions. The first involves the prolonged retention of pathogenic qi that is stagnant and difficult to remove, while the second is a specific ailment that presents with aching and lack of strength, usually affecting either the legs or arms. It is possible that the point name refers to the treatment of these disorders.

An alternate name for this point is 消爍 *xiāo shuò*, which can be rendered as Dispersing Brilliance. 爍, which is the same as 濼 except that it has the fire (火) radical instead of the water radical (水), means brilliant, luminous, and according to some, fire. This name reminds us of the function of the point in dispersing triple burner fire. According to some sources, this is the correct name of the point, while 㵯 *luò* is a mistaken substitute.

臑會

Upper Arm Convergence

TB-13 *(nào huì)*

臑 *nào*: the upper bone of the arm
會 *huì*: to converge, to meet, to join together

Alternate Names

Upper Arm Shu	臑俞	*nào shū*
Upper Arm Bone-Hole	臑髎	*nào liáo*
Upper Arm Intersection	臑交	*nào jiāo*

Classical Location: On the front [i.e., outer] face of the arm, three inches from the tip of the shoulder.
(Systematized Canon)

Point Associations: Intersection-jiaohui point of the hand shao yang triple burner channel and the yang linking vessel.

Explanation of Point Name

The character 臑 *nào* refers to the location of the point on the upper arm, while 會 *huì* denotes the convergence at this point of the triple burner channel and the yang linking vessel. *Essential Questions* states that the hand yang ming connecting vessel meets the triple burner channel at this point. This may further explain why the point is called Upper Arm Convergence.

肩髎

Shoulder Bone-Hole

TB-14 *(jiān liáo)*

肩 *jiān*: shoulder
髎 *liáo*: bone-hole

Classical Location: Above Upper Arm Convergence (TB-13) at the top of the arm at the end of the shoulder. The point is found when the arm is lifted to a slanting position. *(Golden Mirror)*

Point Associations: Intersection-jiaohui point of the hand shao yang triple burner channel and the yang linking vessel.

Explanation of Point Name

This name is a reference to the location of the point.

天髎

Celestial Bone-Hole

TB-15 *(tiān liáo)*

天 *tiān*: celestial, of the heavens, sky; Nature; heaven
髎 *liáo*: bone hole

Alternate Name

    Celestial Hearing   天聽   *tiān tīng*

Classical Location: One inch above Shoulder Bone-Hole (TB-14) in the center of the supraclavicular fossa one inch behind Shoulder Well (GB-21). *(Golden Mirror)*

Point Associations: Intersection-jiaohui point of the hand shao yang triple burner channel and the yang linking vessel.

Explanation of Point Name

The location of this point on the upper body accounts for the epithet "celestial." Its location in a space between bones gives it the name Celestial Bone-Hole.

天牖

Celestial Window

TB-16 *(tiān yǒu)*

天 *tiān*: celestial, of the heavens, sky; Nature; heaven
牖 *yǒu*: window; to enlighten, to teach

Classical Location: At the outer border of the major sinew of the neck, behind Celestial Countenance (SI-17) and in front of Celestial Pillar (BL-10), below the completion bone [i.e., the mastoid process]. *(Great Compendium)*

Explanation of Point Name

This point is located on the head, which is the anatomical parallel of cosmological heaven (天 *tiān*). The eyes and ears are known as the "windows" of the head. The location of this point along with its employment for unblocking qi and opening the portals (the eyes, ears and nose) accounts for the name Celestial Window. Note that TB-16 is located in a region with many other points that share the honorific "celestial."

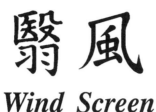

Wind Screen

TB-17 (yì fēng)

翳 *yì*: a screen, to screen, to shade
風 *fēng*: wind

Classical Location: In the depression behind the tip of the ear. When the point is pressed it causes pain in the ear. *(Great Compendium)*

Point Associations: Intersection-jiaohui point of the gall-bladder and triple burner channels.

Explanation of Point Name

This point is located behind the ear, which acts as a screen for the point, shading it and protecting it from the wind. In addition, the point may be utilized to dispel wind, thus screening the body from wind pathogens. The name Wind Screen recalls both ideas.

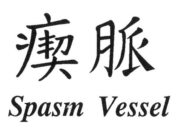

Spasm Vessel

TB-18 (chì mài)

瘛 *chì* (or *jì*): to pull, jerk; spasm
脈 *mài*: vessel, pulse

Alternate Name

Supporting Vessel	資脈	zī mài
Corporal Vessel	體脈	tǐ mài

Classical Location: Behind the base of the ear, at the cyan connecting vessels that resemble a chicken's foot.
(Great Compendium)

Explanation of Point Name

TB-18 is used in the treatment of a disease called 瘈瘲 *chì zòng*, which is tensing or pulling of the muscles immediately followed by relaxation, i.e., clonic spasm. This type of spasm is generally associated with epileptic diseases or psychotic fits. The use of this point in treating this disease is most likely the reason for the name Spasm Vessel.

Also at this location is a blood vessel shaped like a chicken's foot that appears to pull at the ear. A rendering of the point name as Tugging Vessel would correspond to this image.

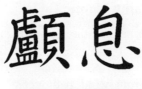

Skull Rest

TB-19 *(lú xí)*
顱 *lú*: skull, cranium,
息 *xí*: to stop, to rest; breath; news

Alternate Names

Skull	顱囟	lú xìn

Classical Location: Between the cyan connecting vessels behind the ear. *(Great Compendium)*

Explanation of Point Name

In classical Chinese 息 *xí* can mean to rest, and fullness or stuffiness. Thus this name could be a reference to an ability to calm the spirit (i.e., allow it to rest), thereby treating fright, spasms, epilepsy and fright palpitations; or it could be a reference to the treatment of clouded head and stuffiness.

It may also be that the point name is a way of indicating the location of the point; when lying on one's side the skull rests on the pillow at this point.

Given that the character 息 *xí* can also mean breath, the name could also be rendered as Skull's Breath. This would be justified because TB-19 is a point on the skull that treats 喘息 (*chuǎn xì*), difficult respiration (dyspnea).

Finally, the ear is where the head receives news (消息 *xiāo xì*), suggesting the translation Skull News.

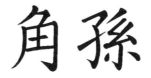

Angle Vertex

TB-20 (*jiǎo sūn*)

角 *jiǎo*: angle, corner; horn; a constellation
孫 *sūn*: grandson; posterity, descendants; a young shoot

Classical Location: Up from Skull Rest (TB-19), at the place above the ear where a hollow appears when the mouth is opened. *(Golden Mirror)*

Point Associations: Intersection-jiaohui point of the hand shao yang triple burner, hand tai yang small intestine and foot shao yang gallbladder channels.

Explanation of Point Name

The location of TB-20 on the head is similar to that of the 角 *jiǎo* (horn) constellation, which occupies a spot on the head of a celestial dragon. 孫 *sūn* in this interpretation refers to the vertex, or end, of the angle (角 *jiǎo*) formed by the triple burner channel at this point just as a grandson is the end of a family line. Thus interpreted the name is locational.

角 *jiǎo* may be a reference to the point's location at the top corner of the ear. A Qing Dynasty dictionary defines 孫 *sūn* as equivalent to 遁 *dùn*, to conceal or to vanish. The channel's seeming disappearance (this branch of the channel ends at TB-20) suggests the name Corner Disappearance.

The character 角 *jiǎo* can also mean "horn" as in the horns of a bull, while 孫 *sūn* can mean a young shoot or sprout. If humans sprouted horns, TB-20 is the spot from which they would grow. Corner Sprout is thus another possible translation of this name.

The character 孫 *sūn* can mean minute or very small, which would correspond to a reference to the minute connecting vessels (called 孫絡 *sūn luò*) in the vicinity of this point. Translating the name as Corner Minute Connecting Vessel would express this meaning.

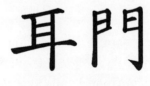

Ear Gate

TB-21 (*ěr mén*)
耳 *ěr*: ear
門 *mén*: gate, door

Classical Location: Around the ear from Angle Vertex (TB-20), in the depression in front of the ear at the [intertragic] notch. *(Golden Mirror)*

Explanation of Point Name

TB-21 is utilized in the treatment of ear disease, and is located at the entrance or gateway of the ear.

和髎

Harmony Bone-Hole

TB-22 *(hé liáo)*

和 *hé:* harmony, peace; to come together
髎 *liáo:* bone-hole

Alternate Names

Grain Bone-Hole	禾髎	*hé liáo*
Harmony Hollow	和空	*hé kōng*
Ear Harmony Bone-Hole	耳和髎	*ěr hé liǎo*

Classical Location: In front of Ear Gate (TB-21) below the sidelock, at the site of the horizontal pulse. *(Golden Mirror)*

Point Associations: Intersection-jiaohui point of the hand shao yang triple burner, hand tai yang small intestine and foot shao yang gallbladder channels.

Explanation of Point Name

The *Spiritual Axis* states that when the kidney is in harmony the ears can hear the five sounds (the kidney opens into the ears). Since this point is employed in treating deafness, it can be said to harmonize the kidney. The rendering of the name as Harmony Bone-Hole is meant to express this idea.

TB-22 is also the intersection-jiaohui point of the gallbladder, small intestine and triple burner channels. It is located in a bone-hole where the channels come together. The point name could therefore be rendered as Uniting Bone-Hole.

In ancient China, the character 和 *hé* was used to describe a gate with banners hanging at both sides. The tufts of hair at the temples where this point is located may be likened to those banners, and translating the point name as Banner-Gate Bone-Hole would express this interpretation.

絲竹空

Silk Bamboo Hole

TB-23 (*sī zhú kōng*)
絲 *sī*: silk
竹 *zhú*: bamboo
空 *kōng*: hole, empty space

Alternate Names

Giant Bone-Hole	巨髎	*jù liáo*
Eye Bone-Hole	目髎	*mù liáo*
Moon Bone-Hole	月髎	*yuè liáo*

Classical Location: In the depression behind the eyebrow.
(Great Compendium)

Explanation of Point Name

The characters 絲竹 *sī zhú*, silk bamboo, refer to a type of bamboo that has tiny leaves. The eyebrow resembles these leaves, and the point is located in a hole at the lateral extremity of the eyebrow. It may therefore be said that the point name refers to the location of the point in the Silk Bamboo Hole.

If TB-22 is rendered as Harmony Bone-Hole then it may be appropriate to translate TB-23 as Strings and Pipes Hole, because 絲 *sī* and 竹 *zhú* (silk and bamboo) refer to stringed and wind instruments respectively. Both points would then have names related to music.

The alternate name Moon Bone-Hole most likely resulted from a mistranscription of the character 目 *mù* (eye) in the alternate name 目髎 *mù liáo*, Eye Bone-Hole, which in turn might have been a mistranscription of an earlier name from the *Systematized Canon*, 巨髎 *jù liáo*, Giant Bone-Hole

Gallbladder Channel
(Foot Shao Yang)

足少陽膽經

瞳子髎

Pupil Bone-Hole

GB-1 *(tóng zǐ liáo)*

瞳 *tóng*: pupil of the eye
子 *zǐ*: noun suffix
髎 *liáo*: bone-hole

Alternate Names

Hind Curve	後曲	*hòu qū*
Greater Yang	太陽	*tài yáng*

Classical Location: Five fen out from the outer canthus. *(Great Compendium)*

Point Associations: Intersection-jiaohui point of the hand tai yang small intestine, hand shao yang triple burner and foot shao yang gallbladder channels.

Explanation of Point Name

This point is named for its position in a depression in the bone just lateral to the eye and level with the pupil, as well as for its utilization in the treatment of eye disorders.

聽會

Auditory Convergence

GB-2 *(tīng huì)*

聽 *tīng*: to hear, to listen
會 *huì*: to converge, to gather; to meet, to join

Alternate Names

Hearing Laughter	聽呵	*tīng hē*
Hind Gate	後關	*hòu guān*
Hinge	機關	*jī guān*

Classical Location: In the depression in front of the ear, where a pulsating vessel can be felt, one inch below Upper Gate (GB-3). The point is found when the mouth is opened. *(Great Compendium)*

Explanation of Point Name

This point is important in the treatment of hearing disorders. Combined with its location in front of the ear, this accounts for the name Auditory Convergence. 關 *guān* in the alternate names for GB-1 and GB-2 could be translated as joint, pass or gate. In all cases it is probably a reference to the mandibular joint (see GB-3).

上關

Upper Gate

GB-3 *(shàng guān)*

上 *shàng*: upper, above; to rise
關 *guān*: gate, pass; joint

Alternate Names

Guest-Host-Person	客主人	*kè zhǔ rén*
Guest-Host	客主	*kè zhǔ*
Guest King	客王	*kè wáng*
Generous Host	容主	*róng zhǔ*
Greater Yang	太陽	*tài yáng*

Classical Location: Above the bone in front of the ear, where a hollow appears when the mouth is opened. *(Great Compendium)*

Point Associations: Intersection-jiaohui point of the foot shao yang gallbladder, hand shao yang triple burner, hand yang ming large intestine and foot yang ming stomach channels.

Explanation of Point Name

The mandibular joint is often referred to in Chinese as the "gate" (關 *guān*). This point, located on the edge of the upper bone of that joint, is called Upper Gate.

The alternate names Guest-Host or Guest-Emperor indicate that the host (or emperor) channel receives the triple burner, large intestine, bladder and stomach channels at GB-3.

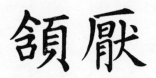

Forehead Fullness

GB-4 *(hàn yàn)*
頷 *hán*: corner of the forehead; chin
厭 *yàn*: full, satiated

Classical Location: On the curved hairline in the upper margin of the temples. *(Systematized Canon)*

Point Associations: Intersection-jiaohui point of the foot shao yang gallbladder, hand shao yang triple burner, hand yang ming large intestine and foot yang ming stomach channels.

Explanation of Point Name

If the jaw is closed tightly, there is a swelling (fullness) at the corner of the forehead. GB-4 is located just above that swelling; hence the name Forehead Fullness.

In rare instances 厭 *yàn* means to close, and can therefore be a mnemonic for remembering that if the jaw is closed tight there is a swelling at the point.

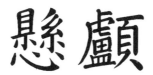

Suspended Skull

GB-5 *(xuán lú)*

懸 *xuán*: to suspend, to hang
顱 *lú*: skull, cranium

Alternate Names

Marrow Hole	髓孔	*suí kǒng*
Marrow Center	髓中	*suí zhōng*
Rice Bite	米嚙	*mǐ niè*
Rice Bite	米齧	*mǐ niè*

Classical Location: On the curved hairline in the middle margin of the temples. *(Systematized Canon)*

Point Associations: Intersection-jiaohui point of the foot shao yang gallbladder, hand shao yang triple burner, foot yang ming stomach and hand yang ming large intestine channels.

Explanation of Point Name

This point is situated as if suspended on the skull between the hairline and the root of the ear, and would furthermore serve as a convenient point from which to suspend someone by their skull. Thus the point is known as Suspended Skull.

Dizziness may resemble the sensation of being hung by the head. The use of this point in treating dizziness may be a further reason for the appellation Suspended Skull.

懸 氂 (厘)

Suspended Tuft

GB-6 *(xuán lí)*

懸 *xuán*: to suspend, to hang
氂 (厘) *lí*: a very small unit of length or weight; minute

Classical Location: On the curved hairline in the lower margin of the temples. *(Systematized Canon)*

Point Associations: Intersection-jiaohui point of the foot shao yang gallbladder, hand shao yang triple burner, hand yang ming large intestine and foot yang ming stomach channels.

Explanation of Point Name

The character 氂 *lí* was originally used to represent the breadth of an ox's hair, and by extension came to have the more general meaning of minute. Because of its original meaning the character is sometimes replaced by its homophone 髦, which means a tuft of hair. Since the hair at the temple must be lifted up (i.e., suspended) in order to locate GB-6, the point is named Suspended Tuft. One source records that the hair at this point is stiff and will "remain suspended" by itself if lifted.

This point is separated from GB-5 by only a small distance (釐 *lí*). The name of this point could be rendered as Slightly Separated from Suspended Skull to reflect this fact.

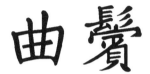

Temporal Hairline Curve

GB-7 *(qū bìn)*
曲 *qū*: curve, bend
鬢 *bìn*: the hair of the temples

Alternate Name

Hair Curve   曲髮   *qū fǎ*

Classical Location: In a depression behind Suspended Tuft (GB-6) in front of the ear behind the curved hairline. A hollow can be felt when the jaw is moved. *(Golden Mirror)*

Point Associations: Intersection-jiaohui point of the foot shao yang gallbladder and foot tai yang bladder channels.

Explanation of Point Name

GB-7 is located at the bottom curve of the temporal hairline, just above the ear. This location accounts for its name.

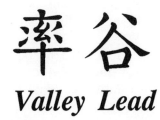

Valley Lead

GB-8 *(shuài gǔ)*

率 *shuài*: to lead
谷 *gǔ*: valley

Alternate Names

Following the Bone	率骨	*shuài gǔ*
Following the Corner	率角	*shuài jiǎo*
Cricket Container	蟀容	*shuài róng*

Classical Location: In the depression one and a half inches within the hairline above the ear. Bite and the point can be felt. *(Great Compendium)*

Point Associations: Intersection-jiaohui point of the foot shao yang gallbladder and foot tai yang bladder channels.

Explanation of Point Name

To find this point one bends the ear in half lengthwise and follows its straight edge past the hairline to the depression (valley) about 1.5 body inches above the tip of the ear. In this way one is "led to the valley."

Of all the "valley" (谷 *gǔ*) points on the body, GB-8 has the topmost location. Considered in this light, the point is the "lead" for all the other valley points.

In Following the Corner and Following the Bone, the character 率 *shuài* is rendered as "following" because the names are locational. In the poetic name Cricket Container 率 has evolved into its homophone 蟀, meaning cricket.

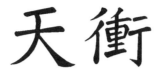

Celestial Hub

GB-9 *(tiān chòng)*

天 *tiān*: celestial, of the heavens, sky; Nature; heaven
衝 *chōng*: surge, rush, flush (沖); thoroughfare;
    a place of importance (a hub)

Alternate Name

Celestial Surge	天沖	*tiān chōng*
Celestial Crossroads	天衢	*tiān qú*

Classical Location: A little over three fen behind Valley Lead (GB-8), two inches within the hairline.
(Golden Mirror)

Point Associations: Intersection-jiaohui point of the foot shao yang gallbladder and foot tai yang bladder channels.

Explanation of Point Name

GB-9 bears the honorific "celestial" due to its location on the head, while "hub" is indicative of its importance as a point of intersection, i.e., an intersection-jiaohui point of the gallbladder and bladder channels. This point is employed in the treatment of disorders that are marked by surges of qi such as headache, wind disease and fright wind. Combined with the point's location on the upper body, this provides a rendering of the point name as Celestial Surge. In this case, the character 衝 *chōng* should be written as 沖 *chōng*, which is more commonly interpreted to mean "surge," though in acupuncture point names the two characters are often used interchangeably (cf. alternate name above).

天衝 *tiān chōng* is also a star name.

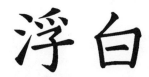

Floating White

GB-10 *(fú bái)*
浮 *fú*: to float, to drift, to rise
白 *bái*: white, pure

Classical Location: Behind the ear, one inch within the hairline. *(Great Compendium)*

Point Associations: Intersection-jiaohui point of the foot shao yang gallbladder and foot tai yang bladder channels.

Explanation of Point Name

The character 浮 *fú*, meaning rising, is a reference to the rising of liver and gallbladder yang qi, while 白 *bái*, meaning white, is the color associated with metal and refers to the point's metal-like function of restraining wood (liver-gallbladder). The point name is therefore a reference to GB-10's use in treating the dizziness and headache that result from hyperactivity of liver yang.

The ideograph 白 *bái* may be taken as a reference to the lung, as this point is utilized in the treatment of various lung disorders such as thoracic fullness with gasping, throat bi and counterflow cough.

頭竅陰

Head Portal Yin

GB-11 *(tóu qiào yīn)*

頭 *tóu*: head
竅 *qiào*: portal, orifice
陰 *yīn*: yin, the complement of yang

Alternate Name

Pillow Bone (Occipital Bone)　　　枕骨　*zhěn gǔ*

Classical Location: Above Completion Bone (GB-12) and below [in front of] the occipital bone, in a hollow felt when the head is turned. *(Great Compendium)*

Point Associations: Intersection-jiaohui point of the foot shao yang gallbladder and foot tai yang bladder channels.

Explanation of Point Name

The word "head" is included in this point name simply to avoid confusion with another point of the same name, Foot Portal Yin (GB-44). The occipital region, where this point is located, is considered to be the yin portion of the head. GB-11 is employed in the treatment of diseases related to the five portals of the five viscera, i.e., the eyes (eye pain from taxation jaundice), ears (deafness, tinnitus), mouth (bitter taste), nose (nasal congestion) and tongue (stiffness). Due to the point's location in a yin region and to its use in the treatment of disorders of the portals (which, being associated with the viscera, can also be seen to be related to yin), the point is known as Head Portal Yin.

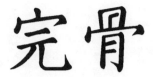

Completion Bone

GB-12 *(wán gǔ)*
完 *wán*: completed, finished
骨 *gǔ*: bone

Classical Location: Four fen into the hair at the back of the ear. *(Systematized Canon)*

Point Associations: Intersection-jiaohui point of the foot shao yang gallbladder and foot tai yang bladder channels.

Explanation of Point Name

The term 完骨 *wán gǔ* is the traditional name for the mastoid process, which is the bony protuberance just behind the ear. This point is located at the edge of that process and is thus named for its location.

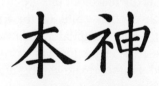

Root Spirit

GB-13 *(běn shén)*
本 *běn*: root, origin, source
神 *shén*: spirit

Alternate Name

Rib Bone-Hole 肋髎 *lè liáo*

Classical Location: One inch and five fen to the side of Deviating Turn (BL-4), directly above the ears, four fen within the hairline. *(Great Compendium)*

Point Associations: Intersection-jiaohui point of the foot shao yang gallbladder channel and the yang linking vessel.

Explanation of Point Name

GB-13 is utilized in treating spirit disorders, and treating the spirit is known as treating the source (root) of a disease. The chapter of the *Spiritual Axis* that discusses this aspect of treatment is called by the same name as GB-13; Root Spirit. Locationally, GB-13 may be called Root Spirit because the brain is the root of the spirit; the point, located on the head (near the brain), is used in treating spirit disorders.

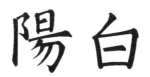

Yang White

GB-14 (*yáng bái*)
陽 *yáng*: yang, the complement of yin
白 *bái*: white, pure, clear

Classical Location: One inch above the eyebrow, on a line with the pupil. *(Great Compendium)*

Point Associations: Intersection-jiaohui point of the shao yang gallbladder and triple burner, yang ming large intestine and stomach channels, and the yang linking vessel.

Explanation of Point Name

Because this point is situated on the head, which is associated with yang, and is furthermore the meeting point of five yang channels, the character 陽 *yáng* is included in its appellation. The character 白 *bái*, in addition to meaning "white," also has an extended meaning of "clear." This point is employed in the treatment of eye diseases and thus helps to make things clear. The name Yang White recalls not only the point's location on the head, but as well its relationship to the yang channels, and its ability to treat eye diseases.

Four Whites (四白 *sì bái*: ST-2) is also located near the eye. Readers may wish to refer to the discussion of that point for further information concerning the meaning of white in relation to the eye.

頭臨泣

Head Overlooking Tears

GB-15 *(tóu lín qì)*
頭 *tóu*: head
臨 *lín*: to overlook, to face towards; to arrive at
泣 *qì*: tear

Classical Location: In the depression five fen into the hair, directly above the eyes. The point is found by having the patient look straight forward. *(Great Compendium)*

Point Associations: Intersection-jiaohui point of the foot shao yang gallbladder and foot tai yang bladder channels and the yang linking vessel.

Explanation of Point Name

The word "head" is included in the name of this point in order to avoid confusion with another point of similar name, Foot Overlooking Tears (GB-41). Since GB-15 "overlooks" the eye, the place that tears come from, it may be called Head Overlooking Tears.

GB-15 may be used to treat diseases of the eye and thus "overlooks" the eyes (and tears, which are the liquid of the eyes). 臨 *lín*, which means to overlook, also has an extended meaning of supervision, or, as in this case, treatment. This is especially meaningful in light of the line from the *Ode of a Hundred Patterns:* "[If there is] tearing, needle Overlooking Tears (GB-15) and Head Corner (ST-8)." Rendering the point name as Treating Tears would reflect this idea.

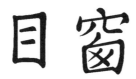

Eye Window

GB-16 *(mù chuāng)*
目 *mù*: eye
窗 *chuāng*: window

Alternate Name

Arriving at Splendor　　　至榮　　*zhì róng*

Classical Location: One and a half inches behind Overlooking Tears (GB-15). *(Great Compendium)*

Point Associations: Intersection-jiaohui point of the foot shao yang gallbladder channel and the yang linking vessel.

Explanation of Point Name

This point is located directly above the eye and treats eye diseases. The appellation Eye Window reveals both its location and its function.

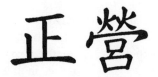

Upright Construction

GB-17 (zhèng yíng)

正 zhèng: right, upright, true, straight
營 yíng: the former half of construction-blood, nourishment; to manage, to regulate

Classical Location: One and one half inches behind Eye Window (GB-16). (Great Compendium)

Point Associations: Intersection-jiaohui point of the foot shao yang gallbladder channel and yang linking vessel.

Explanation of Point Name

The character 正 zhèng refers to the point's location right at the top of the head, while 營 yíng may be considered as an indication of the point's ability to reach construction-blood (營血 yíng xuè) and thereby nourish the eyes and the spirit.

In geographical nomenclature 營 yíng refers to the lines that demarcate the east-west, i.e., horizontal direction. (楚辭.離牙南北爲經, 東西爲營) GB-17 is located on the horizontal line that crosses exactly (正 zhèng) at the top of the head and thus could be named for its location.

正營 *zhèng yíng* also can mean fear or solicitude. This name may therefore be indicative of the use of GB-17 for quieting the spirit and easing palpitations.

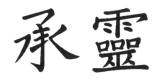

Spirit Support

GB-18 *(chéng líng)*

承 *chéng*: to support; to contain; to receive
靈 *líng*: spirit; ingenious

Classical Location: One inch and five fen behind Upright Construction (GB-17). *(Great Compendium)*

Point Associations: Intersection-jiaohui point of the foot shao yang gallbladder channel and yang linking vessel.

Explanation of Point Name

GB-17 is located at the place the ancient Chinese termed the "cover of the celestial spirit." Whether the name should be translated as Support Spirit, Receive Spirit or Contain Spirit is not entirely clear. 承 *chéng*, in this case, means "to support" in most Chinese sources.

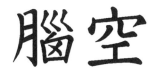

Brain Hollow

GB-19 *(nǎo kōng)*

腦 *nǎo*: brain
空 *kōng*: empty, spacious

Alternate Name

Temple Region 顳顬 *niè rú*

Classical Location: One inch and five fen behind Spirit Support (GB-18), in the depression on either side beneath the occipital bone. *(Great Compendium)*

Point Associations: Intersection-jiaohui point of the foot shao yang gallbladder channel and the yang linking vessel.

Explanation of Point Name

Located in a depression (空 *kōng*) in the "brain bone" (skull), this point treats diseases of the brain such as epileptic diseases and headache. The appellation Brain Hollow serves as a reminder of both the location and function of the point.

The fact that GB-19 is called Brain Hollow and GB-18 is called Spirit Support shows that the ancient Chinese realized the relationship of the brain to what they termed disorders of the spirit. Many points on the governing vessel, gallbladder and bladder channels are used to treat psychiatric (i.e., spirit) disorders because these three channels traverse the head.

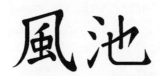

Wind Pool

GB-20 *(fēng chí)*
風 *fēng*: wind
池 *chí*: pool, pond

Alternate Name

Heat Mansion 熱府 *rè fǔ*

Classical Location: In the depression within the hairline behind the ear and the temple region, below Brain Hollow (GB-19). If the point is pressed a sensation is felt in the ear. *(Great Compendium)*

Point Associations: Intersection-jiaohui point of the foot shao yang gallbladder, hand shao yang triple burner channels and the yang linking vessel.

Explanation of Point Name

The depression in which GB-20 is located resembles a pool in the landscape of the body. Wind pathogens are said to collect in this depression, and the point is used in the treatment of wind disease. Thus it is known as Wind Pool.

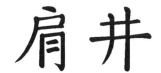

Shoulder Well

GB-21 *(jiān jǐng)*

肩 *jiān*: shoulder
井 *jǐng*: a well

Alternate Name

Shoulder Well 膊井 *bó jǐng*

Classical Location: In the depression above Empty Basin (ST-12), in front of the great bone. *(Systematized Canon)*

Point Associations: Intersection-jiaohui point of the foot shao yang gallbladder, the hand shao yang triple burner, and the foot yang ming stomach channels and the yang linking vessel.

Explanation of Point Name

This point is located in a depression on the shoulder that could be said to resemble a well (i.e., a depression). In addition, the bone structure of the shoulder is reminiscent of the external framework of a well.

淵腋

Armpit Abyss

GB-22 (yuān yè)
淵 yuān: abyss, deep pool
腋 yè: armpit

Alternate Names

Abyss Humor	淵液	yuán yè
Humor Abyss	液淵	yè yuán
Armpit Gate	掖門	yè mén
Humor Gate	液門	yè mén
Spring Armpit	泉腋 (涇)	quán yè
Spring Humor	泉液	quán yè

Classical Location: In the depression three inches below the armpit. The point is found with the arm raised.
(Great Compendium)

Explanation of Point Name

This point is called Armpit Abyss due to its location in the deep abyss of the armpit. Note that the character 淵 has the water radical (three dots on the left hand side), which is appropriate because the armpit is often a place of copious perspiration.

The alternate names for GB-22 center around the characters 液 *yè* (humor, i.e., fluids) and its homophone 腋 (armpit), with the addition of the characters 淵 *yuān* (abyss) and 泉 *quán* (spring), both of which indicate a source of water. The names provide a good example of the variations that can develop over time, especially given the oral tradition of Chinese medicine and the large number of homophones in the Chinese language.

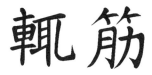

Sinew Seat

GB-23 *(zhé jīn)*

輒 *zhé*: the two seats of an ancient chariot;
 the sides of the chariot just above the wheels
筋 *jīn*: sinew

Alternate Names

Spirit Light	神光	*shén guāng*
Gallbladder Mu	膽募	*dǎn mù*

Classical Location: Three inches down from the armpit and one inch forward. *(Systematized Canon)*

Point Associations: Intersection-jiaohui point of the foot shao yang gallbladder and foot tai yang bladder.

Explanation of Point Name

GB-23 is located below the armpit on the side of the rib cage. The shape of the rib cage is said to resemble the sides of a chariot in the area above the wheels. In fact, the intercostal muscles are sometimes called 軶筋 *zhé jīn*. The point rides within these sinews as if they were the seats of a chariot, and derives its name from its location in these muscles.

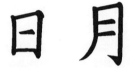

Sun and Moon

GB-24 *(rì yuè)*
日 *rì*: sun; day
月 *yuè*: moon; month

Alternate Names

Spirit Light	神光	*shén guāng*
Gallbladder Mu	膽募	*dǎn mù*

Classical Location: Five fen below Cycle Gate (LV-14). *(Great Compendium)*

Point Associations: Alarm-mu point of the gallbladder; intersection-jiaohui point of the foot shao yang gallbladder and foot tai yin spleen channels, and the yang linking vessel.

Explanation of Point Name

The sun represents yang and the moon yin. GB-24 represents the meeting of yin and yang in two ways. First, it is an intersection-jiaohui point of the foot shao yang and foot tai yin channels. Second, as stated in the *Classic of Difficult Issues,* 67th Difficulty: "alarm-mu points are located on the yin [side of the body]." Thus alarm-mu points are yin in nature, while this particular one is located on a yang channel.

Classical Chinese texts call the left eye sun and the right eye moon. The eyes are associated with the liver, and, through exterior-interior relationship, with the gallbladder. This name Sun and Moon reflects the relation of GB-24 to the eyes by way of association with the liver.

The gallbladder governs decision making, and this point can facilitate clarity of thought. The Chinese word for "clear" is 明 *míng*, which is a composite made up of the characters for sun (日) and moon (月). Thus, just as the sun and moon make things clear on earth, this point can help to make things clear in the psyche.

Both the liver and the gallbladder are associated with the wood phase, in turn associated with east. The sun and moon rising in the east can be correlated to the gallbladder and liver, and provide another association for the naming of this point as Sun and Moon.

The alternate names for GB-23 and GB-24 show us that disagreement exists as to which is the alarm-mu point of the gallbladder. Most sources list GB-24, but the *Great Compendium of Acupuncture and Moxibustion* lists GB-23.

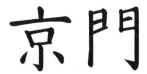

Capital Gate

GB-25 (*jīng mén*)
京 *jīng*: capital city; hill
門 *mén*: gate, door

Alternate Names

Qi Mansion	氣府	qì fǔ
Qi Shu	氣俞	qì shū
Kidney Mu	腎募	shèn mù

Classical Location: From Sun and Moon (GB-24) toward the ilium, in the low back, in the region of the free ribs on either side of the spine, five fen above, and nine and a half inches either side of the navel. The patient should lie on his side, bend the top leg, straighten the bottom leg, and raise the arm to facilitate point location. *(Golden Mirror)*

Point Associations: Alarm-mu point of the kidney.

Explanation of Point Name

A capital is an important gathering place, as is an alarm-mu point. Here 京 *jīng* refers to GB-25 as the kidney alarm-mu. 門 *mén*, gate, identifies an acupoint. In *Selected Explanations of Point Names* 京 *jīng* is said to include the meaning of 原 *yuán*, source, in ancient Chinese. GB-25 is the alarm-mu point of the kidney, a gathering point for kidney qi. Because the kidney is the root of prenatal source qi, the point name could be translated as Source Gate, indicating that GB-25 is like a gate to the body's source qi.

The chest is like a hill in the bodily landscape. GB-25 is located on the edge of the chest and is metaphorically a gate to the chest. Thus the name Hill Gate.

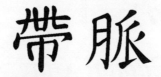

Girdling Vessel

GB-26 (dài mài)

帶 *dài*: girdle, belt; to lead, take in one's charge; to carry
脈 *mài* (*mo*): vessel (of blood and qi); pulse

Classical Location: In the depression one inch and eight fen below the region of the free ribs, two inches above the navel, seven and a half inches either side of the midline. *(Great Compendium)*

Point Associations: Intersection-jiaohui point of the foot shao yang gallbladder channel and the girdling vessel.

Explanation of Point Name

This point is called Girdling Vessel because it is a major point on the girdling vessel and is utilized in treating diseases of that vessel. The girdling vessel itself is so named because it encircles the body like a belt and takes charge of the conception, governing and penetrating vessels.

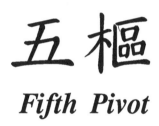

Fifth Pivot

GB-27 *(Wŭ shū)*

五 *wŭ*: five, fifth

樞 *shū*: pivot, axis, central point; indispensable, cardinal

Classical Location: Three inches below Girdling Vessel (GB-26), five inches and five fen to the side of Waterway (ST-28). *(Great Compendium)*

Point Associations: Intersection-jiaohui point of the foot shao yang gallbladder channel and the girdling vessel.

Explanation of Point Name

Each of the five positions has a particular number associated with it. Five is the number associated with the center.

GB-27 can be considered the central point of the abdominal points on the gallbladder channel, and is also located at a level central to the body as a whole. 樞 *shū*, meaning pivot, refers to the fact that the body turns or pivots at this point. Since 樞 also has meanings of indispensable or central, it reinforces the connotations of 五 *wǔ*, five.

GB-27 is an intersection-jiaohui point of the gallbladder channel and the girdling vessel. Since the girdling vessel wraps around the center of the body, and a place of intersection is in fact a pivot of sorts, the point's location on the girdling vessel can be said to account for it being named Fifth (i.e., central) Pivot.

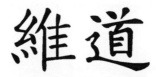

Linking Path

GB-28 *(wéi dào)*
維 *wéi*: to link, to hold together; to protect
道 *dào*: road, path, way; to lead, to guide

Alternate Name

Outer Pivot   外樞   *wài shū*

Classical Location: Five inches and three fen below Camphorwood Gate (LV-13). *(Great Compendium)*

Point Associations: Intersection-jiaohui point of the foot shao yang gallbladder channel and the girdling vessel.

Explanation of Point Name

This gallbladder channel point is an intersection-jiaohui point of the girdling vessel. 道 *dào*, meaning path, can be considered a reference to the girdling vessel. The character 維 *wéi*, which can mean to protect or to link, expresses two functions of that vessel, i.e., protecting and linking the yin and yang channels. For these reasons the name could be either Protective Path or Linking Path.

居髎

Squatting Bone-Hole

GB-29 *(jū liáo)*
居 *jū*: to sit, to squat; to reside, to dwell
髎 *liáo*: bone-hole

Classical Location: Eight inches and three fen below Camphorwood Gate (LV-13), in the depression above the ilium. *(Great Compendium)*

Point Associations: Intersection-jiaohui point of the foot shao yang gallbladder channel and the yang motility vessel.

Explanation of Point Name

This bone-hole (in this case a depression between two bones) becomes visible in a sitting or squatting position, calling to mind the name Squatting Bone-Hole. GB-29 can also be seen to "reside" (居 *jū*) at a bone-hole. The rendering Bone-Hole Residence reflects this idea.

環跳

Jumping Round

GB-30 *(huán tiào)*
環 *huán*: ring, circle; to encircle; turn
跳 *tiào*: to jump, to leap

Alternate Names

Round Valley	環谷	*huán gǔ*
Divided Center	分中	*fēn zhōng*
Hip Joint	髀樞	*bì shū*
Buttocks Pressing	髀壓	*bì yā*
Kneecap	臏骨	*bìn gǔ*
Hip Bone	骻骨	*kuà gǔ*
Pivot Center	樞中	*shū zhōng*
Pivot Union Center	樞合中	*shū hé zhōng*

Classical Location: With the patient lying on his side with his bottom leg stretched out and his top leg bent, the point is found in the hip joint. The left hand shakes the leg as the right hand feels for the point. *(Great Compendium)*

Point Associations: Intersection-jiaohui point of the foot shao yang gallbladder and foot tai yang bladder channels; one of the nine needles for returning yang.

Explanation of Point Name

The part of the body where this point is found is pivotal for jumping and turning movements, i.e., for Jumping Round. When a person squats down in preparation for a jump, a semi-circular (round) depression appears at this point; hence the name Jumping Round. After treatment at this point, the patient whose mobility was limited can once again jump and turn.

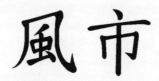

Wind Market

GB-31 (*fēng shì*)
風 *fēng*: wind
市 *shì*: market, fair, city

Classical Location: Between the two sinews on the outer side above knee, at the end of the middle finger when the hand is placed on the thigh. *(Great Compendium)*

Explanation of Point Name

Wind disorders can be treated by applying acupuncture or moxibustion at this point. Furthermore, wind qi may gather in this area like people gathering at a market or fair. Thus the point is known as Wind Market.

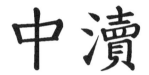

Central River

GB-32 *(zhōng dú)*

中 *zhōng*: center, central
瀆 *dú*: river, ditch, drain

Classical Location: On the thigh, five inches above the knee, in the parting of the flesh. *(Great Compendium)*

Explanation of Point Name

Qi flows in the channels like water in a river. The gallbladder channel is in a central position relative to the other two yang channels on the lower limbs. The name Central River can be seen to represent the gallbladder channel as a whole. Or, GB-32 may be called Central River because the gallbladder channel communicates with the triple burner channel (both belong to the shao yang). The triple burner is referred to in the *Spiritual Axis* as 中瀆 *zhōng dú*, "the central river." Because this point is located in the center of a groove in the muscles that resembles a ditch (瀆 *dú*); the point name could also be rendered as Central Ditch.

膝陽關

Knee Yang Joint

GB-33 *(xī yáng guān)*

膝 *xī*: knee
陽 *yáng*: yang, the complement of yin
關 *guān*: gate; passage; joint

Alternate Names

Joint Yang	關陽	*guān yáng*
Joint Mound	關陵	*guān líng*
Yang Mound	陽陵	*yáng líng*
Cold Mansion	寒府	*hán fǔ*

Classical Location: Three inches above Yang Mound Spring (GB-34), in the depression lateral to Calf's Nose (ST-35). *(Great Compendium)*

Explanation of Point Name

This point is located at the knee joint on the yang aspect of the leg; it is therefore called Yang Joint. The word knee is included simply to distinguish the point from another which is also called 陽關 *yáng guān*, Lumbar Yang Pass (GV-3).

陽陵泉

Yang Mound Spring

GB-34 *(yáng líng quán)*

陽 *yáng*: yang, the complement of yin
陵 *líng*: mound, burial mound
泉 *quán*: spring, fountain

Alternate Names

Yang Mound	陽陵	*yáng líng*
Yang's Mound Spring	陽之陵泉	*yáng zhī líng quán*
Sinew Convergence	筋會	*jīn huì*

Classical Location: One inch below the knee, in the depression on the outer face of the shin. The point is found in squatting posture. *(Great Compendium)*

Point Associations: Uniting-he (earth) point. Meeting-hui point of the sinews.

Explanation of Point Name

GB-34 is located in a depression next to a protuberance or "mound;" thus it is a "mound spring." It may be that "mound" is also a reference to GB-34 as the earth point of the gallbladder channel, as mounds are made of earth. Located on the yang aspect of the leg, opposite to Yin Mound Spring (SP-9); it is therefore called Yang Mound Spring.

GB-34 is the meeting-hui point of the sinews and thus moistens the sinews like a spring moistens the land. While this explanation is useful, it is probably wrong. The meeting-hui points were first discussed in the *Classic of Difficult Issues*, a later text than either the *Inner Canon* or the *Systematized Canon*, both of which mention this name.

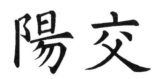

Yang Intersection

GB-35 (*yáng jiāo*)

陽 *yáng*: yang, the complement of yin
交 *jiāo*: to intersect, to meet; to hand over

Alternate Names

Divergent Yang	別陽	*bié yáng*
Leg Bone-Hole	足髎	*zú liáo*
Leg Bone-Hole	足節	*zú liáo*
Leg Hollow	足空	*zú kōng*

Classical Location: Seven inches above the outer ankle, in the parting of the flesh among the three yang channels. *(Great Compendium)*

Point Associations: Cleft-xi point of the yang linking channel; intersection-jiaohui point of the foot shao yang gallbladder and the yang linking vessel.

Explanation of Point Name

GB-35 is the cleft-xi point of the yang linking vessel as well as the intersection-jiaohui point of that vessel and the gallbladder channel. The name Yang Intersection recalls these facts.

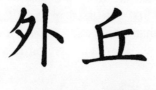

Outer Hill

GB-36 *(wài qiū)*
外 *wài*: outer, outside
丘 *qiū*: hill, mound

Classical Location: Seven inches above the outer anklebone. *(Great Compendium)*

Point Associations: Cleft-xi point of the gallbladder channel.

Explanation of Point Name

This point is named Outer Hill because of its location on the outer aspect of the leg in a fleshy area that resembles a hill (the calf). Note that the calf is surrounded by points whose names include references to hills, mountains, mounds, and valleys, such as Yang Mound Spring (GB-34), Yin Valley (KI-10), Yin Mound Spring (SP-9), Leaking Valley (SP-7), Mountain Support (BL-57) and Outer Hill (GB-36).

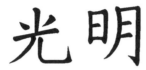

Bright Light

GB-37 *(guāng míng)*

光 *guāng*: light, brightness
明 *míng*: clear, bright; acute (of eyesight)

Classical Location: Five inches above the outer ankle.
(Great Compendium)

Point Associations: Connecting-luo point of the gallbladder channel connecting to the liver channel.

Explanation of Point Name

Both the characters 光 *guāng* and 明 *míng* are often used to describe the eyes (e.g., 道藏： 左目神,字英明,右目神,字玄光). GB-37 is the connecting-luo point of the gallbladder channel, i.e., the spot where the connecting vessel that joins to the liver leaves the main channel. Because of this connection (the liver opens at the eyes), GB-37 is useful in treating eye diseases. It is able to restore the light of the eyes, and is therefore called Bright Light.

陽輔

Yang Assistance

GB-38 *(yáng fǔ)*

陽 *yáng*: yang, the complement of yin
輔 *fǔ*: to assist, to support;
    pole attached to a cart to keep it from upsetting

Alternate Names

Severed Bone	絶骨	*jué gǔ*
Parting of the Flesh	分肉	*fēn ròu*
Parting Space	分間	*fēn jiān*

Classical Location: Four inches above the outer ankle, in front of the assisting bone, three fen from the edge of the bone, seven inches above Hill Ruins (GB-40).
(Great Compendium)

Point Associations: River-jing (fire) point.

Explanation of Point Name

GB-38 is on the yang aspect of the leg in front of the fibula, which in Chinese is called the 輔骨 *fǔ gǔ*, literally, "assisting bone." Thus the point is called Yang Assistance.

懸鐘

Suspended Bell

GB-39 *(jué gǔ)*

懸 *xuán*: to suspend, to hang
鐘 *zhōng*: bell; clock; handleless cup

Alternate Names

| Severed Bone | 絕骨 | *jué gǔ* |
| Marrow Convergence | 髓會 | *suí huì* |

Classical Location: At the pulsating vessel three inches above the outer ankle; feel for the tip of the bone. *(Great Compendium)*

Point Associations: Meeting-hui point of the marrow.

Explanation of Point Name

The outer anklebone appears like a bell hung from this point, providing the image of Suspended Bell. In ancient China, children often wore foot bells at the level of this point. The other name for this point, of equally common usage, is 絕骨 *jué gǔ*, Severed Bone. This name is a reference to the prominence at the distal end of the fibula where the point is located. In fact, this whole area of the leg is called 絕骨.

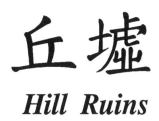

Hill Ruins

GB-40 *(qiū xū)*
丘 *qiū*: hill, hillock, mound
墟 *xū*: old burial grounds; ruins; wasteland

Alternate Name

| Hill Ruins | 坵墟 | *qiū xū* |

Classical Location: In the depression below the lower outer anklebone, three inches from [Foot] Overlooking Tears (GB-41). *(Systematized Canon)*

Point Associations: Source-yuan point of the gallbladder channel.

Explanation of Point Name

The character 丘 *qiū* here describes the mound of the outer anklebone, while 墟 *xū* may be a reference to the many protuberances and depressions in the vicinity of the ankle where the point is located, causing the area to resemble ancient burial grounds or ruins.

Since both characters in this name can mean mound, it could be interpreted simply as a reference to the protuberance of the anklebone. In that case translating the name as Mound would be sufficient.

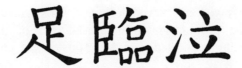

Foot Overlooking Tears

GB-41 *(zú lín qì)*
足 *zú*: foot
臨 *lín*: to overlook, to face toward; to arrive at
泣 *qì*: tears; to weep (silent tears)

Classical Location: In the depression behind and between the base joints of the little toe and the one next to it, one inch and five fen from Pinched Ravine (GB-43).
(Great Compendium)

Point Associations: Stream-shu (wood) point.

Explanation of Point Name

Near this point, a branch of the gallbladder channel leaves the main channel to connect with the liver channel at Large Pile (LV-1). Because the liver opens into the eyes, this connection, combined with the fact that the gallbladder channel originates at the outer edge of the eye, enables the point to treat eye disorders such as pain in the outer canthus, dry eyes and visual dizziness.

The name Overlooking Tears is therefore a reference to the functions of this point as regards the eyes. The word foot is included in the name to distinguish this point from another of similar name, Head Overlooking Tears (GB-15).

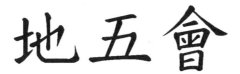

Earth Fivefold Convergence

GB-42 (dì wǔ huì)

地 *dì*: earth, ground
五 *wǔ*: five, fifth
會 *huì*: to converge, to meet

Alternate Names

Earth Five	地五	*dì wǔ*
Pinched Ravine	夾谿	*jiā xī*

Classical Location: In the depression behind and between the base joints of the little toe and the one next to it, one inch from Pinched Ravine (GB-43). *(Golden Mirror)*

Explanation of Point Name

The character 地 *dì* , meaning earth or ground, may here be considered as a reference to this point's location on the foot, i.e., the point of contact between the body and the ground. The ideogram 五 *wǔ* may be a reference to the five toes collectively or the fifth toe specifically, while 會

huì , meaning meeting or gathering, could be symbolic of the gathering together of the five toes, i.e., the foot, again indicating the location of the point.

It may be significant that 五會 *wǔ huì*, as well as constituting a part of this point name, is also an alternate name for 百會 *bǎi huì*, Hundred Convergences (GV-20). While it is unclear here what the phrase five convergences actually means, unless it is a reference to the five toes, it is more clear as regards Fivefold Convergence (GV-20), where the six yang channels intersect with the governing vessel. Thus "five," like the "hundred" in Hundred Convergences, can be construed to mean many. It seems more than mere coincidence that there is a Fivefold Convergence at both the top and bottom of the body.

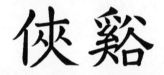

Pinched Ravine

GB-43 *(xiá xī)*
俠 *xiá*: bold, generous
谿 (溪) *xī*: ravine, mountain stream gully

Alternate Name

> Pinched Ravine　　夾谿　　*jiā xī*

Classical Location: In front of the base joints of the little toe and the one next to it, in the depression in the fork of the bones. *(Great Compendium)*

Point Associations: Spring-ying (water) point.

Explanation of Point Name

As in the case of 俠白 *xiá bái* (LU-4), 俠 *xiá* may be interpreted as meaning 夾 *jiā*, which means to pinch from both sides or to insert between. The ideogram 谿 *xī* (or its homophone 溪) refers to cleft-like grooves in the body. GB-43 is pinched in the groove between the fourth and fifth toes; therefore it is named Pinched Ravine. (夾白 is, in fact, an alternate name for this point.)

Some sources say 俠 *xiá* is a substitute for 狹 *xiá*, meaning narrow. Considered in this light a rendering of the point name as Narrow Ravine is also possible.

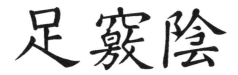

Foot Portal Yin

GB-44 *(zú qiào yīn)*
足 *zú*: foot, (lower) leg
竅 *qiào*: portal, orifice
陰 *yīn*: yin, the complement of yang

Classical Location: On the outer side of the toe next to the little toe, the width of a Chinese leek leaf away from the corner of the nail. *(Great Compendium)*

Point Associations: Well-jing (metal) point.

Explanation of Point Name

As was true with Head Portal Yin (GB-11), the name of this point may be a reference to its use in the treatment of diseases of the eyes, mouth, nose and tongue, which are the portals of the five viscera (yin). The word foot distinguishes this point from its namesake on the head.

This point is the opening to the foot jue yin liver channel, where qi passes from the end of the gallbladder channel to the beginning of the liver channel during its daily cycle. Because the character 竅 *qiào* indicates an opening, and the liver channel is associated with yin, the name of this point could also be rendered as Opening to Yin.

Liver Channel
(Foot Jue Yin)

足厥陰肝經

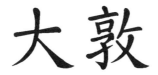

Large Pile

LV-1 *(dà dūn)*

大 *dà*: large, great, major
敦 *dūn*: to pile up; a hill; thick

Alternate Names

Great Favorableness	大順	*dà shùn*
Water Spring	水泉	*shuǐ quán*

Classical Location: On the great toe, a little more than the width of a Chinese leek leaf away from the nail, on the outer side amid the "three hairs." *(Golden Mirror)*

Point Associations: Well-jing (wood) point.

Explanation of Point Name

LV-1 is the wood point of the wood channel. Since wood restrains earth this point can be used to treat an overabundance (i.e., a Large Pile) of earth. The point name reminds us of this function. This explanation is supported by a line in *Essential Questions* where an excess of earth is called a 敦阜 *dūn fù*, mound.

This point is located in the thick flesh of the large toe, which could be said to resemble a Large Pile.

行間

Moving Between

LV-2 *(xíng jiān)*

行 *xíng*: to walk, to move
間 *jiān*: between; a space

Classical Location: On the web of the great toe, in the depression where the pulsating vessel may be sensed through palpation. *(Great Compendium)*

Point Associations: Spring-ying (fire) point.

Explanation of Point Name

The channel arrives at this point after passing between the two toes; hence it is called Moving Between. Another interpretation of this name claims that the name contains the character 行 *xíng*, meaning to move or to walk, because this point is pivotal for walking and has the function of moving qi and resolving stagnation. 間 *jiān*, meaning between, refers to the point's location between the toes.

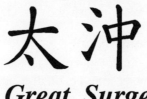

Great Surge

LV-3 *(tài chōng)*

太 *tài*: great, supreme; too, excessive
沖 *chōng*: surge, rush; flush; empty;
    thoroughfare, key position, hub (衝)

Alternate Name

Great Thoroughfare	太衝	*tài chōng*
Large Surge	大沖	*dà chōng*

Classical Location: One and a half to two inches below the base of the great toe, in the depression where the pulsating vessel can be felt. *(Great Compendium)*

Point Associations: Stream-shu (earth) and source-yuan point.

Explanation of Point Name

The character 太 *tài* is similar to 大 *dà* in both form and meaning. Here it is a reference to the large toe. The ideograph 沖 *chōng* refers to the surging of the pulse located at this point.

Essential Questions calls LV-3 the place where "the penetrating vessel (沖脈 *chōng mài*) and the kidney channel show great (大 *dà*) exuberance," and states that this is the reason that the point is called 太沖 *tài chōng*.

LV-3 is the source-yuan point of the liver channel. It can be said to be in a key position where the source qi gathers or along a thoroughfare of qi activity. For these reasons, Great Thoroughfare or Supreme Position would also be appropriate renderings for this name.

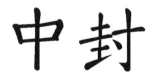

Mound Center

LV-4 *(zhōng fēng)*
中 *zhōng*: center, central
封 *fēng*: mound, heap; to seal, to block

Alternate Name

Suspended Spring   懸泉   *xuán quán*

Classical Location: One inch in front of the inner ankle-bone, in the depression between the sinews.
(Great Compendium)

Point Associations: River-jing (metal) point.

Explanation of Point Name

The character 中 *zhōng* is a reminder that the point is located in the middle of the two sinews, while 封 *fēng* may be a reference to both the mound of flesh formed by the sinews and the fact that the point is "sealed" within the sinews. Mound Center and Sealed Center are therefore both acceptable translations of this name.

蠡溝

Woodworm Canal

LV-5 *(lǐ gōu)*

蠡 *lí*: a wood-boring worm; a gourd; *lí*: ladle
溝 *gōu*: canal, ditch, channel

Alternate Name

Intersection Apparatus   交儀   *jiāo yí*

Classical Location: Five inches above the inner anklebone.
(Great Compendium)

Point Associations: Connecting-luo point of the foot jue yin liver channel, connecting with the foot shao yang gallbladder channel.

Explanation of Point Name

LV-5 is the connecting-luo point of the liver channel and as such connects the liver and gallbladder channels. The point may therefore be named Woodworm Canal in reference to the connecting vessel that joins the two wood channels. The alternate name Intersection Apparatus supports this interpretation.

The character 蠡 *lí* can also mean ladle and in this respect may be seen to resemble the hollow formed by the space between the bone and flesh of the calf. That area also looks like a ditch (溝 *gōu*), and thus a rendering of the point name as Ladle Ditch could be preferred.

The character 蠡 *lí* can also mean gourd and could thus represent the gastrocnemius muscle, which can be said to resemble a gourd. A rendering of the point name as Gourd Ditch would highlight the point's location in the groove next to the calf muscle.

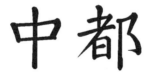

Central Metropolis

LV-6 *(zhōng dū)*
中 *zhōng*: center, middle, central
都 *dū*: metropolis, capital, market

Alternate Names

Central Cleft	中郄	*zhōng xī*
Supreme Yin	太陰	*tài yīn*
Great Yin	大陰	*dà yīn*

Classical Location: Seven inches above the inner anklebone, at the midpoint of the shinbone, parallel to the shao yin. *(Great Compendium)*

Point Associations: Cleft-xi point of the liver channel.

Explanation of Point Name

This point is the cleft-xi point of the liver channel, at which qi and blood gather just as people gather in a large metropolis (都 *dū*). The character 中 *zhōng*, meaning center, is probably a reference to the point's central location along the length of the shinbone, or to the fact that the point is found in the middle of a hollow.

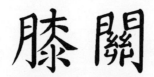

Knee Joint

LV-7 *(xī guān)*

膝 *xī*: knee
關 *guān*: joint; gate, pass, passageway

Classical Location: In the depression two inches below the Inner Eye of the Knee (M-LE-16). *(Great Compendium)*

Explanation of Point Name

This point is located near, and treats diseases affecting, the knee. Thus the name could be rendered as either Knee Joint or Passageway to the Knee, depending on which meaning of 關 *guān* is chosen.

曲泉

Spring at the Bend

LV-8 *(qū quán)*

曲 *qū*: bend, curve, curved
泉 *quán*: spring, water source

Classical Location: On the inside of the knee in the depression above the larger sinew and below the smaller sinew. When the knee is flexed the point is found at the end of the horizontal crease. *(Great Compendium)*

Point Associations: Uniting-he (water) point.

Explanation of Point Name

The character 泉 *quán*, meaning spring, is here a reference to this point being the water point of the liver channel. Because this "spring" is located at the bend in the knee, the point is called Spring at the Bend. Three nearby points contain the word 泉 spring: Yin Mound Spring (SP-9), Yang Mound Spring (G-34), Spring at the Bend (LV-8). All three are uniting-he points.

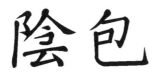

Yin Bladder

LV-9 *(yīn bāo)*

陰 *yīn*: yin, the complement of yang
包 *bāo*: to wrap, to envelope; bag, sack

Alternate Name

Yin Bladder 陰胞 *yīn bāo*

Classical Location: Four inches above the knee, between the two sinews on the inner face of the thigh. The point is found with the leg flexed. *(Great Compendium)*

Explanation of Point Name

The character 包 *bāo*, meaning to wrap or envelope, may here be considered as a reference to either the urinary bladder or the womb, disorders of which may be treated through this point, while 陰 *yīn* indicates the point's position on a yin channel. The alternate name for this point uses the character 胞 *bāo*, which is the same as 包 but for the addition of the flesh radical (月 *rù*) on the left, indicating that it is a body part.

足五里

Foot Five Li

LV-10 *(zú wǔ lǐ)*
足 *zú*: foot, (lower) leg
五 *wǔ*: five, fifth
里 *lǐ*: a measure of distance (360 paces); village

Classical Location: Three inches below Surging Qi (ST-30) on the inside of the thigh, where a pulsating vessel can be felt. *(Great Compendium)*

Explanation of Point Name

The character 里 *lǐ* can be construed as having the same meaning as 理 *lǐ*, i.e., to rectify, because these two characters were not always clearly distinguished in classical Chinese. Five (五 *wǔ*) may be a synonym for center, since in five-phase theory five corresponds to earth and the central position. It could also reference the five viscera. The name reflects LV-10's ability to rectify both the center and the viscera.

If 里 *lǐ* is taken to mean a village or ward, the name can be interpreted as a place. This highlights LV-10 as the fifth point from Cycle Gate (LV-14), the channel's end.

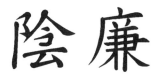

Yin Corner

LV-11 *(yīn lián)*
陰 *yīn*: yin, the complement of yang
廉 *lián*: angle, corner, side, ridge

Classical Location: Below Goat Arrow (LV-12 alternate name), two inches from Surging Qi (ST-30), at the pulsating vessel. *(Great Compendium)*

Explanation of Point Name
The point is located on the yin aspect of the leg at the inner angle or corner of the groin; hence the name.

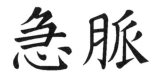

Urgent Pulse

LV-12 *(jí mài)*
急 *jí*: urgent, hasty; anxious; acute
脈 *mài (mò)*: vessel; pulse

Alternate Name

Goat Arrow   羊矢   *yáng shǐ*

Classical Location: Above Yin Corner (LI-11) and the genitals, two and a half inches either side of the midline. A hardness can be dimly felt under pressure and hard pressure will produce pain that radiates up and down.
(Golden Mirror)

Explanation of Point Name

This point name is described in *Essential Questions* as being derived from the nature of the pulse at the point when the liver channel is struck by pathogenic cold.

The alternate name 羊矢 *yáng shǐ*, Goat Arrow, is derived from the hard arrow-shaped sinew located just below the point.

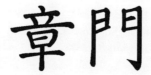

Camphorwood Gate

LV-13 *(zhāng mén)*

章 *zhāng*: complete (an essay); a chapter; a strain of
    music; the flat area on top of a hill
門 *mén*: gate, door

Alternate Names

Rear Camphorwood Gate	後章門	*hòu zhāng mén*
Elbow Tip	肘尖	*zhǒu jiān*
Long Level	長平	*cháng píng*
Lateral Costal Bone-Hole	脅窌	*xié liáo*

Free Ribs	季肋	*jì lè*
Free Ribs	季脅	*jì xié*
Lard Bone-Hole	肪髎	*fáng liáo*
Spleen Mu	脾募	*pí mù*

Classical Location: In the region of the free ribs, two inches above the navel and six inches either side of the midline. The point is found with the patient on her side; with top leg bent and bottom leg extended. Also, the point is located where the tip of the elbow touches.
(Great Compendium)

Point Associations: Alarm-mu point of the spleen; intersection-jiaohui point of the foot jue yin liver and foot shao yang gallbladder channels; meeting-hui point of the five viscera.

Explanation of Point Name

The character 章 *zhāng* was originally used to denote the camphor laurel tree and, by extension, any valuable lumber. This point is an intersection-jiaohui point of the two wood channels as well as being the alarm-mu point of the spleen (earth). It is the point where wood receives earth. In *The Book of History* (史記) it is stated that: "When wood receives the virtue of earth, it becomes a thousand pieces of valuable lumber (木稟土德而成千章之材)." Thus Camphorwood Door is one possible rendering of this point name.

The ideogram 章 *zhāng* can also be used to describe the flat area at the top of a hill. LV-13 is located just below the rib cage in an area that can be said to resemble this geological formation. The character 門 *mén*, meaning gate, is in this case a metaphor for an acupuncture point.

章 *zhāng* can have the same meaning as 障 *zhàng*, which represents a screen or veil. The rib cage screens the viscera and this point is like a gateway (門 *mén*) past that screen through which the physician can treat diseases of those organs. Thus the point name could also be rendered Screen Gate. In support of this interpretation is the Forty-fifth Difficulty in the *Classic of Difficult Issues*, in which Camphorwood Gate (LV-13) is designated as the meeting-hui point of the viscera.

期門

Cycle Gate

LV-14 *(qí mén)*

期 *qí*: period, cycle; one hundred years; expect; one year
門 *mén*: gate, door

Alternate Name

Liver Mu   肝募   *gān mù*

Classical Location: Two ribs directly below the nipple, one inch and five fen to the side of Not Contained (ST-19). *(Great Compendium)*

Point Associations: Alarm-mu point of the liver, intersection-jiaohui point of the foot tai yin spleen channel, foot jue yin liver channel, and yin linking vessel.

Explanation of Point Name

LV-14 is the last point in the channel cycle, which begins anew at Cloud Gate (LU-2). This point is thus a gateway (門) in the qi cycle much as the end of one year (期) is a gateway to the next. The name Cycle Gate conveys this idea.

Conception Vessel

任脈

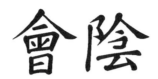

Meeting of Yin

CV-1 *(huì yīn)*
會 *huì*: meeting, convergence
陰 *yīn*: yin, the complement of yang

Alternate Names

Screen	屏翳	*píng yì*
Flat Screen	平翳	*píng yì*
Lower Extreme	下極	*xià jí*
Metal Gate	金門	*jīn mén*
Seabed	海底	*hǎi dǐ*
Ghost Store	鬼藏	*guǐ cáng*
Lower Yin Divergence	下陰別	*xià yīn bié*

Classical Location: Between the anterior and posterior yin. *(Great Compendium)*

Point Associations: Intersection-jiaohui point of the conception, governing, and penetrating vessels; the eleventh of the thirteen ghost points.

Explanation of Point Name

This point is located halfway between the anterior and posterior yins, the genitals and anus (前陰 *qián yīn*, anterior yin, refers to the genitals; 後陰 *hòu yīn*, posterior yin, refers to the anus). Hence it is called Meeting of Yin.

CV-1 is the intersection-jiaohui point of the governing, conception and penetrating vessels. The name Meeting of Yin is reminiscent of the fact that CV-1 is an intersection-jiaohui point on a yin vessel.

Hundred Convergences (GV-20), located at the top of the head, is a point at which yang qi gathers (i.e., a meeting of yang). CV-1 is GV-20's anatomical opposite, and is a point a which yin qi gathers; hence it is called Meeting of Yin. The alternate names Seabed and Lower Extreme highlight the yin nature of the point.

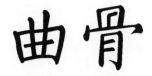

Curved Bone

CV-2 (*qū gǔ*)
曲 *qū*: curved, bent
骨 *gǔ*: bone

Alternate Names

Crooked Bone	屈骨	*qū gǔ*
Crooked Bone's End	曲骨端	*qū gǔ duān*
Curved Bone's End	曲骨端	*qū gǔ duān*
Return Bone	回骨	*huí gǔ*
Urinary Bladder	尿胞	*niào bāo*
Marrow Shu	髓俞	*suí shū*

Classical Location: Directly above Meeting of Yin (CV-1), above the transverse bone, in the depression at the pubic hairline where the pulsating vessel can be felt, five inches below the navel. *(Golden Mirror)*

Point Associations: Intersection-jiaohui point of the foot jue yin liver channel and the conception vessel.

Explanation of Point Name

The location of CV-2 just above the curvature of the pubic bone accounts for its name. The alternate names are similarly derived from the location of the point.

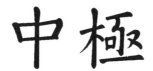

Central Pole

CV-3 *(zhōng jí)*

中 *zhōng*: center, central
極 *jí*: pole (as in polar opposites), extreme

Alternate Names

Qi Source	氣原	*qì yuán*
Qi Fish	氣魚	*qì yú*
Jade Spring	玉泉	*yù quán*
Bladder Mu	膀胱募	*páng guāng mù*

Classical Location: Directly above Curved Bone (CV-2) four inches below the navel. *(Golden Mirror)*

Point Associations: Alarm-mu point of the bladder; intersection-jiaohui point of the three yin channels of the foot (liver, spleen and kidney) and the conception vessel.

Explanation of Point Name

CV-3 is in the middle of the body on both a vertical and horizontal axis. Its name is the same as the Chinese name for the North Star, which is in the center of the sky.

The character 中 *zhōng* may be a reference to the center, i.e., central burner, while 極 *jí* can be considered as a substitute for its homophone 急, which means acute or urgent. A rendering of the point name as Urgent Center would reflect the point's effectiveness in the treatment of acute abdominal pain.

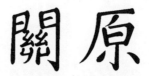

Origin Pass

CV-4 (*guān yuán*)

關 *guān*: pass, passageway, gate; critical juncture; to lock in
原 *yuán*: origin, original, source

Alternate Names

Source Pass	關原	*guān yuán*
Cinnabar Field	丹田	*dān tián*
Triple Intersection	三結交	*sān jié jiāo*
Origin of Huang	肓之原	*huāng zhī yuán*
Lower Huang	下肓	*xià huāng*
Lower Regulator	下紀	*xià jì*
Great Sea	大海	*dà hǎi*
Great Reservoir	大涃	*dà kùn*
Great Central Pole	大中極	*dà zhōng jí*

Infant's Door	子戶	zǐ hù
Infant's Palace	子宮	zǐ gōng
Infant's Place	子處	zǐ chù
Infant's Intestine	子腸	zǐ cháng
Fifth City	五城	wǔ chéng
Second Gate	次門	cì mén
Blood Chamber	血室	xuè shì
Sea of Blood	血海	xuè hǎi
Crux Disinhibitor	利機	lì jī
Life Gate	命門	mìng mén
Kunlun Mountains	昆侖	kūn lún
Fallen Sauce	垂漿	chuí jiāng
Junior Pivot	持樞	chí shū
Bladder Gate	胞門	bāo mén
Sea of Qi	氣海	qì hǎi
Delivery Gate	產門	chǎn mén
Navel	脖胦	bó yāng
Urine	溺水	niào shuǐ
Essential Dew	精露	jīng lù

Classical Location: Three inches below the navel. *(Great Compendium)*

Point Associations: Alarm-mu point of the small intestine; intersection-jiaohui point of the three foot yin channels (spleen, liver and kidney) and the conception vessel.

Explanation of Point Name

Depending on which meaning of the character 關 *guān* is considered, CV-4 is a "passageway of original qi," the "critical juncture of original yang and original yin," or the place where "original qi is stored [locked in]." The rendering of this name as Origin Pass is an attempt to include all these ideas.

The plethora of alternate names for this point are a result of it being the site of the uterus (i.e., blood chamber), the cinnabar field (*dān tián*), and the life gate fire.

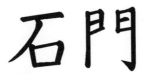

Stone Gate

CV-5 *(shí mén)*

石 *shí*: stone
門 *mén*: gate, door

Alternate Names

Cinnabar Field	丹田	*dān tián*
Crux Disinhibitor	利機	*lì jī*
Life Gate	命門	*mìng mén*
Shu Gate	圊	*shū mén*
Infertility	絶孕	*juě yùn*
Essential Dew	精露	*jīng lù*
Triple Burner Mu	三焦募	*sān jiāo mù*

Classical Location: Directly above Origin Pass (CV-4), two inches below the navel. *(Golden Mirror)*

Point Associations: Alarm-mu point of the triple burner.

Explanation of Point Name

CV-5 is effective in treating stone conglomerations (石瘕 *shí jiǎ*), which are stone-like masses in the lower abdomen. The point is a gate through which these conglomerations can be treated; hence the name Stone Gate.

A place where crops cannot grow is called a stone field (石田 *shí tián*), and a woman who is not able to give birth is called a stone woman (石女 *shí nú*). Needling this point can prevent conception; therefore the point is called

Stone Gate. The alternate name Infertility supports this explanation.

Stone Gate is the name of a mountain, and is also an ancient place name.

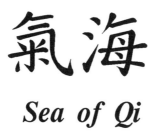

Sea of Qi

CV-6 (qì hǎi)
氣 qì: qi, breath
海 hǎi: sea

Alternate Names

Lower Sea of Qi	下氣海	xià qì hǎi
Lower Huang	下肓	xià huāng
Huang Origin	肓之原	huāng zhī yuán
Navel	脖胦	bó yāng
Small Navel	季胦	jì yāng

Classical Location: In the depression one and a half inches below the navel. *(Great Compendium)*

Explanation of Point Name

This area serves as a reservoir of qi for the whole of the body. It is the place from which qi emanates and to which it returns and is thus the Sea of Qi.

In Taoist meditation practices the breath is brought to this area and the qi is stored there. The delineation between qi and breath is unclear in Chinese, an ambiguity preserved by the name Sea of Qi.

The three alternate names for CV-6 that contain the word 肓 *huāng* stem from a line of the *Inner Canon* which states that the huang has its origin in the area below the navel.

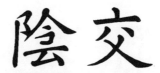

Yin Intersection

CV-7 (*yīn jiāo*)

陰 *yīn*: yin, the complement of yang
交 *jiāo*: intersection

Alternate Names

Small Pass	小關	*xiǎo guān*
Scarce Pass	少關	*shào guān*
Cinnabar Field	丹田	*dān tián*
Horizontal Door	橫戶	*héng hù*

Classical Location: One inch below the umbilicus, even with the upper border of the bladder. *(Great Compendium)*

Point Associations: Intersection-jiaohui point of the conception and penetrating vessels and the kidney channel.

Explanation of Point Name

CV-7 is called Yin Intersection because it is located on the yin side of the body and is also the intersection-jiaohui point of three yin vessels (the kidney channel, the conception vessel and the penetrating vessel). Note that the Chinese word for intersection is 交會 *jiāo huì*, the first character of which is also the second character in the point name.

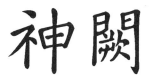

Spirit Gate

CV-8 *(shén què)*

神 *shén*: spirit

闕 *què*: a watch tower on either side of a palace gate, a gate; a palace

Alternate Names

Life Stem	命蒂	*mìng dì*
Qi Union	氣合	*qì hé*
Qi Abode	氣舍	*qì shè*
Linking Convergence	維會	*wéi huì*
Center of the Navel	臍中	*qí zhōng*

Classical Location: In the center of the navel.
(Great Compendium)

Explanation of Point Name

The character 闕 *què* is a symbol for an empty space that serves as a gate; it is considered interchangeable with 缺 *què*, meaning a gap. The spirit enters and leaves through CV-8, the Spirit Gate.

The navel is said to be the residence of the Supreme Unity (太乙 *tài yǐ*), the source of life. For this reason, this point name could be rendered as Spirit's Palace.

Originally, the name of CV-8 was Qi Abode, which may have been chosen on the basis of the statement in the *Taoist Storehouse* (道藏) that "the qi of later heaven (i.e., postnatal qi) resides at the navel." Its name was later changed to avoid confusion with ST-11, which is also called Qi Abode.

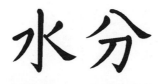

Water Divide

CV-9 *(shuī fēn)*

水 *shuǐ*: water
分 *fēn*: divide, part, separate

Alternate Names

Divided Waters	分水	*fēn shuǐ*
Central Guard	中守	*zhōng shǒu*

Classical Location: Directly above Spirit Gate (CV-8), one inch above the navel. *(Golden Mirror)*

Explanation of Point Name

This point is located in the region of lower opening of the small intestine, which functions in separating the clear and the turbid, drawing off fluid from the digesta and sending it to the bladder, leaving the solid waste to be conveyed to the large intestine. CV-9 is employed in the treatment of water swelling. For both of these reasons CV-9 is called Water Divide. Its clinical functions also explain the alternate names.

下脘

Lower Venter

CV-10 *(xià wǎn)*

下 *xià*: lower, below; to descend
脘 *wǎn (guǎn)*: venter

Alternate Name

Lower Duct	下管	xià guǎn
Dark Gate	幽門	yōu mén

Classical Location: Directly above Water Divide (CV-9), two inches above the navel. *(Golden Mirror)*

Point Associations: Intersection-jiaohui point of the foot tai yin spleen channel and the conception vessel.

Explanation of Point Name

The *Elucidation of Characters* (説文解字) says, "Venter means the stomach bowel," (脘, 胃府也) while modern Chinese medical dictionaries define the word as meaning the physical aspect of the stomach, including the lower portion of the esophagus and the upper part of the duodenum. The venter is divided into three sections: upper, middle and lower. CV-10 is located at the lower border of the stomach and is thus called Lower Venter.

建里

Interior Strengthening

CV-11 (jiàn lǐ)

建 *jiàn*: to establish, to erect; to stand
里 *lǐ*: a measure of distance; a small hamlet

Classical Location: Directly above Lower Venter (CV-10), three inches above the navel. *(Great Compendium)*

Explanation of Point Name

The most meaningful interpretation of this point name relies on the assumption that both ideograms are substitutes for homophones. In ancient times the character 里 *lǐ* was often used to convey the meaning inherent in its homophone 裡, which means inner or inside, while 建 *jiàn* was often used in place of its homophone 健, meaning healthy or to strengthen. Considered in this light the point name may be rendered as Interior Strengthening, which is indicative of CV-11's function of strengthening the central burner.

CV-11 occupies an established position in the neighborhood of the stomach, between Upper Venter (CV-10) and Lower Venter (CV-12). Since the meaning of the character 里 *lǐ* can be extended to express the idea of place, the name of this point can also be rendered as Established Place.

Since this point stands in the center of the internal path of digesta, the point name could be rendered as Center Stand.

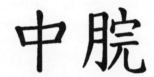

Central Venter

CV-12 *(zhōng wǎn)*

中 *zhōng*: center, central, middle
脘 *wǎn (guǎn)*: venter

Alternate Names

Central Duct	中管	*zhōng guǎn*
Venter	胃脘	*wèi wǎn*
Upper Regulator	上紀	*shàng jì*
Supreme Granary	太倉	*tài cāng*
Stomach Mu	胃募	*wèi mù*

Classical Location: Directly above Interior Strengthening (CV-11), four inches above the navel, midway between the navel and the bone that covers the heart. *(Golden Mirror)*

Point Associations: Intersection-jiaohui point of the hand tai yang small intestine, hand shao yang triple burner, and foot yang ming stomach channels, and the conception vessel; alarm-mu point of the stomach; one of the nine needles for returning yang; meeting-hui point of the bowels.

Explanation of Point Name

While the character 脘 *wǎn* is a certain reference to the venter, 中 *zhōng* can refer either to the point's location at the center of the venter, or to its location halfway between the navel and the xiphoid process.

This point is also called 太倉 *tài cāng*, Supreme Granary, in reference to a line from the *Spiritual Axis* that reads, "The stomach is the Supreme Granary." (胃者，太倉.) *The Classic of Difficult Issues* also refers to CV-12 by this name: "The bowels meet at the Supreme Granary." (府會，太倉.)

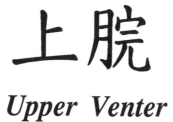

Upper Venter

CV-13 *(shàng wǎn)*
上 *shàng*: above, upper
脘 *wǎn (guǎn)*: venter

Alternate Names

Upper Duct	上管	*shàng guǎn*
Upper Regulator	上紀	*shàng jì*
Venter	胃脘	*wèi wǎn*
Stomach Duct	胃管	*wèi guǎn*

Classical Location: Directly above Central Venter (CV-12), five inches above the navel. *(Golden Mirror)*

-315-

Point Associations: Intersection-jiaohui point of the foot yang ming stomach and hand tai yang small intestine channels and the conception vessel.

Explanation of Point Name

CV-13 is located at the upper opening of the stomach; hence the name Upper Venter.

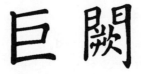

Great Tower Gate

CV-14 *(jù què)*
巨 *jù*: great, gigantic
闕 *què*: gate tower (watch towers located on either side of a palace gate); a palace

Alternate Name

| Heart Mu | 心募 | *xīn mù* |

Classical Location: Directly above the umbilicus, two inches below the joining of the ribs. *(Golden Mirror)*

Point Associations: Alarm-mu point of the heart.

Explanation of Point Name

The space below the breastbone can be seen to be shaped like a gate, while the rib cage on either side forms the watch towers for that gate. The honorific great is applied to points related to the commanding organ (the heart). As CV-14 is the alarm-mu point of the heart, the name Great

Tower Gate is thus indicative of a route of access to that viscus.

The character 闕 *què* can indicate a palace as a whole as well as the more specific reference to a palace gate tower. Because alarm-mu points are places where qi collects much as officials gather at a palace, the point name could also be rendered as Great Palace.

A 巨闕 *jù què* was a type of sword in ancient China. Its shape resembled the breastbone, below which CV-14 is located.

The xiphoid process is also called 巨闕 *jù què* in some cases. The name of this point is in this respect locational in nature.

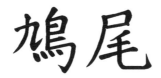

Turtledove Tail

CV-15 (*jiū wěi*)
鳩 *jiū*: turtledove
尾 *wěi*: tail

Alternate Names

Tail Screen	尾翳	*wěi yì*
Spirit Mansion	神府	*shén fǔ*
Anterior Breast	臆前	*yì qián*
Breastbone	𩩲骬	*hé gān*
Breastbone	𩩲𩩲	*hé hé*

Classical Location: One inch above Great Tower Gate (CV-14). *(Golden Mirror)*

Point Associations: Connecting-luo point of the conception vessel.

Explanation of Point Name

Viewed from the front, the entire are of the chest can be said to resemble a turtledove. The area above the breastbone is the turtledove's head, the breastbone is its back, the costal regions are its wings and the area in which CV-15 is located is the turtledove's tail. Alternately the breastbone can be seen as the center of a turtledove's tail (it is sometimes called "turtledove's tail") with the ribs being the feathers that spread out left and right. In either case the point takes its name from its location just inferior to the breastbone. This metaphor becomes even more intricate when one considers the turtledove's habit of pulling in its tail and leaving a space similar to the one where CV-15 is located. This parallels the idea of the "hidden bone" (i.e., the xiphoid process) at the location of this point.

Ingestion of turtledove tail was an ancient folk cure for esophageal constriction. The name of this point may be derived from the fact that this disorder manifests in the area of CV-15.

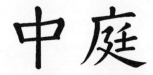

Center Palace

CV-16 (zhōng tíng)

中 *zhōng*: center, central, middle
庭 *tíng*: court, courtyard; palace

Classical Location: In the depression one inch directly above Turtledove's Tail (CV-15). *(Golden Mirror)*

Explanation of Point Name

The chest is the abode of the heart; the heart is the sovereign organ (emperor). The sternum and rib cage are like a palace that surrounds and protects the emperor. At the center of this area is CV-16, the Center Palace.

A Taoist text, *Canon of the Yellow Court,* (黃庭內景經), names the central cinnabar field (or heart field) the central palace: "The three fields are the upper [or] celestial field, the central [or] heart field, and the lower [or] cinnabar field. The upper palace receives the essential qi from below, the central palace receives essential qi from above, and the lower palace receives essential qi from the center." CV-16 is in the region of the central cinnabar field and is thus named Central Palace.

Within the palace of the rib cage is the Jade Hall (CV-18); CV-16 is like a courtyard in front of that hall. The word central can refer to both the the midline location and a central position in the upper burner. The name could thus be rendered as Central Courtyard in keeping with these ideas.

The Spirit Courtyard (CV-24) is above (on the head) and the Inner Courtyard (ST-44) is below (on the foot). CV-16 then is the Central Courtyard.

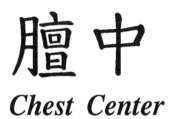

Chest Center

CV-17 *(dàn zhōng)*
膻 *dàn*: the central area of the chest
中 *zhōng*: center, middle

Alternate Names

Chest Hall	胸堂	*xiōng táng*
Upper Sea of Qi	上氣海	*shàng qì hǎi*
The Source	元見	*yuán jiàn*
Original Child	元兒	*yuán ér*

Classical Location: One inch and six fen directly above Central Palace (CV-16). *(Golden Mirror)*

Point Associations: Meeting-hui point of qi; intersection-jiaohui point of the foot tai yin spleen, foot shao yin kidney, hand tai yang small intestine, and hand shao yang triple burner channels and the conception vessel; alarm-mu point of the pericardium.

Explanation of Point Name

This point is named after its location in the center of the chest. The *Spiritual Axis* calls this area of the body the "palace of the heart governor [pericardium]."(心主之宮城.) This may explain the imperial nature of the point names in the region.

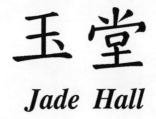

Jade Hall

CV-18 *(yù táng)*

玉 *yù*: jade
堂 *táng*: hall; palace; a hall within a palace

Alternate Name

| Jade's Beauty | 玉英 | *yù yīng* |

Classical Location: In the depression one inch and six fen directly above Chest Center (CV-17). *(Golden Mirror)*

Explanation of Point Name

The heart is the sovereign viscus and resides within the palace hall. With the Purple Palace (CV-19) above and the Central Palace (CV-16) below, the Jade Hall completes the imperial landscape.

Some Taoist texts refer to the lung as the Jade Hall. ("肺爲玉堂宮" *The Canon of the Yellow Court* 黃庭內景經.) This point is located on the sternum above the lung; hence the name. Jade Hall was also the name of a Han dynasty palace.

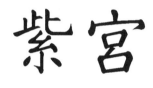

Purple Palace

CV-19 *(zǐ gōng)*

紫 *zǐ*: purple
宮 *gōng*: palace

Classical Location: In the depression one inch and six fen directly above Jade Hall (CV-18). *(Golden Mirror)*

Explanation of Point Name

The Chinese generally consider yellow to be the imperial color, though the color purple is sometimes also associated with royalty, as in the terms 紫宸 *(zǐ chén)*, the palace, and 紫禁城 *(zǐ jìn chéng)*, the Forbidden City. The abode of the heart, sovereign among viscera, is thus, by analogy, called the Purple Palace.

The phrase 紫宮 *zǐ góng*, Purple Palace, could also be a reference to heaven. In evidence of this, it has been said that: " Tai Yi (太乙, the Supreme Unity) resides in the

Purple Palace.'' (淮南子: 紫宮者,太乙之居也.) As heaven rules man, the heart rules the body. Hence the residence of the heart is called the Purple Palace.

We can also see purple as the color of blood. The heart, which commands the blood, resides in the Purple Palace. Also of note, Purple Palace is the name of a star that is a part of the Celestial Emperor Constellation.

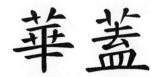

Florid Canopy

CV-20 *(huá gài)*
華 *huá*: flower, flowery; glory
蓋 *gài*: cover, canopy

Classical Location: In the depression one inch and six fen directly above Purple Palace (CV-19). *(Golden Mirror)*

Explanation of Point Name

Many early Taoist and medical texts describe the lung as the florid canopy or parasol, which can be taken as a symbol of the lung's position in the body in relation to the other organs. *Essential Questions* tells us that ''the lung is the canopy of the five viscera and the six bowels.'' (肺者五藏 六腑之蓋也.) CV-20 is located at the level of the upper extreme of the lung and is employed in treating disorders of that viscus such as dyspnea and cough. Its name is therefore derived from its close relationship to the lung.

Florid Canopy, 華蓋 *huá gài*, is also the name of a star.

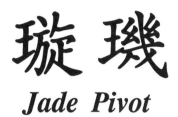

Jade Pivot

CV-21 *(xuán jī)*

璇 *xuán*: a kind of fine jade

璣 *jī*: a (non-globular) pearl; astronomical instrument gear

Alternate Name

Turning Pivot 旋機 *xuán jī*

Classical Location: In the depression one inch directly above Florid Canopy (CV-20). *(Golden Mirror)*

Explanation of Point Name

The combination 璇璣 *xuán jī* names an ancient astronomical instrument that turns on a pivot, much as the head turns on the neck. Thus the point is named after its location at the bottom of the neck.

The first four stars of the big dipper form the bowl of the dipper the last three form the handle. The second and third stars are called 璇 *xuán* and 璣 *jī* respectively. The dip at the top of the sternum resembles the bowl of the dipper. CV-21 is located in the area that corresponds to the bottom of the dipper formed by the stars 璇 and 璣 . To picture this, simply imagine the collar bone as the handle of the dipper and CV-21 as the bottom of the bowl.

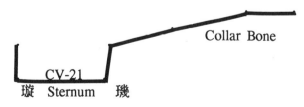

Collar Bone

CV-21

璇 Sternum 璣

璇璣 *xuán jī* is also the name of a particular palindrome that was embroidered on satin in the 4th century A.D. It was done by a woman for her husband (who had been banished to Tartary), and it consisted of 840 characters, which could be read the same backwards as forwards.

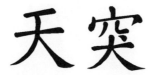

Celestial Chimney

CV-22 *(tiān tú)*

天 *tiān*: celestial, of the heavens, sky; Nature; heaven
突 *tú*: a chimney; to protrude; abrupt, sudden;
    to dash forward

Alternate Names

| Celestial Alarm | 天瞿 | *tiān qú* |
| Jade Door | 玉戶 | *yù hù* |

Classical Location: One inch above Jade Pivot (CV-21). *(Golden Mirror)*

Point Associations: Intersection-jiaohui point of the yin linking and conception vessels.

Explanation of Point Name

The windpipe is like the chimney of the upper burner, which is associated with heaven in the cosmology of the body. This point is located at the bottom of the windpipe and is thus called Celestial Chimney. Alternately, the two bony protrusions on either side of CV-22 allow for the rendering of this point name as Celestial Protrusion.

During respiration celestial qi (天氣 *tiān qì*) dashes by this point into the lung, and when this point is needled qi rushes forth. For these reasons the name could also be rendered as Celestial Rush.

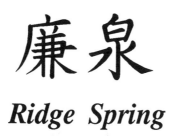

Ridge Spring

CV-23 *(lián quán)*
廉 *lián*: ridge; corner; aspect
泉 *quán*: spring (as a mountain spring)

Alternate Names

Tongue Root	舌本	*shé běn*
Root Pool	本池	*běn chí*
Larynx Center	喉中	*hóu zhōng*

Classical Location: When the head is tilted back, the point is directly above Celestial Chimney (CV-22), midway between the chin and the Adam's apple, below the root of the tongue. Find the point in supine posture. *(Golden Mirror)*

Point Associations: Intersection-jiaohui point of the yin linking and conception vessels.

Explanation of Point Name

This point is located above the ridge of the Adam's apple and just below the tongue, where fluids flow forth as though from a spring. Thus it is known as Ridge Spring.

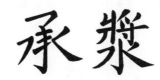

Sauce Receptacle

CV-24 (chéng jiāng)
承 *chéng*: to receive; to support
漿 *jiāng*: sauce, juice, rich fluid

Alternate Names

Heavy Sauce	重漿	*zhòng jiàng*
Suspended Sauce	懸漿	*xuán jiāng*
Celestial Pool	天池	*tiān chí*
Ghost Market	鬼市	*guǐ shì*

Classical Location: When the mouth is open, the point is in the center of the depression beneath the protrusion of the lower lip. *(Great Compendium)*

Point Associations: Intersection-jiaohui point of the foot yang ming stomach and hand yang ming large intestine channels and the conception and governing vessels; the eighth of the thirteen ghost points.

Explanation of Point Name

If food dribbles from the mouth, some of it may collect at this point. Hence the name Sauce Receptacle.

Governing Vessel

督脈

長強

Long Strong

GV-1 *(cháng qiáng)*

長 *cháng*: long (in space or time);
  zhǎng: to grow; to excel; to lead
強 *qiáng*: strong, forceful; stiff

Alternate Names

Jue Bone	厥骨	*jué gǔ*
Peg Bone	橛骨	*jué gǔ*
End Bone	偏骨	*piān gǔ*
Sacral Bone	骨骶	*gǔ dǐ*
End of Sacral Spine	脊骶端	*jí dǐ duān*
Sacrum Above	骶上	*dǐ shàng*
Hollow Below
the Tailbone	尾骨下空	*wěi gǔ xià kōng*
Tail Kingfisher Bone	尾翠骨	*wěi cuì gǔ*
Tail Maggot Bone	尾蛆骨	*wěi qū gǔ*
Fish Tail	魚尾	*yú wěi*
Tortoise Tail	龜尾	*guī wěi*
Tortoise Tail
Long Border	龜尾長疆	*guī wěi cháng jiāng*
Tail Palm	尾櫚	*wěi lú*
Qi Cleft	氣郄	*qì xī*

Yin Cleft	陰郄	*yīn xī*
Yin Cleft of Qi	氣之陰郄	*qì zhī yīn xī*
Cao's Ravine Road	曹溪路	*cáo xī lù*
River Cart Road	河車路	*hé chē lù*
Dragon Tiger	龍虎	*lóng hǔ*
Dragon & Tiger Point	龍虎穴	*lóng hǔ xuè*
Heavenward-Looking		
Summit	朝天巔	*cháo tiān diān*
Stairway to Heaven	上天梯	*shàng tiān tī*
Three Fen From		
the Gate	三分閭	*sān fēn lǘ*
Damage Mountain	傷山	*shāng shān*
That's It	爲之	*wéi zhī*

Classical Location: Three fen below the tip of the tail bone. The point is found in prostrate posture.
(Great Compendium)

Point Associations: Connecting-luo point of the governing vessel connecting to the conception vessel; intersection-jiaohui point of the foot shao yin kidney and foot shao yang gallbladder channels and the governing vessel.

Explanation of Point Name

Being associated with yang, the governing vessel is both long and strong. As this is the first point on the vessel, it can represent the entirety of it. Thus it is known as Long Strong.

The kidney is the organ of strength. GV-1 can be used to extend the strength of the kidney since it treats seminal emission, premature ejaculation, and impotence. Thus the name of this point could also be rendered as Strength Extender. In addition, needling of this point can cause the penis to become "long and strong."

The governing vessel can be said to lead the yang of the body. If the governing vessel is weak, the whole body is weak. If it is replete, the spine is stiff. By treating such conditions, GV-1 controls or leads the strength of the entire body. If the character 長 is read as *zhǎng*, the point name could be rendered as Strength Leader.

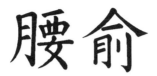

Lumbar Shu

GV-2 (*yāo shū*)

腰 *yāo*: lumbus, lower back; kidney; waist
俞 *shū*: a general term for acupuncture points

Alternate Names

Lumbar Birth	腰產	*yāo chàn*
Lumbar Pillar	腰柱	*yāo zhù*
Lumbar Door	腰戶	*yāo hù*
Marrow Hole	髓空	*suí kǒng*
Marrow Hole	髓孔	*suí kǒng*
Marrow Shu	髓俞	*suí shū*
Marrow Mansion	髓府	*suí fǔ*
Back Fresh	背鮮	*bèi xiān*
Back's Resolution	背解	*bèi jiě*

Classical Location: Below the twenty-first vertebra.
(Golden Mirror)

Explanation of Point Name

This point is most probably called Lumbar Shu because it is located among the lumbar vertebrae and treats low back pain.

In common speech, 腰 *yāo*, which in Chinese medicine normally refers to the lumbus, also means kidneys. This point is employed in the treatment of kidney disorders such as urinary incontinence and low back pain and may have been named in accordance with its relationship to the kidney.

腰陽關

Lumbar Yang Pass

GV-3 (yāo yáng guān)
腰 yāo: lumbus, lower back; kidney; waist
陽 yáng: yang, the complement of yin
關 guān: pass, passageway; gate; joint

Classical Location: Below the sixteenth vertebra.
(Golden Mirror)

Explanation of Point Name

The yang qi of the governing vessel travels up the spine, passing through GV-3 on its way to the life gate. Thus the point is called Lumbar Yang Pass. The word lumbar is included in the name of this point simply to avoid confusion with another point also known as 陽關 *yáng guān*, (Knee) Yang Joint (GB-33).

GV-3 is situated between the two large intestine associated-shu points; applying moxibustion at this point spreads yang qi through the abdomen. The point functions, in these respects, as a passageway for yang qi; thus its name could be rendered as Yang Passageway.

Located on the back (yang) side of the body, GV-3 is used to treat the lumbar joints, allowing free movement of the lower back. Thus the name of this point could also be rendered, like its namesake (GB-33), as Lower Back Yang Joint.

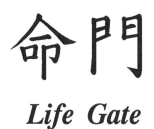

Life Gate

GV-4 *(mìng mén)*

命 *mìng*: life; fate; command
門 *mén*: gate, door

Alternate Names

Palace of Essence	精宮	*jīng gōng*
Bamboo Stick	竹杖	*zhú zhàng*
Connected	屬累	*shǔ lèi*

Classical Location: Below the fourteenth vertebra.
(Golden Mirror)

Explanation of Point Name

A long-standing belief amongst the Chinese is that the life essence is located in the area below the navel, which is called the life gate. *The Classic of Difficult Issues* calls this location "the area between the two kidneys." It is also known as the Cinnabar Field (丹田 *dān tián*) and the Jade Capital (玉都 *yù dū*). The life gate is sometimes equated with the womb in females and the palace of essence in males. It is the sea of blood and essence. GV-4 is located between the kidney shu points on the back side of this region, and is considered to be a major point in influencing the life gate.

懸樞

Suspended Pivot

GV-5 *(xuán shū)*

懸 *xuán*: to suspend, to hang; space
樞 *shū*: pivot, axis

Classical Location: Below the thirteenth vertebra. *(Golden Mirror)*

Explanation of Point Name

GV-5 is located at a point on the spine that is pivotal in bending and twisting motions. It is furthermore "suspended" in the space between the first and second lumbar vertebrae; hence the name Suspended Pivot.

The point is also "suspended" within the central burner, between the two associated-shu points of the triple burner. It forms a "suspended pivot" in the triple burner system.

脊中

Spinal Center

GV-6 *(jǐ zhōng)*

脊 *jǐ* (or *jī*): the spine
中 *zhōng*: center, central, middle

Alternate Names

Spine Pillar	脊柱	*jí zhù*
Spine Shu	脊俞	*jí shū*
Spirit Gathering	神宗	*shén zōng*

Classical Location: Below the eleventh vertebra.
(Golden Mirror)

Explanation of Point Name

This point is located half way up the spine and is thus called Spinal Center.

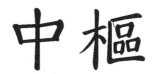

Central Pivot

GV-7 *(zhōng shū)*

中 *zhōng*: center, central, middle
樞 *shū*: pivot, axis

Classical Location: Below the tenth vertebra.
(Golden Mirror)

Explanation of Point Name

GV-7 is a point of rotation in the center of the spine. Thus it is called Central Pivot. Note that the point's name contains the "pivot" (樞 *shū*) of Suspended Pivot (GV-5), and the "center" (中 *zhōng*) of Spine's Center (GV-6). These three points are similar in both name and function.

筋縮

Sinew Contraction

GV-8 (*jīn suō*)

筋 *jīn*: sinew, tendon
縮 *suō*: to contract, to shrink

Alternate Name

Sinew Binder   筋束   *jīn shù*

Classical Location: Below the ninth vertebra.
(Golden Mirror)

Explanation of Point Name

GV-8 is situated between the two liver associated-shu points. The liver governs the sinews and this point, by virtue of its proximity to the associated-shu points of the liver, is effective in treating sinew disorders such as spasms, hypertonicity and contracture. Thus the point is named Sinew Contraction.

至陽

Extremity of Yang

GV-9 (*zhì yáng*)

至 *zhì*: extreme; to reach, to arrive
陽 *yáng*: yang, the complement of yin

Alternate Name

Bottom of the Lung 肺底 *fèi dǐ*

Classical Location: Below the seventh vertebra.
(Golden Mirror)

Explanation of Point Name

GV-9 is located on the upper back, which is the most yang aspect of the body; it is on the governing vessel, which is the commander of yang qi; and it is positioned below the seventh vertebra, seven being a number associated with yang. For all of these reasons the point is considered to be yang within yang, or the "extremity of yang."

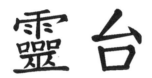

Spirit Tower

GV-10 *(líng tái)*

靈 *líng*: spirit, supernatural
台 *tái*: terrace, platform, tower

Classical Location: Below the sixth vertebra.
(Golden Mirror)

Explanation of Point Name

Wen Wang, an emperor of the Zhou Dynasty, built a tower he called 靈台 *líng tái*, the Spirit Tower, from which he could look out over all his territory. The term 靈台 has by extension come to mean the faculties of reason, or the mind. In Chinese thought the heart and mind are nearly synonymous, thus 靈台 is also representative of the heart. The *Jin Canon* confirms this interpretation in a passage that states: "Taoist texts consider the heart to be the Spirit Tower." (道經則以心爲靈台.) This point is located just below the associated-shu point of the heart; the heart stores the spirit. It is the association of this point with the heart that results in its name Spirit Tower.

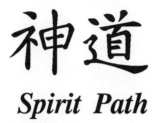

Spirit Path

GV-11 *(shén dào)*
神 *shén*: spirit
道 *dào*: path, road, way

Alternate Name

Visceral Shu   臟兪   *zàng zhū*

Classical Location: Below the fifth vertebra.
(Golden Mirror)

Explanation of Point Name

GV-11 is located between the two associated-shu points of the heart; the heart can be treated though this point. Because the heart stores the spirit, GV-11 can be said to be a path to the spirit or a "spirit path."

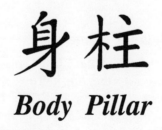

Body Pillar

GV-12 *(shēn zhù)*
身 *shēn*: body; person
柱 *zhù*: pillar, post; support

Alternate Names

Wisdom's Advantage Hair	智利毛	*zhì lì máo*
Wisdom's Advantage Qi	知利氣	*zhī lì qì*
Wisdom's Advantage Armor	知利介	*zhī lì jiè*
Dust Qi	塵氣	*chén qì*

Classical Location: Below the third vertebra.
(Golden Mirror)

Explanation of Point Name

This point is located between the shoulder blades, below the third thoracic vertebra. As a part of the "pillar" of the spine, it provides support for the body. The name Body Pillar refers to both the spine in general and to this point on the spine in particular.

GV-12 is located between the lung associated-shu points and opposite to CV-17, the meeting-hui point of qi. Lung qi is crucial for the support of the body, as is qi in general. The name Body Pillar may thus be a metaphor emphasizing this point's relationship to qi, the pillar of the body.

In the alternate names the characters 智 *zhì*, wisdom, and 知 *zhī*, knowledge, are both rendered as wisdom. Though today the two carry different meanings, in ancient times 知 was used to express both knowledge and wisdom.

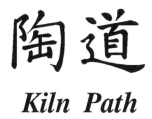

Kiln Path

GV-13 *(táo dào)*
陶 *táo*: kiln; pleased or happy
道 *dào*: path, road, way

Classical Location: Below the first vertebra.
(Golden Mirror)

Point Associations: Intersection-jiaohui point of the governing vessel and the foot tai yang bladder channel.

Explanation of Point Name

The character 陶 is used to represent a kiln, which the spinous processes may be said to resemble. This point lies on the path to the kiln-like protuberance of the first cervical vertebra; thus it is called Kiln Path.

If the word kiln is taken as a metaphor for fire (i.e., yang qi), then the point name is indicative of GV-14's location on the pathway of yang qi (i.e., the governing vessel).

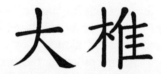

Great Hammer

GV-14 *(dà zhuī)*
大 *dà*: great, big, large
椎 *zhuī*: hammer, mallet; vertebra

Alternate Name

      Hundred Taxations   百勞   *bǎi láo*

Classical Location: Above the first vertebra.
(Golden Mirror)

Point Associations: Intersection-jiaohui point of the six yang channels and the governing vessel.

Explanation of Point Name

The Chinese call the vertebrae "spine hammers" by virtue of their similarity in shape to the carpenter's tool. The most prominent one, the seventh cervical, was traditionally called the "great hammer." GV-14 takes its name from its position just below this vertebra.

Do not mistake the alternate name Hundred Taxations for (M-HN-30), a non-channel point with the same name.

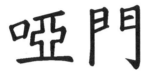

Mute's Gate

GV-15 *(yǎ mén)*

啞 *yǎ*: a mute
門 *mén*: gate, door

Alternate Names

Loss-of-Voice Gate	瘖門	*yīn mén*
Tongue Root	舌根	*shé gēn*
Tongue Swelling	舌腫	*shé zhǒng*
Opposite the Tongue	橫舌	*héng shé*
Tongue's Horizontal	舌橫	*shé héng*
Tongue Repression	舌厭	*shé yàn*
Repressed Tongue	厭舌	*yàn shé*

Classical Location: In the depression at the center of the back of the neck, five fen within the hairline. The point is found with the head lifted. *(Great Compendium)*

Point Associations: Intersection-jiaohui point of the governing vessel and the yang linking vessel; one of the nine needles for returning yang.

Explanation of Point Name

This point connects with the root of the tongue and treats voice disorders. It is a gate to the voice and is thus known as Mute's Gate.

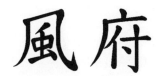

Wind Mansion

GV-16 *(fēng fǔ)*

風 *fēng*: wind

府 *fǔ*: mansion, palace; storehouse, treasury

Alternate Names

Tongue Root	舌本	*shé běn*
Root of Preoccupation	思本	*sī běn*
Cao's Ravine	曹谿	*cáo xī*
Clearheadedness	惺惺	*xīng xīng*
Ghost Hole	鬼穴	*guǐ xuè*
Ghost Forest	鬼林	*guǐ lín*
Ghost Pillow	鬼枕	*guǐ zhěn*

Classical Location: One inch above the hairline at the back of the neck; in the depression between the two large sinews. The flesh at the point rises when the patient speaks and sinks back when he ceases talking. *(Great Compendium)*

Point Associations: Intersection-jiaohui point of the yang motility and governing vessels; the sixth of the thirteen ghost points.

Explanation of Point Name

This point is used to treat wind disorders such as wind strike, stiff neck, headache, aversion to cold, visual dizziness, hemiplegia, head wind and wind cold. It treats both endogenous or exogenous wind, especially when that wind affects the brain. GV-16 is further considered to be a point at which wind pathogens enter the body. Hence it is the Wind Mansion.

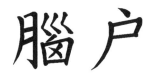

Brain's Door

GV-17 *(nǎo hù)*
腦 *nǎo*: brain
戸 *hù*: door, household

Alternate Names

Skull Union	合顱	*hé lú*
Circumference Wind	匝風	*zā fēng*
West Wind	西風	*xī fēng*
Meeting of the Forehead	會額	*huì é*

Classical Location: One and a half inches directly above Wind Mansion (GV-16), on the pillow bone.
(Golden Mirror)

Point Associations: Intersection-jiaohui point of the foot tai yang bladder channel and the governing vessel.

Explanation of Point Name

GV-17 is located on the ''pillow bone'' (occipital bone), directly behind the brain. It is called Brain's Door because of its location and its use in the treatment of epilepsy and dizziness, i.e., disorders of the brain.

強間

Unyielding Space

GV-18 *(qiáng jiān)*

強 *qiáng*: unyielding, stiff; forceful, strong
間 *jiān*: a space; between, among, in the middle of

Alternate Name

Great Feather   大羽   *dà yǔ*

Classical Location: One inch and five fen directly above Brain's Door (GV-17). *(Golden Mirror)*

Explanation of Point Name

The character 間 *jiān* refers to the point's location in a depression (space) between the occipital bone and the parietal bone, while 強 *qiáng* may refer to either the hard, unyielding bone of the skull or the point's use in the treatment of stiff neck. Thus the name is rendered as Unyielding Space.

If 強 *qiáng* is taken as a reference to the point's ability to strengthen the brain (treating epilepsy, headache, madness, and visual dizziness), then the name could be rendered as Strengthening Space.

The 強 *qiáng* derives its meaning of strength from its radical 弓 *gōng*, which represents the archer's bow. When joined by a line, GV-17, GV-18 and GV-19 form a bow, with GV-18 in the middle. If we accept the assertion made by some sources that this reasoning accounts for the name, the rendering Center of the Bow would be appropriate.

後頂

Behind the Vertex

GV-19 *(hòu dǐng)*

後 *hòu*: behind; after
頂 *dǐng*: crown of the head, the vertex

Alternate Names

Intersection Hub	交衝	*jiāo chōng*
Intersection Surge	交沖	*jiāo chōng*

Classical Location: One inch and five fen directly above Unyielding Space (GV-18). *(Golden Mirror)*

Explanation of Point Name

This point is named for its location posterior to the vertex of the head.

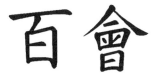

Hundred Convergences

GV-20 *(bǎi huì)*

百 *bǎi*: one hundred
會 *huì*: meeting, convergence

Alternate Names

Three Yang	三陽	*sān yáng*
Fivefold Convergence	五會	*wǔ huì*
Three Yang Fivefold Convergence		
	三陽五會 (涇)	*sān yáng wǔ huì*
Linking Convergence	維會	*wéi huì*
Mountain Top	巔上	*diān shàng*
Ridge Top	嶺上	*lǐng shàng*
Ridge Top Celestial Fullness		
	嶺上天滿	*lǐng shàng tiān mǎn*
Celestial Fullness	天滿	*tiān mǎn*
Mud Ball Palace	泥丸宮	*ní wán gōng*

Classical Location: One inch and five fen directly above Behind the Vertex (GV-19), in the depression that is in line with the apex of the ear. *(Golden Mirror)*

Point Associations: This point is the intersection-jiaohui point of the six yang channels and governing vessel *(Great Compendium)*. Most earlier sources list this point only as an intersection-jiaohui point of the foot tai yin bladder channel and the governing vessel.

Explanation of Point Name

According to the *Classic of Difficult Issues,* yang converges at the head. GV-20 is the intersection-jiaohui point of the six yang channels and the governing vessel. In Chinese the number one hundred stands for many; thus the meeting of many channels is called Hundred Convergences. Further, the numerous bones of the skull all meet at this point.

A passage in the text *Taoist Storehouse* (道藏) refers to the head as the most important part of the body, and further states that it is the meeting place of the hundred spirits. As the uppermost point on the head GV-20 represents the place of convergence of the hundred spirits, or Hundred Convergences.

The numerative hundred may also be a reference to this point's effectiveness "treating the hundred diseases," as is stated in the *Life-Promoting Canon*.

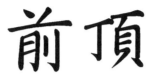

Before the Vertex

GV-21 *(qián dǐng)*

前 *qián*: before, in front of
頂 *dǐng*: crown of the head, vertex

Classical Location: One inch and five fen directly in front of Hundred Convergences (GV-20). *(Golden Mirror)*

Explanation of Point Name

This point is named for its location anterior to the vertex of the head.

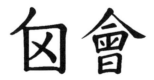

Fontanel Meeting

GV-22 *(xìn huì)*

囟 *xìn*: fontanel
會 *huì*: meeting, convergence

Alternate Names

Fontanel Gate	囟門	*xìn mén*
Top of the Fontanel	囟上	*xìn shàng*
Hundred Convergences of the Forehead	前頭百會	*qián tóu bǎi huì*
Ghost Gate	鬼門	*guǐ mén*
Vertex Gate	頂門	*dǐng mén*

Classical Location: One inch and five fen directly in front of Before the Vertex (GV-21). *(Golden Mirror)*

Explanation of Point Name

This point is located at the junction of the cranial fontanels in infants, and is the meeting place of channel qi and of the bones. Thus it is called Fontanel Meeting.

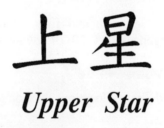

Upper Star

GV-23 *(shàng xīng)*

上 *shàng*: upper, top; to rise
星 *xīng*: star

Alternate Names

Bright Hall	明堂	*míng táng*
Spirit Hall	神堂	*shén táng*
Ghost Hall	鬼堂	*guǐ táng*
Hall of Fame	名堂	*míng táng*

Classical Location: Behind Spirit Court (GV-24) in the depression one inch within the hairline; it can contain a bean. *(Great Compendium)*

Point Associations: The tenth of the thirteen ghost points.

Explanation of Point Name

The word 星 *xīng*, meaning star, was probably chosen for this point name because stars are located in the heavens and thus parallel the position of the head relative to the body. Furthermore, a star "is the essence of the myriad things." This point is located on the front and top (both yang) part of the head (also yang) and is thus, like a star, the essence of yang qi. The adjective "upper" is most likely a reference to the point's location on the top of the head.

The essence of the five viscera is reflected in the eyes and the point treats eye disorders. A star being the "essence of the myriad things," the point's name also denotes function.

The alternate names Bright Hall and Spirit Hall can be considered indicative of GV-23's ability to treat eye disorders because brightness of the eyes reflects the spirit.

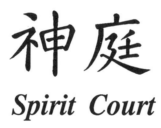

Spirit Court

GV-24 *(shén tíng)*

神 *shén*: spirit
庭 *tíng*: court, courtyard; hall; palace

Alternate Name

      Hairline   髮際   *fǎ jì*

Classical Location: Directly above the nose, five fen within the hairline. *(Great Compendium)*

Point Associations: Intersection-jiaohui point of the foot tai yang bladder and foot yang ming stomach channels and the governing vessel.

Explanation of Point Name

The face is the "court of the spirit" (續博物志： "面者，神之庭也 "). Because this point is located above the face and is utilized in treating various disorders of the head, forehead, eyes and nose, its name may be rendered as Spirit Court. A further validation for this rendering refers to the fact that the center of the brain, where the original spirit is stored, is called the "upper cinnabar field" (上丹田) and, alternately, the "upper court" (上庭). Thus Spirit Court is located near the brain and treats spirit disorders.

The *Compendium of Materia Medica* (本草綱目) states that "the brain is the palace (府 *fŭ*) of the original spirit." This point is used to treat the brain, and, because the characters 府 *fŭ* and 庭 *tíng* are sometimes synonymous, its name may be translated as Spirit Palace.

If 庭 *tíng* is taken in its sense of "courtyard," then there is a connection between GV-23 and GV-24. GV-23 is known as the Spirit Hall (alternate name), and GV-24, the place in front of the spirit hall, is the Spirit Court.

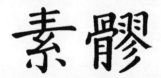

White Bone-Hole

GV-25 *(sù liáo)*

素 *sù*: pure, simple, plain; white;
    the original nature of things; common
髎 *liáo*: bone-hole

Alternate Names

Nose Tip	準頭	*zhŭn tóu*
Nose Tip	鼻準	*bí zhŭn*
Center of the Face	正面	*zhèng miàn*

| Face Center | 面正 | *miàn zhèng* |
| King of Face | 面王 | *miàn wáng* |

Classical Location: At the very tip of the nose.
(Great Compendium)

Explanation of Point Name

The ideograph 素 *sù* can mean white, the color associated with the lung. As this point is located on the tip of the nose, which is portal of the lung, the name may be rendered as White Bone-Hole.

The character 素 *sù* carries a meaning of emptiness, like a hole. The term 素手 *sù shǒu*, for example, means empty-handed (素 *sù*: empty, 手 *shǒu*: hand). The hole at the tip of the nose may therefore be called Empty Bone-Hole.

This point is located at the tip of the nose, which is in the center of the face. Thus GV-25 has the alternate names of Nose Tip and Center of the Face. This is the natural arrangement of things, so the name of the point may also be translated as Original Bone-Hole.

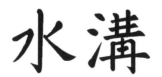

Water Trough

GV-26 (*shuǐ gōu*)
水 *shuǐ*: water
溝 *gōu*: trough, ditch

Alternate Names

| Human Center | 人中 | *rén zhōng* |
| Nose Human Center | 鼻人中 | *bí rén zhōng* |

Ghost Palace	鬼宮	*guǐ gōng*
Ghost Reception Room	鬼客廳	*guǐ kè tīng*
Ghost Market	鬼市	*guǐ shì*

Classical Location: In the depression close to the nostrils at the center of the trough below the nose.
(Great Compendium)

Point Associations: Intersection-jiaohui point of the hand yang ming large intestine and foot yang ming stomach channels with the governing vessel; first of the thirteen ghost points.

Explanation of Point Name

This point is located below the nose in the center of the philtrum. The philtrum resembles a "water trough" or drain.

This point is just as frequently referenced by its alternate name 人中 *rén zhōng*, Human Center. The three basic components of the Chinese universe are Heaven (天), Man (人) and Earth (地). The nose receives the five qi from heaven and the mouth receives the five sapors from the earth. Located between the nose and the mouth, GV-26 can thus be likened to humankind, which stands in the center, between heaven and earth.

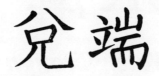

Extremity of the Mouth

GV-27 *(duì duān)*
兑 *duì*: the 58th trigram of the *Book of Changes*;
  to exchange, to barter; to weigh
端 *duān*: end, extremity; proper, upright

Alternate Names

Upper Extremity of the Lip
唇上端 *chún shàng duān*
Mouth Means Edge 兌通兌 *duì tōng duì*
Bone Strengthener 壯骨 *zhuàng gǔ*

Classical Location: At the peak of the upper lip.
(Great Compendium)

Explanation of Point Name

The *Book of Changes* states that "兌 *duì* is the mouth"
(兌爲口也). This point is located on the upper border of
the upper lip, thus its name may be rendered as Extremity
of the Mouth.

Some sources suggest that the character 兌 *duì* is a substitute for 銳 *ruì*, meaning a sharp edge, which can be taken
as a description of the border of the upper lip. The character 端 *duān*, meaning end, may then refer to the end of
the Governing Vessel just after this point.

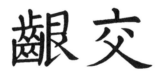

Gum Intersection

GV-28 *(yín jiāo)*
齦 *yín*: the gums
交 *jiāo*: intersection

Alternate Names

Gum Crevice Sinew Center
齦縫筋中 *yín fèng jīn zhōng*

Extremity Intersection   斷交   *duàn jiāo*

Classical Location: In the cleft above the teeth.
(Golden Mirror)

Point Associations: Intersection-jiaohui point of the conception and governing vessels and the foot yang ming stomach channel.

Explanation of Point Name

This point is located on the gums where they join with the frenulum of the upper lip. It is also the intersection-jiaohui point of the conception and governing vessels and the stomach channel, giving it the name Gum Intersection.

Appendix A

Glossary of Single Characters

The characters that occur in the primary acupuncture point names are here listed in pinyin alphabetical order. A list of English equivalents accompanies each entry. Following this is information that either relates to the etymology of the character or is relevant to its usage in Chinese medicine. Etymology is not included for every entry, but is limited to characters likely to be of particular interest to students of Chinese medicine where simple, reliable information is available. The final item accompanying each entry is a list of all point names that contain the character. This listing enables the reader to compare point names that contain the same character and to make deductions about the usage of that character in the different names.

āi 哀 grief, sorrow; to lament, commiserate.

腹哀　fù āi　Abdominal Lament　SP-16

bá (bó) 白 white; clear; bright.
The character is a pictograph of the sun （日） rising. The line at the top of the character represents a ray of light at dawn. The idea of whiteness and brightness is derived from the color of eastern sky as the sun rises. In the acupuncture point names this character often implies some connection with metal, as white is the color associated with that phase.

俠白　xiá bái　Guarding White　LU-4
四白　sì bái　Four Whites　ST-2
隱白　yǐn bái　Hidden White　SP-1
太白　tài bái　Supreme White　SP-3
白環俞　bái huán shū　White Ring Shu　BL-30

-353-

浮白　fú bái　Floating White　GB-10
陽白　yáng bái　Yang White　GB-14

băi 百 one hundred.
In Chinese the word one hundred can represent the idea of
many or all. Phrases such as the hundred diseases, the hundred surnames and the hundred flowers exemplify this use
of the character 百.

百會　băi huì　Hundred Convergences　GV-20

bāo 胞 placenta; bladder; cell; born of the same parents.
This character is composed of a flesh radical （肉 modified
to 月）combined with the character 　包, meaning bag or
sack. It was invented to take the place of 包 *bāo* when
that character began to take on more abstract meanings (see
包 *bāo* below).

胞肓　bāo huāng　Bladder Huang　BL-53

bāo 包 to wrap, to include; a bag, a parcel; to guarantee,
to contract.
This character is a pictorial representation of a fetus in the
womb. It originally represented gestation, but later took on
the more general meaning of to wrap or embrace.

大包　dà bāo　Great Embracement　SP-21
陰包　yīn bāo　Yin Bladder　LV-9

běn 本 root, stem; basis, origin, source, foundation;
volume (of books).
This pictograph derives its meaning through being a representation of a tree （木）with the horizontal line at the bottom representing the ground and the vertical line extending
below it emphasizing the roots. 本 *běn* is used in Chinese
medicine to denote the root of disease as opposed to the
branches.

本神　běn shén　Root Spirit　GB-13

bí 鼻 nose.

犢鼻　dú bí　Calf's Nose　ST-35

bì (bèi) 臂 arm; upper arm.

臂臑　bì nào　Upper Arm　LI-14

bì 髀 buttocks, thigh, the lateral aspect of the groin.

髀關　bì guān　Thigh Joint　ST-31

biān 邊 side; margin, edge, rim, brim; border, frontier, boundary; limit, bound.

秩邊　zhì biān　Sequential Limit　BL-54

bīn 賓 guest, visitor; obey, submit.

築賓　zhú bīn　Guest House　KI-9

bìn 鬢 temples; hair of the temples.

曲鬢　qū bìn　Temporal Hairline Curve　GB-7

bǐng 秉 grasp, hold; control, preside over.
This character is composed of the old form of the character for hand shown grasping a sheaf of grain 禾.

秉風　bǐng fēng　Grasping the Wind　SI-12

bù 不 not, a negative particle.

不容　bù róng　Not Contained　ST-19

bù 步 step, pace; walk, go on foot; stage, phase, step; an ancient. unit of length equivalent to five chi　（尺）
This character is composed of the ideograph 止 *zhǐ,* to stop, and the same character turned upside down, which then means to go. Stopping and going describes walking or taking steps.

步廊　bù láng　Corridor Walk　KI-22

cān 參 counsel; consult; participate; intervene; consider; compare; impeach, report against; mix, admix; visit a superior; reach, penetrate to. Pronounced *cēn*: uneven. Pronounced *shēn*: the 21st constellation of the zodiac; ginseng

仆參 pū cān Subservient Visitor BL-61

cāng 倉 a granary.
The modern form of this character is said to be formed from a contraction of the food radical 食 *shí* and either a 口 *kǒu*, meaning mouth, or a 口 *wéi*, representing a storeroom. In its old form the entirety of the character more closely resembled a mouth.

地倉 dì cāng Earth Granary ST-4
胃倉 wèi cāng Stomach Granary BL-50

cáng 藏 hide, conceal; store, hoard. Pronounced *zàng:* storehouse; Tibet.
It is from this character that 臟 *zàng*, meaning viscus, solid organ, was derived through the addition of a flesh radical (肉 i.e., 月). In older texts the usage of the two characters is not clearly distinguished, and 藏 is often used where 臟 is meant.

神藏 shén cáng Spirit Storehouse KI-25

chā 差 to err, error, mistake; discrepancy, deviation, difference; unlike. Pronounced *chāi*: send, depute on official business; servant of an official. Pronounced *cī*: uneven, irregular; go wrong

曲差 qū chā Deviating Turn BL-4

cháng 長 long (of space or time); profitable; excelling. Pronounced *zhǎng*: grow, increase; excel; old, senior; show respect for age. Pronounced *zhàng*: remainder, surplus.

長強 cháng qiáng Long Strong GV-1

cháng 腸 bowels, intestines; affections, feelings.

大腸俞 dà cháng shū Large Intestine Shu BL-25
小腸俞 xiǎo cháng shū Small Intestine Shu BL-27

chē (jū) 車 cart, carriage, chariot, (any vehicle); apparatus for lifting water. Pronounced *jū*: chariot in Chinese chess, equivalent to the rook in Western chess
The vertical line in this character represents the axle running through the two wheels 二 and the cart 日 . The character is a bird's eye view of a chariot. When found as a radical in other characters it generally indicates transportation or movement.

頰車 jiá chē Jawbone ST-6

chéng 承 hold, contain, support; receive, inherit; contract for, undertake; continue; confess, acknowledge; please, flatter; meet.
In the point names this character usually means to support, to receive, or to assume responsibility.

承泣 chéng qì Tear Container ST-1
承滿 chéng mǎn Assuming Fullness ST-20
承光 chéng guāng Light Guard BL-6
承扶 chéng fú Support BL-36
承筋 chéng jīn Sinew Support BL-56
承山 chéng shān Mountain Support BL-57
承靈 chéng líng Spirit Support GB-18
承漿 chéng jiāng Sauce Receptacle CV-24

chí 池 pool, pond; moat; cistern.
Points containing the character 池 *chí* in their names are located in wide, bowl-like depressions. Note that the character is composed with the water radical.

曲池 qū chí Pool at the Bend LI-11
天池 tiān chí Celestial Pool PC-1
陽池 yáng chí Yang Pool TB-4
風池 fēng chí Wind Pool GB-20

chǐ 尺 cubit, foot, 10 cun 寸 (Chinese inches), the equivalent of 0.3581 meters, or 14.1 inches; a foot rule; the area from the cubit pulse (the most proximal of the three pulses) to LU-5, which measures one cubit.

In the Zhou Dynasty a 尺 was the equivalent of about 20 centimeters, it grew in length to about 35 centimeters sometime after that.

尺澤 chǐ zé Cubit Marsh LU-5

chì (qì , jì) 瘛 a jerking or tugging spasm, as in the term 瘛瘲 (chì zòng, clonic spasm), meaning jerking spasm alternating with relaxation.

瘛脈 chì mài Spasm Vessel TB-18

chōng 沖 surge, soar, dash against; pour out; infuse; wander, digress; weak, young; complacent, agreeable; empty.

The characters 沖 and 衝 are now essentially two forms of the same word. In earlier times the former carried mainly the meaning of to flush or to surge, while the latter meant a thoroughfare or place of key importance. In Chinese medicine these characters are used to describe the penetrating vessel (沖脈 chōng mài) and the surging of counterflow qi (沖氣 chōng qì).

氣沖 qì chōng Surging Qi ST-30
沖陽 chōng yáng Surging Yang ST-42
沖門 chōng mén Surging Gate SP-12
少沖 shào chōng Lesser Surge HT-9
太沖 tài chōng Supreme Surge LV-3

chōng 衝 rush against, clash; thoroughfare. (see 沖 ch⁻ong above.)

眉衝 méi chōng Eyebrow Ascension BL-3
中衝 zhōng chōng Central Hub PC-9
關衝 guān chōng Passage Hub TB-1
天衝 tiān chòng Celestial Hub GB-9

chù 處 place; office, department; to dwell, abide in, rest on. Pronounced *chǔ:* manage, handle; settle, judge, punish

五處 wǔ chù Fifth Place BL-5

chuāng 窗 window, shutter.

膺窗 yīng chuāng Breast Window ST-16
天窗 tiān chuāng Celestial Window SI-16
目窗 mù chuāng Eye Window GB-16

cì 次 next in order, secondary; inferior, lower; series; a time, occasion. (measure word for events); a place, halting place; to camp; reach, arrive; by, amidst

次髎 cì liáo Second Bone-Hole BL-32

dà 大 large; full-grown; great.
Originally a picture of a grown person with arms and legs extended, this character came to mean large, great or big. It is often synonymous with 太 *tài,* supreme, most, greatest.

大迎 dà yíng Great Reception ST-5
大巨 dà jù Great Gigantic ST-27
大都 dà dū Great Metropolis SP-2
大橫 dà hèng Great Horizontal SP-15
大包 dà bāo Great Embracement SP-21
大杼 dà zhù Great Shuttle BL-11
大腸俞 dà cháng shū Large Intestine Shu BL-25
大鐘 dà zhōng Large Goblet KI-4
大赫 dà hè Great Manifestation KI-12
大陵 dà líng Great Mound PC-7
大敦 dà dūn Large Pile LV-1
大椎 dà zhuī Great Hammer GV-14

dài 帶 girdle, belt, sash, tape; bear, carry; involve; lead.
帶脈 dài mài Girdling Vessel GB-26

dǎn 膽 gallbladder.
膽俞 dǎn shū Gallbladder Shu BL-19

dān 膻 center of chest.

膻中 dàn zhōng Chest Center CV-17

dào 道 road, way, path; The Way, The Tao; religion; speak, tell.
This character is formed of a 首 *shǒu,* meaning head, along with the radical that means to go. The original meaning was to go at the head, to lead. By extension it came to mean a road or way in both the physical and abstract sense.

水道 shuǐ dào Waterway ST-28
靈道 líng dào Spirit Pathway HT-4
維道 wéi dào Linking Path GB-28
神道 shén dào Spirit Path GV-11
陶道 táo dào Kiln Path GV-13

dì 地 earth, land; place, locality; territory; position, rank, situation.
In Chinese cosmology, philosophy and medicine, 地 is used in the sense of Earth as opposed to Man （人） or Heaven （天）. "Earth" as in the five phases (i.e., soil or dirt, the substance of earth) is represented in Chinese by a different character, 土 *tǔ.* When interpreting the point names, however, the Chinese often claim that 地 also can be thought of as relating to the earth phase.

地倉 dì cāng Earth Granary ST-4
地機 dì jī Earth's Crux SP-8
地五會 dì wǔ huì Earth Fivefold Convergence GB-42

dǐng 頂 the top, topmost; very; to wear on the head; to push against, to butt (with the head); opposing.

後頂 hòu dǐng Behind the Vertex GV-19
前頂 qián dǐng Before the Vertex GV-21

dǐng 鼎 a vessel supported on a tripod base, usually of bronze with two ears; a sacrificial vessel symbolizing imperial power.

天鼎　tiān dǐng　Celestial Tripod　LI-17

dòu 竇 hole, drain, sluice; sinus; corrupt practice.

食竇　shí dòu　Food Hole　SP-17

dū 督 oversee, superintend; reprove; viceroy or governor general; governing vessel; center; middle seam of the back of a coat.

The governing vessel (督脈 *dū mài*) is so called because it oversees or superintends the yang of the body.

督俞　dū shū　Governing Shu　BL-16

dū 都 city, metropolis, capital; elegant, refined. Pronounced *dōu*: all, entire.

The right portion of the character 都 is a modification of the character 邑 *yì*, which means a district or province. The left portion is a phonetic element.

大都　dà dū　Great Metropolis　SP-2
陰都　yīn dū　Yin Metropolis　KI-19
中都　zhōng dū　Central Metropolis　LV-6

dú 瀆 river; ditch, sluice, drain.

The four great rivers of China, known as 四瀆 *sì dú*, are the Yangtze 長江, Yellow River 黃河, the Huai 淮, and the Ji 濟.

四瀆　sì dú　Four Rivers　TB-9
中瀆　zhōng dú　Central River　GB-32

dú 犢 calf; sacrificial animal.

犢鼻　dú bí　Calf's Nose　ST-35

duān 端 beginning, end, extremity; clue, reason, pretext; principle, doctrine.

兌端　duì duān　Extremity of the Mouth　GV-27

duì 兌 to exchange, to weigh; the 58th trigram of the book of changes. Pronounced *yuè*: speak; gratify; rejoice.

This character is made up of a the divided breath 八 coming from the mouth 口 . The bottom part represents the two legs of a person. The character most directly means to speak. Because one can gratify others by speaking it has taken on an extended meaning of to gratify. A modern borrowing of the character resulted in its meaning of to exchange. It does not inherently mean mouth or hole, but is sometimes (especially as relates to the point names) interpreted to imply such. The following quotation from Lao Tzu illustrates the interpretation of 兑 *duì* as representing a hole or aperture: "Stop its apertures (兑), close its doors, and one's whole life is without toil. Open its apertures (兑) and be busy about its affairs, and one's whole life is beyond redemption."
(From the *Wisdom of Laotse,* translated by Lin Yutang)

厲兑　lì duì　Severe Mouth　ST-45
兑端　duì duān　Extremity of the Mouth　GV-27

dūn 敦　honest, sincere; generous; esteem; regard as important.

大敦　dà dūn　Large Pile　LV-1

ěr 耳　ear; fungus; soft, pliable; a final particle.
This is a pictograph of the external ear.

耳門　ěr mén　Ear Gate　TB-21

èr 二　two, second, twice, twofold, dual, duality.

二間　èr jiān　Second Space　LI-2

fáng 房　house, building; room, chamber; a wife or concubine.

庫房　kù fáng　Storeroom　ST-14

fēi 飛　fly; go quickly; high and lofty.

飛揚　fēi yáng　Taking Flight　BL-58

fèi 肺 lung.

肺兪   fèi shū   Lung Shu   BL-13

fēn 分 divide, share, separate, distinguish; one tenth of a Chinese inch; one tenth of a 錢 *qián* (measure of weight). Pronounced *fèn*: a share, helping, part.

附分   fù fēn   Attached Branch   BL-41
水分   shuī fēn   Water Divide   CV-9

fēng 封 a seal; a measure word for letters; boundary, dike; a mound; to heap; to appoint to an office or territory, bestow honors or nobility upon.

神封   shén fēng   Spirit Seal   KI-23
中封   zhōng fēng   Mound Center   LV-4

fēng 風 wind.
This character is much altered from its ancient form. Some modern sources claim that it is composed of the element 气 *qì* , meaning vapor, surrounding the central part, which represents insects. The meaning of the character is thus said to be derived from the idea that when pestilential winds blow, insects are born. It is used in Chinese medicine to represent wind pathogens - "the hundred diseases are born of wind." *(Essential Questions)*

秉風   bǐng fēng   Grasping the Wind   SI-12
風門   fēng mén   Wind Gate   BL-12
翳風   yì fēng   Wind Screen   TB-17
風池   fēng chí   Wind Pool   GB-20
風市   fēng shì   Wind Market   GB-31
風府   fēng fǔ   Wind Mansion   GV-16

fēng 豐 abundant, fruitful, luxuriant, bountiful.

豐隆   fēng lóng   Bountiful Bulge   ST-40

fū 跗 instep, the dorsum of the foot.

跗陽   fū yáng   Instep Yang   BL-59

fú 浮 to float, drift; light; insubstantial, fleeting, frivolous; excessive.

In Chinese medicine a floating pulse is represented by this character. 浮 furthermore describes the upward and outward movement of rootless yang, which is a form of kidney yang vacuity characterized by a floating pulse.

浮郄 fú xī Superficial Cleft BL-38
浮白 fú bái Floating White GB-10

fú 伏 prostrate; to lay low, wait in ambush; hidden, latent; to yield, suffer; humble.

伏兔 fú tù Crouching Rabbit ST-32

fú 扶 to support, hold up, prop up, help.

扶突 fú tú Protuberance Assistant LI-18
承扶 chéng fú Support BL-36

fǔ 輔 poles attached to a cart to keep it from upsetting; to help, support, guide; territory around the capital.

陽輔 yáng fǔ Yang Assistance GB-38

fǔ 府 storehouse, treasury; palace, mansion; prefecture, officer. governing a prefecture

This character was originally used to denote the bowels (hollow organs), although in this sense it is now written as 腑, being distinguished by the addition of the flesh radical 肉 （月）．

中府 zhōng fǔ Central Treasury LU-1
天府 tiān fǔ Celestial Storehouse LU-3
府舍 fǔ shè Bowel Abode SP-13
少府 shào fǔ Lesser Mansion HT-8
俞府 shū fǔ Shu Mansion KI-27
風府 fēng fǔ Wind Mansion GV-16

fù 附 near to; adhere to; dependent upon; be possessed (by a spirit); append, add to.

附分 fù fēn Attached Branch BL-41

附分　fù fēn　Attached Branch　BL-41

fù 腹 abdomen.

腹結　fù jié　Abdominal Bind　SP-14
腹哀　fù āi　Abdominal Lament　SP-16

fù 復 to return; to repeat; to reply; again, repeatedly.

復溜　fù liū　Recover Flow　KI-7

gài 蓋 to cover, hide; a lid, cover; to build, erect; now.

華蓋　huá gài　Florid Canopy　CV-20

gān 肝 liver.

肝俞　gān shū　Liver Shu　BL-18

gāng 綱 headrope of a net; outline; principle.

陽綱　yáng gāng　Yang Headrope　BL-48

gāo 膏 paste, ointment, plaster; fat, grease; rich, unctuous, sleek; 膏肓 *gāo huāng,* the region below the heart and above the diaphragm.

膏肓俞　gāo huāng shū　Gao Huang Shu　BL-43

gé 膈 diaphragm; any separating membrane.
膈 incorporates the flesh radical 肉（月）and is akin in meaning to 隔 *gé,* which means to separate, divide or partition.　The two characters are sometimes used interchangeably in older texts.

膈俞　gé shū　Diaphragm Shu　BL-17
膈關　gé guān　Diaphragm Pass　BL-46

gēn 根 root.
The radical is 木 *mù,* wood, while 艮 *gēn* is here a phonetic element.　In acupuncture this character is used to denote the roots of the channels as opposed to the bindings. The roots are at the ends of the four extremities and the

bindings are at the head, face, chest, and abdomen.

乳根　rŭ gēn　Breast Root　ST-18

gōng 宮 palace; temple.

聽宮　tīng gōng　Auditory Palace　SI-19
勞宮　láo gōng　Palace of Toil　PC-8
紫宮　zĭ gōng　Purple Palace　CV-19

gōng 公 public; just, fair, equal; duke; sir, gentleman; husband's father; male.

公孫　gōng sūn　Yellow Emperor　SP-4

gōu 溝 water-course, drain, ditch, aqueduct.

支溝　zhī gōu　Branch Ditch　TB-6
蠡溝　lĭ gōu　Woodworm Canal　LV-5
水溝　shuĭ gōu　Water Trough　GV-26

gŭ 骨 bone.
This character is a radical for words relating to the skeletal structure. The upper part is a stylized rendition of a pictograph of a skull and the shoulder bones, while the bottom part is the flesh radical 肉 （月） .

巨骨　jù gŭ　Great Bone　LI-16
腕骨　wàn gŭ　Wrist Bone　SI-4
京骨　jīng gŭ　Capital Bone　BL-64
束骨　shù gŭ　Bundle Bone　BL-65
橫骨　héng gŭ　Pubic Bone　KI-11
完骨　wán gŭ　Completion Bone　GB-12
絶骨　jué gŭ　Severed Bone　GB-39
曲骨　qū gŭ　Curved Bone　CV-2

gŭ 谷 valley, ravine.
谷 is often used as a substitute for 穀 gŭ, meaning grain. It is also employed as a radical, as in 谿, meaning ravine. According to *Essential Questions,* a "large meeting of the flesh" is called a valley (谷 gŭ) and a "small meeting of the flesh" is called a ravine (谿 xī). Most points contain-

ing 谷 are located in large, fleshy depressions, often, a juncture of two or more sinews and/or bones.

合谷 hé gǔ Union Valley LI-4
陷谷 xiàn gǔ Sunken Valley ST-43
漏谷 lòu gǔ Leaking Valley SP-7
前谷 qián gǔ Front Valley SI-2
陽谷 yáng gǔ Yang Valley SI-5
通谷 tōng gǔ Valley Passage BL-66
然谷 rán gǔ Blazing Valley KI-2
陰谷 yīn gǔ Yin Valley KI-10
通谷 tóng gǔ Open Valley KI-20
率谷 shuài gǔ Valley Lead GB-8

guān 關 frontier pass or gate; a customs house; to shut, close; to connect, implicate, involve; crisis, juncture. Pronounced *wān*: to bend (a bow).

The character 關 *guān* can usually be considered to mean joint when it is part of a point name that is located at a joint. Otherwise it may mean pass, passageway, a gate or to connect. In addition, 關 is in some respects similar to its radical 門 *mén,* meaning gate, in that they can both be poetic representations of acupuncture points, i.e., places where qi enters and exits.

下關 xià guān Below the Joint ST-7
關門 guān mén Pass Gate ST-22
髀關 bì guān Thigh Joint ST-31
關元俞 guān yuán shū Origin Pass Shu BL-26
膈關 gé guān Diaphragm Pass BL-46
石關 shí guān Stone Pass KI-18
內關 nèi guān Inner Pass PC-6
關衝 guān chōng Passage Hub TB-1
外關 wài guān Outer Pass TB-5
上關 shàng guān Upper Gate GB-3
膝陽關 xī yáng guān Knee Yang Joint GB-33
膝關 xī guān Knee Joint LV-7
關元 guān yuán Origin Pass CV-4
腰陽關 yāo yáng guān Lumbar Yang Pass GV-3

guāng 胱 urinary bladder.
This character is generally found as a part of the term 膀胱 *páng guāng,* which means urinary bladder.

膀胱俞 páng guāng shū Bladder Shu BL-28

guāng 光 light, brightness, to illuminate; glossy; favor; smooth, naked, bare; alone.
In ancient times this character was composed of the character for twenty on the top （廿） and that for fire （火） on the bottom. Thus it stood for the brightness of twenty fires.

承光 chéng guāng Light Guard BL-6
光明 guāng míng Bright Light GB-37

guī 歸 marriage of a woman; return, revert, restore to; send back to; belong to.

歸來 guī lái Return ST-29

hǎi 海 sea, ocean, maritime.
The left part of this character is the water radical and the right part is phonetic. The phonetic may be said to carry some meaning if its lower part 母 *mǔ* is considered. That character means mother and is a picture (much clearer in the old script) of a woman （女） with the breasts emphasized. The mother figure is a fitting metaphor for the sea because it nourishes and engenders life. This accords well with the use of the word sea in Chinese medicine.

血海 xuè hǎi Sea of Blood SP-10
少海 shào hǎi Lesser Sea HT-3
小海 xiǎo hǎi Small Sea SI-8
氣海俞 qì hǎi shū Sea-of-Qi Shu BL-24
照海 zhào hǎi Shining Sea KI-6
氣海 qì hǎi Sea of Qi CV-6

hàn 頷 chin; jaws; to nod.

頷厭 hàn yàn Forehead Fullness GB-4

hé 和 harmony, peace; harmonize, reconcile; kindly; mild. Pronounced *huò*: mix, blend. Pronounced *hè* or *hán*: with, together.

The character 和 *hé* was originally written as 龢 and was a representation of musical pipes. Its current meanings of harmony, etc., have been derived through extension of this fact.

和髎 hé liáo Harmony Bone-Hole TB-22

hé 禾 corn, rice; growing grain; crops.

禾髎 hé liáo Grain Bone-Hole LI-19

hé 合 to shut, close, enclose; to join, gather together, unite; pair; to tally, agree, accord.

This character is formed of a triangle positioned above a mouth (口 *kǒu*). The triangle represents the union of many elements, as the three sides unite to form the triangle. The mouth below the triangle lends the character the additional meaning of whole or combined, because the mouth, as the element united, represents many voices speaking together in harmony. Its meanings of union, to join, accord, etc., are all derived from this idea.

合谷 hé gǔ Union Valley LI-4
合陽 hé yáng Yang Union BL-55

hè 赫 bright, luminous, glorious; awe-inspiring; red.

大赫 dà hè Great Manifestation KI-12

héng 横 crosswise, horizontal; east to west; at right angles to; sideways.

大横 dà hèng Great Horizontal SP-15
横骨 héng gǔ Pubic Bone KI-11

hòu 後 behind, after (in space and time); the back of; descendants, posterity.

後溪 hòu xī Back Ravine SI-3

後項　hòu dǐng　Behind the Vertex　GV-19

hù 戶 door; household; family; individual.
This character is the representation of a one-leafed door (c.f. 門 *mén,* a two-leafed door).

氣戶　qì hù　Qi Door　ST-13
魄戶　pò hù　Po Door　BL-42
腦戶　nǎo hù　Brain's Door　GV-17

huá 滑 to slip, slide; slippery, glossy, smooth; cunning, subtle.
This character is made up of the water radical on the left and a bone (骨) on the right. The meanings slippery and glossy are thus derived from the idea of a wet bone. This character is used to describe both the slippery pulse and glossy tongue that are associated with the damp pathogen in Chinese medicine.

滑肉門　huá ròu mén　Slippery Flesh Gate　ST-24

huá 華 flower, blossom; flowery, variegated; glory, splendor.

華蓋　huá gài　Florid Canopy　CV-20

huán 環 bracelet; ring, circle; to encircle.

白環俞　bái huàn shū　White Ring Shu　BL-30
環跳　huán tiào　Jumping Round　GB-30

huāng 肓 the region between the heart and diaphragm, the vitals.

膏肓俞　gāo huāng shū　Gao Huang Shu　BL-43
肓門　huāng mén　Huang Gate　BL-51
胞肓　bāo huāng　Bladder Huang　BL-53
肓俞　huāng shū　Huang Shu　KI-16

huì 會 meet, assemble, converge; understand; know how to. Pronounced *huǐ*: a short while. Pronounced *kuài*: calculate.

The triangular portion at the top of this character means to meet (see 合 *hé* above) and the bottom, 曰 *yuè*, means to speak. The central part of the character represents a door. The character thus derives its meaning of to meet from the concept of people gathering at a door to converse.

會陽　huì yáng　Meeting of Yang　BL-35
會宗　huì zōng　Convergence and Gathering　TB-7
臑會　nào huì　Upper Arm Convergence　TB-13
聽會　tīng huì　Auditory Convergence　GB-2
地五會　dì wǔ huì　Earth Fivefold Convergence　GB-42
會陰　huì yīn　Meeting of Yin　CV-1
百會　bǎi huì　Hundred Convergences　GV-20
囟會　xìn huì　Fontanel Meeting　GV-22

hún 魂 hun, soul.

The *hún* is the part of the spirit that rises to heaven after death, though in general usage the word often refers to the spiritual faculties. In *Spiritual Axis* it is said that *hún* follows the movement of the spirit （隨神往來者） and is stored in the liver. The *hún* is yang in nature whereas its counterpart, the 魄 *pò,* is yin. The characters for *hún* and *pò* both incorporate the character 鬼 *guǐ* on the right side. This character means ghost or devil. The top part represents the head of a person while the bottom part represents the body of a ghost. The angular figure in the lower right corner represents the movement of the ghost as it comes and goes. (See also 魄 *pò.*)

魂門　hún mén　Hun Gate　BL-47

jī 璣 a pearl (that is not quite globular); the pivotal gear of an astronomical instrument.

璇璣　xuán jī　Jade Pivot　CV-21

jī 箕 winnowing basket; dustpan.

箕門　jī mén　Winnower Gate　SP-11

jī 機 machine, loom, trigger; changes and motions; moving power; origin; opportunity; secret, occult; cunning.

地機 dì jī Earth's Crux SP-8

jí 極 ridgepole; utmost point, pole; extremely.

極泉 jí quán Highest Spring HT-1
中極 zhōng jí Central Pole CV-3

jí 急 anxious; hurried, hasty; urgent, rapid; emergency; acute.

急脈 jí mài Urgent Pulse LV-12

jǐ 脊 spine, ridge.

脊中 jǐ zhōng Spinal Center GV-6

jì 際 border, boundary, limit; between; time or occasion; while, at a time when.

魚際 yú jì Fish Border LU-10

jiá 頰 jaw; cheek.

頰車 jiá chē Jawbone ST-6

jiān 肩 shoulder; sustain; competent to.
This character originally consisted of a curved line, representing the arm, extending out of the flesh （肉）. Over time the line changed into a 尸 and the 肉 became 月.

肩髃 jiān yú Shoulder Bone LI-15
肩眞 jiān zhēn True Shoulder SI-9
肩外俞 jiān wài shū Outer Shoulder Shu SI-14
肩中俞 jiān zhōng shū Central Shoulder Shu SI-15
肩髎 jiān liáo Shoulder Bone-Hole TB-14
肩井 jiān jǐng Shoulder Well GB-21

jiān 間 space; between, among; to divide, separate, part.
The character 間 is made of 門 *mén* and 日 *rì*. 門 is a picture of a traditional Chinese two-winged door and 日 is

a squared drawing of the sun. The character's meanings of space and between are thus derived from the idea of sunlight streaming in through the space between the two leaves of a door.

二間　èr jiān　Second Space　LI-2
三間　sān jiān　Third Space　LI-3
間使　jiān shǐ　Intermediary Courier　PC-5
行間　xíng jiān　Moving Between　LV-2
強間　qiáng jiān　Unyielding Space　GV-18

jiàn 建　to erect, establish, found. C.f. 健 : strong, strengthen; constant, regular.

建里　jiàn lǐ　Interior Strengthening　CV-11

jiāng 漿　thick fluid, paste.

承漿　chéng jiāng　Sauce Receptacle　CV-24

jiāo 交　to commit to, hand to, deliver, pay; to exchange, barter; to communicate, intersect; intertwine, intercourse.

三陰交　sān yīn jiāo　Three Yin Intersection　SP-6
交信　jiāo xìn　Intersection Reach　KI-8
陽交　yáng jiāo　Yang Intersection　GB-35
陰交　yīn jiāo　Yin Intersection　CV-7
齦交　yín jiāo　Gum Intersection　GV-28

jiāo 焦　burn, scorch; vexed, anxious.
In Chinese medicine this character means 1) the burnt smell that is associated with the heart *(Classic of Difficult Issues)*; 2) emaciated, as is seen in the facial complexion of an old man *(Essential Questions)*; 3) burner, as in triple burner; 4) scorch (the effect of heat on the organs); 5) parched, as of the tongue.

三焦俞　sān jiāo shū　Triple Burner Shu　BL-22

jiǎo 角　horn (of an animal); corner, angle.

角孫　jiǎo sūn　Angle Vertex　TB-20

jié 結 knot, tie, bind; cohesion, coagulation, to congeal; to contract, give bond for; bear fruit, finish.

腹結 fù jié Abdominal Bind SP-14

jiě 解 to release, untie, divide, separate, to explain.

解溪 jiě xī Ravine Divide ST-41

jīn 金 metal; gold.
The top portion of this character is a modified form of the character 今 jīn and is in this case a phonetic element. The lower portion is a pictograph of two nuggets of gold lying beneath the earth （土）. The character may refer specifically to gold, generally to metal, or to the metal phase of the five phases.

金門 jīn mén Metal Gate BL-63

jīn 筋 sinew, tendon, ligament; veins (visible through the skin).
This character is made up of 竹 zhú, bamboo, 肉 ròu （月 rù), flesh or muscles, and 力 lì, strength. It thus indicates fibrous (i.e., bamboo-like) flesh that imparts strength. The word sinews is used to express this concept in English because it is as ambiguous as the Chinese word, and may apply equally to tendons, ligaments, and muscle.

承筋 chéng jīn Sinew Support BL-56
輒筋 zhé jīn Sinew Seat GB-23
筋縮 jīn suō Sinew Contraction GV-8

jīng 京 capital, metropolis; great, exalted; elevated.
This character is a contraction of the character 高 gao, meaning high. The bottom was changed to 小 xiǎo, which means small, but the meaning of high or elevated remained. All modern meanings of the character are derived through extension.

京骨 jīng gǔ Capital Bone BL-64
京門 jīng mén Capital Gate GB-25

jīng 睛 eye, pupil.

睛明 jīng míng Bright Eyes BL-1

jīng 經 channel, to pass through, the warp of a fabric.

The character 經 *jīng* is especially important in acupuncture as it is the character used to refer to the channels. It carries a plethora of meanings, reflected in the components of the character. The left portion of 經 is the thread radical 糸 *mì*, which is found as a part of many characters that denote string-like objects. The right portion of the character is 巠 *jīng*, which is here employed as both a phonetic and meaning element. 巠 is the character used by geomancers to denote the flow of water underground. The top line of 巠 represents the ground, while the three curved lines beneath it represent the flow of water. The 工 on the bottom of the character is a corruption of the original phonetic element 壬 *tíng*, which also adds meaning to the character as a representation of a man with his ear to the ground (i.e., listening for water). Understood through its construction the character 經 can thus be said to represent the flow of a subterranean river, and is used in this sense within the field of acupuncture to represent both the channels and the river-jing points, where qi flows like water in a river.

The actual dictionary definitions of this character are slightly different, having been derived through extension. The original meaning assigned to it is the warp of a fabric and, by extension, any type of line that runs lengthwise, such as meridians and lines of longitude (and, again, the channels). By extension of this idea it also means an invariable rule, a standard or a constant, as in the terms 月經 *yuè jīng,* the menses, and 經書 *jīng shū,* a classic text or canon. Used as a verb, it means to pass. All these notions reflect the combined meanings of 糸 and 巠.

經渠 jīng qú Channel Ditch LU-8

jǐng 井 a water well.

The pictograph 井 *jǐng* comes to mean a well through it being a representation of the ancient arrangement of agricultural fields, in which eight families each tended one plot of land adjoining a common field, located in the center of the eight plots. This central plot contained a well that was shared by all eight adjoining households. The character 井 was originally written as 丼 , the dot in the center representing the well and the surrounding divisions representing the familial fields. It is used in acupuncture to refer to the well-jing points.

天井　tiān jǐng　Celestial Well　TB-10
肩井　jiān jǐng　Shoulder Well　GB-21

jiū 鳩 turtle dove; pigeon; collect assemble.

鳩尾　jiū wěi　Turtledove Tail　CV-15

jū 居 dwell, remain; be in (a state or circumstance); sit; bent on, determined; unkindly.

居髎　jū liáo　Squatting Bone-Hole　GB-29

jù 巨 a carpenter's square (now written 矩 *jǔ*); chief, great, very; numerous.
This character is a pictorial representation of a carpenter's square. It is a tool that is larger (i.e., greater) than the 工 *gōng,* which is also a carpenter's square. The principle meaning of the character, great, is derived from this fact.

巨骨　jù gǔ　Great Bone　LI-16
巨髎　jù liáo　Great Bone-Hole　ST-3
大巨　dà jù　Great Gigantic　ST-27
上巨虛　shàng jù xū　Upper Great Hollow　ST-37
下巨虛　xià jù xū　Lower Great Hollow　ST-39
巨闕　jù què　Great Tower Gate　CV-14

jué 厥 he, she or it; bend, flex; go the wrong way.
Within the field of Chinese medicine this character has three meanings: 1) counterflow qi rising from the abdomen to the chest and throat, 2) fainting (sudden collapse), 3) inversion counterflow of qi from the extremities, leaving the hands and feet cold. In addition, the character is a part of the name of the jue yin channels (pericardium and liver).

厥陰俞　jué yīn shū　Jue Yin Shu　BL-14

kōng 空 empty; nothingness; insincere; impoverished.
Note that the top of the character is the radical for hole,
the character used to represent acupuncture points, *xuè,* 穴 .
The bottom, 工 *gōng,* is phonetic.

絲竹空　sī zhú kōng　Silk Bamboo Hole　TB-23
腦空　nǎo kōng　Brain Hollow　GB-19

kǒng 孔 opening, hold; touch-hole; hole of a wind-
instrument; penetrate; great, very; peacock; Confucius
(whose surname was Kong, and whose English name is the
Latin transcription of 孔夫子 *kǒng fū zǐ,* Master Kong).

孔最　kǒng zuì　Collection Hole　LU-6

kǒu 口 mouth, opening; speech.

條口　tiáo kǒu　Ribbon Opening　ST-38

kù 庫 treasury, storehouse; granary; armory.

庫房　kù fáng　Storeroom　ST-14

kūn 昆 elder brother; posterity; afterward; together, a multitude; interchangeable with 崑 , as in 崑崙 the Kunlun
(Koulkun) mountains of Tibet.

昆侖　kūn lún　Kunlun Mountains　BL-60

lái 來 come.

歸來　guī lái　Return　ST-29

láng 廊 veranda, porch, corridor.

步廊　bù láng　Corridor Walk　KI-22

láo 勞 to labor, toil, strain, tax; weary; to give trouble to.
The strength radical （力） gives this character its meaning.
In Chinese medicine it is the five taxations （五勞 *wǔ láo*),
diseases of overstrain.

勞宮 láo gōng Palace of Toil PC-8

lǎo 老 old, venerable (term of honor and respect).

養老 yǎng lǎo Nursing the Aged SI-6

lěng 冷 cold, frigid.
This character is differentiated from 寒 *hán,* the character for cold in classical Chinese. Where 寒 describes the cold of the eight parameters and the cold pathogen, 冷 is primarily used to describe the sensation of cold, as in counterflow frigidity of the limbs. 冷 is the manifestation of 寒.

清冷淵 qīng lěng yuān Clear Cold Abyss TB-11

lí 厘（釐） the thousandth part of a 兩 liang (Chinese ounce); the thousandth part of a 尺 chi (Chinese foot).

懸厘 xuán lí Suspended Tuft GB-6

lí 蠡 a wood-boring insect; worm-eaten. Pronounced *lí :* calabash.

蠡溝 lǐ gōu Woodworm Canal LV-5

lǐ 里 a Chinese measure of distance equal to about 1/3 of a mile; a small hamlet.
This character is composed of radicals for field (田 *tián*) and earth (土 *tǔ*). It originally represented the agricultural fields that were set up in the fashion of a tic-tac-toe board, eight families farming the eight fields surrounding a common field and well (see 井 *jǐng* above). The character later became a representation of a unit of length equal to the side of one of these fields, and further took on the meaning of a small village or a ward of a city (originally the eight families sharing the common well).
In classical Chinese medical texts the character 里 was often used to represent the meanings of the presumably relatively newer characters 理 *lǐ*, to rectify or regulate, and 裡 *lǐ*, inner or inside. As regards the acupuncture point names, different renderings of the character 里 such as Chinese

mile, ward or interior could be considered appropriate depending on the point in question. In each case in this text the transliteration "li" has been employed so that the connections between the various point names that include this character are more obvious.

手三里　shǒu sān lǐ　Arm Three Li　LI-10
手五里　shǒu wǔ lǐ　Arm Five Li　LI-13
足三里　zú sān lǐ　Leg Three Li　ST-36
通里　tōng lǐ　Connecting Li　HT-5
足五里　zú wǔ lǐ　Foot Five Li　LV-10
建里　jiàn lǐ　Interior Strengthening　CV-11

lì 厲　whetstone, to grind; harsh, severe, stern; to discipline; to oppress; to cross water wearing clothes.

厲兌　lì duì　Severe Mouth　ST-45

lì 歷　calculate; the calendar; pass through; in order, successive.

偏歷　piān lì　Veering Passageway　LI-6

lián 廉　pure, modest, incorrupt; not avaricious; inexpensive; angle, corner, ridge; investigate, examine.

下廉　xià lián　Lower Ridge　LI-8
上廉　shàng lián　Upper Ridge　LI-9
陰廉　yīn lián　Yin Corner　LV-11
廉泉　lián quán　Ridge Spring　CV-23

liáng 梁　bridge over a brook; beam, joist; ridge.

梁門　liáng mén　Beam Gate　ST-21
梁丘　liáng qiū　Beam Hill　ST-34

liáo 髎　bone-hole.
This character is constructed of bone radical on the left
（骨）and a phonetic element on the right. It is used to describe crevices and holes in or between bones. The character 窌 is sometimes used as a substitute for 髎. The meaning is the same.

肘髎　zhǒu liáo　Elbow Bone-Hole　LI-12
禾髎　hé liáo　Grain Bone-Hole　LI-19
巨髎　jù liáo　Great Bone-Hole　ST-3
顴髎　quán liáo　Cheek Bone-Hole　SI-18
上髎　shàng liáo　Upper Bone-Hole　BL-31
次髎　cì liáo　Second Bone-Hole　BL-32
中髎　zhōng liáo　Central Bone-Hole　BL-33
下髎　xià liáo　Lower Bone-Hole　BL-34
肩髎　jiān liáo　Shoulder Bone-Hole　TB-14
天髎　tiān liáo　Celestial Bone-Hole　TB-15
和髎　hé liáo　Harmony Bone-Hole　TB-22
瞳子髎　tóng zǐ liáo　Pupil Bone-Hole　GB-1
居髎　jū liáo　Squatting Bone-Hole　GB-29
素髎　sù liáo　White Bone-Hole　GV-25

liè 列 arrange, order, enumerate, classify; a file or rank.

列缺　liè quē　Broken Sequence　LU-7

lín 臨 descend; overlook, come to; near to, on the point of.

頭臨泣　tóu lín qì　Head Overlooking Tears　GB-15
足臨泣　zú lín qì　Foot Overlooking Tears　GB-41

líng 陵 mound, tumulus (burial mound), barrow.

外陵　wài líng　Outer Mound　ST-26
陰陵泉　yīn líng quán　Yin Mound Spring　SP-9
大陵　dà líng　Great Mound　PC-7
陽陵泉　yáng líng quán　Yang Mound Spring　GB-34

líng 靈 spirit, ingenious, efficacious.
This character has the rain radical 雨 *yǔ* on top. The three squares in the center originally stood for rain drops, while the bottom of the character represented sorcerers dancing for rain. Since it was the spirits that were being supplicated for rain, the character eventually took on the meaning of spirit. In Chinese medicine 靈 *líng* carries much the same meanings as 神 *shén,* but, as indicated by its relationship to water (rain), 靈 *líng* is relatively yin in nature.

青靈 qīng líng Cyan Spirit HT-2
靈道 líng dào Spirit Pathway HT-4
靈墟 líng xū Spirit Ruins KI-24
承靈 chéng líng Spirit Support GB-18
靈台 líng tái Spirit Tower GV-10

liū 溜 to slip, slide, skate; to slink, sneak; to stroll; smooth, glossy; current, stream.
In classical Chinese this character was often used to express ideas now more associated with the characters 留 , to remain or dwell, and 流 , to flow, both pronounced *liú* .

溫溜 wēn liù Warm Dwelling LI-7
復溜 fù liū Recover Flow KI-7

lóng 隆 eminent, surpassing; abundant, prosperous; to exalt, magnify.

豐隆 fēng lóng Bountiful Bulge ST-40

lòu 漏 leak, drip; disclose; a funnel, colander, sieve; leave out, omit.

漏谷 lòu gǔ Leaking Valley SP-7

lú 顱 skull; forehead.

顱息 lú xí Skull Rest TB-19
懸顱 xuán lú Suspended Skull GB-5

lǚ 膂 backbone; muscles of the back; strength.

中膂俞 zhōng lǚ shū Central Backbone Shu BL-29

lún 侖 to arrange; to think; same as 崙 *lún,* as in 崑崙 , the Kunlun (Koulkun) Mountains of Tibet.

昆侖 kūn lún Kunlun Mountains BL-60

luò 濼 a river in Shandong; a riverbed.
In Chinese medicine this character is pronounced *luò* or *pò* and denotes a disease characterized by pain and/or weakness (especially in the lower leg).

消濼 xiāo luò Dispersing Riverbed TB-12

luò 絡 unreeled silk, hemp, cotton fiber; a cord; to spin silk; mesh, connect, continuous; connecting vessels; the stringy pith of citrus fruits, the fibrous mesh of the loofah. This character is composed of the silk radical （糸） on the left and a phonetic element on the right. Its various associations of stringy fibers led to its extended meaning of to enmesh and to connect. In Chinese medicine this character is used as a both verb and a noun. As a noun it refers primarily to the various connecting vessels （絡脈 *luò mài*), while as a verb it means to enmesh, as the connecting vessels enmesh the whole body, or to connect, as the primary channels all home to their related organ and connect to the organ of their yin-yang related pair.

絡卻 luò què Declining Connection BL-8
三陽絡 sān yáng luò Three Yang Connection TB-8

mài (mò) 脈 vessel, vein; pulse.

申脈 shēn mài Extending Vessel BL-62
瘈脈 chì mài Spasm Vessel TB-18
帶脈 dài mài Girdling Vessel GB-26
急脈 jí mài Urgent Pulse LV-12

mǎn 滿 full, to fill; satisfied, self-sufficient; the whole, complete.

承滿 chéng mǎn Assuming Fullness ST-20
四滿 sì mǎn Fourfold Fullness KI-14

méi 眉 eyebrow.

眉衝 méi chōng Eyebrow Ascension BL-3

mén 門 gate, door, opening.
This character is a picture of a two-leafed door or gate. In the point names it is usually a poetic way of indicating a place where qi enters and exits; i.e., an acupuncture point.

雲門 yún mén Cloud Gate LU-2

梁門　liáng mén　Beam Gate　ST-21
關門　guān mén　Pass Gate　ST-22
滑肉門　huá ròu mén　Slippery Flesh Gate　ST-24
箕門　jī mén　Winnower Gate　SP-11
沖門　chōng mén　Surging Gate　SP-12
神門　shén mén　Spirit Gate　HT-7
風門　fēng mén　Wind Gate　BL-12
殷門　yīn mén　Gate of Abundance　BL-37
魂門　hún mén　Hun Gate　BL-47
肓門　huāng mén　Huang Gate　BL-51
金門　jīn mén　Metal Gate　BL-63
幽門　yōu mén　Dark Gate　KI-21
郄門　xī mén　Cleft Gate　PC-4
液門　yè mén　Humor Gate　TB-2
耳門　ěr mén　Ear Gate　TB-21
京門　jīng mén　Capital Gate　GB-25
章門　zhāng mén　Camphorwood Gate　LV-13
期門　qí mén　Cycle Gate　LV-14
石門　shí mén　Stone Gate　CV-5
命門　mìng mén　Life Gate　GV-4
瘂門　yǎ mén　Mute's Gate　GV-15

míng 明 bright, clear; intelligent; to understand; the name of a Chinese imperial dynasty.
This character is made up of the sun radical, 日 *rì*, and the moon radical, 月 *yuè*. Its various shades of meaning are derived from this fact. It is the character used in referring to the yang ming channels (large intestine and stomach).

睛明　jīng míng　Bright Eyes　BL-1
光明　guāng míng　Bright Light　GB-37

mìng 命 command, decree; fate, destiny; life; to name.

命門　mìng mén　Life Gate　GV-4

mù 目 eye.
This character is a picture of the eye.

目窗　mù chuāng　Eye Window　GB-16

nǎo 腦 brain.

腦空　nǎo kōng　Brain Hollow　GB-19
腦戶　nǎo hù　Brain's Door　GV-17

nào 臑 upper arm.

臂臑　bì nào　Upper Arm　LI-14
臑俞　nào shū　Upper Arm Shu　SI-10
臑會　nào huì　Upper Arm Convergence　TB-13

nèi 内 inside, inward; specifically inner body.
This character represents entering into (入 rù, to enter) a bordered region (represented by the open-ended square). It is largely synonymous with 裡 lǐ, which means interior in the sense of the eight parameters.

内庭　nèi tíng　Inner Court　ST-44
内關　nèi guān　Inner Pass　PC-6

páng 膀 urinary bladder.
膀胱 páng guāng is usually found in this combination, meaning urinary bladder.

膀胱俞　páng guāng shū　Bladder Shu　BL-28

pén 盆 basin, tub, pot, bowl.
The radical 皿 min, a dish, gives this character its meaning. 分 fēn is phonetic.

缺盆　quē pén　Empty Basin　ST-12

pí 脾 spleen.

脾俞　pí shū　Spleen Shu　BL-20

piān 偏 to one side, off center; slant, lean, veer; partial, prejudiced.

偏歷　piān lì　Veering Passageway　LI-6

pò 魄 po, soul.

In general usage, 魄 *pò* is the part of the human spirit that remains after death. It is yin in nature and thus does not rise to heaven but either becomes a ghost or returns to the earth. In Chinese medicine the *pò* is said to be stored in the lung. It is intimately connected to essence (yin), whereas its counterpart, 魂 *hún*, is related to spirit (yang). (See also 魂 *hún*)

魄戶 pò hù Po Door BL-42

pú 僕 servant, slave.

僕參 pú cān Subservient Visitor BL-61

qí 期 period, date, deadline; a fixed date; a month; expect; one hundred years. Pronounced *jī*: a full year.

期門 qí mén Cycle Gate LV-14

qì 氣 qi (ch'i); gas, smell; breath; weather; manner, air; the active aspect of matter in the body.

This character is composed of the vapor radical (气) enclosing the radical for rice or grain (米). It is said to be a picture of fumes wafting up from a batch of fermenting rice. Qi is therefore a smell or gas, and, by extension, something that moves yet cannot be seen and is detected only by the effects it has on other things. It is used to describe things that in English we would loosely call forces or influences, e.g, 天氣 *tiān qì*, celestial forces or influences (the weather); 力氣 *lì qì*, strength or force; 氣勢 *qì shì*, momentum. In medicine it denotes forces within the body, e.g., 元氣 *yuán qì*, original qi, 精氣 *jīng qì*, essential qi, and 正氣 *zhèng qì*, correct qi, as well as influences outside of it such as 濕氣 *shī qì*, damp qi and 癘氣 *lì qì*, pestilential qi.

氣舍 qì shè Qi Abode ST-11
氣戶 qì hù Qi Door ST-13
氣沖 qì chōng Surging Qi ST-30
氣海俞 qì hǎi shū Sea-of-Qi Shu BL-24

氣穴　qì xuè　Qi Point　KI-13
氣海　qì hǎi　Sea of Qi　CV-6

qì 泣 weep (silent tears).

承泣　chéng qì　Tear Container　ST-1
頭臨泣　tóu lín qì　Head Overlooking Tears　GB-15
足臨泣　zú lín qì　Foot Overlooking Tears　GB-41

qián 前 before, formerly; in front of.

前谷　qián gǔ　Front Valley　SI-2
前頂　qián dǐng　Before the Vertex　GV-21

qiáng 強 strong, strengthen; stiff, rigid; better, superior. Pronounced *qiǎng*: to force, compel, insist

This character was originally written as 彊. The radical is 弓 *gōng,* meaning an archer's bow, while the right hand portion of the character serves as a phonetic element. This phonetic contributes some meaning to the character because it consists of two fields （田） and their boundaries. The character's meaning of strength comes from the concept of a bow strong enough to shoot an arrow over two fields. The right hand part of the character changed to its present form because the old character was too tiresome to write.

長強　cháng qiáng　Long Strong　GV-1
強間　qiáng jiān　Unyielding Space　GV-18

qiào 竅 hole, cavity.

Note the hole radical, 穴 *xuè,* which is used to represent acupuncture points, at the top of this character. 竅 is the character used in Chinese medicine to represent the portals of the five viscera (i.e., the tongue is the portal of the heart, the nose is the portal of the lung, etc.).

頭竅陰　tóu qiào yīn　Head Portal Yin　GB-11
足竅陰　zú qiào yīn　Foot Portal Yin　GB-44

qīng 清 clear, pure; fresh, cool.

This character is used in medicine to denote the concept of clearing, as in clearing heat. The water radical gives the character meaning, while the right portion is phonetic.

清冷淵　qīng lěng yuān　Clear Cold Abyss　TB-11

qīng 青 green, blue, black, cyan.

青靈　qīng líng　Cyan Spirit　HT-2

qiū 丘 hill, hillock.
This character appears in a number of point names as it is a convenient guide to locations on the landscape of the body.

梁丘　liáng qiū　Beam Hill　ST-34
商丘　shāng qiū　Shang Hill　SP-5
外丘　wài qiū　Outer Hill　GB-36
丘墟　qiū xū　Hill Ruins　GB-40

qū 曲 bent, crooked, winding; wrong, false; obscure, little known. Pronounced *qǔ*: song, plays; minutiae, trifles
This character occurs in several point names as it is a convenient description of the numerous bends, crooks, turns and curves encountered when traversing the landscape of the body.

曲池　qū chí　Pool at the Bend　LI-11
曲垣　qū yuán　Crooked Wall　SI-13
曲差　qū chā　Deviating Turn　BL-4
商曲　shāng qū　Shang Bend　KI-17
曲澤　qū zé　Marsh at the Bend　PC-3
曲鬢　qū bìn　Temporal Hairline Curve　GB-7
曲泉　qū quán　Spring at the Bend　LV-8
曲骨　qū gǔ　Curved Bone　CV-2

qú 渠 drain, gutter; circular rim of a wheel; great, ample.

經渠　jīng qú　Channel Ditch　LU-8

quán 顴 cheek-bone, the area of the cheek around the cheek bone.

顴髎　quán liáo　Cheek Bone-Hole　SI-18

quán 泉 spring, fountain.
The ancient form of this character was clearly a picture of water flowing out from the ground. The modern character consists of a 白 *bái,* white, above a 水 *shuǐ,* water. One can imagine the character as picturing the pure (white) water of a mountain spring. Though not consistent with the true etymology of the character, this explanation of the modern adaptation is of useful mnemonic value. The use of this character in the point names can be attributed to its poetic value in describing origins (i.e., springs), and the flowing nature of qi at acupuncture points.

陰陵泉　yīn líng quán　Yin Mound Spring　SP-9
極泉　jí quán　Highest Spring　HT-1
涌泉　yǒng quǎn　Gushing Spring　KI-1
水泉　shuǐ quán　Water Spring　KI-5
天泉　tiān quán　Celestial Spring　PC-2
陽陵泉　yáng líng quán　Yang Mound Spring　GB-34
曲泉　qū quán　Spring at the Bend　LV-8
廉泉　lián quán　Ridge Spring　CV-23

quē 缺 broken, defective; a deficiency, vacancy; an official post.

列缺　liè quē　Broken Sequence　LU-7
缺盆　quē pén　Empty Basin　ST-12

què 闕 the look-out tower above a gate; an imperial city, palace; deficiency; to omit.

神闕　shén què　Spirit Gate　CV-8
巨闕　jù què　Great Tower Gate　CV-14

què 卻 but, yet still; reject, decline, withdraw.

絡卻　luò què　Declining Connection　BL-8

rán 然 burn, blaze; yes, certainly, really; still, nevertheless, but; although; on the other hand.

然谷　rán gǔ　Blazing Valley　KI-2

rén 人 human being, humankind; person, man.
This is a pictograph of a person, with emphasis on the legs.

人迎　rén yíng　Man's Prognosis　ST-9
人中　rén zhōng　Human Center　GV-26

rì 日 sun; day, daily.
This is a picture of the sun. It was originally a circle with a dot in the center, but was squared for ease in writing and the line extended for clarity.

日月　rì yuè　Sun and Moon　GB-24

róng 榮 glory, splendor, luster; flourishing, prosperous; beautiful.

周榮　zhōu róng　All-Round Flourishing　SP-20

róng 容 appearance, countenance, manner; allow, permit; endure; forgive; contain; admit; easy.
This character is a valley (谷 gǔ) with a cover over it. A valley is open and one can see all within it, but 容 is a covered valley, and hence means to shut up or contain. By extension, the character also means the countenance that hides (or reveals) the emotions of the heart.

不容　bù róng　Not Contained　ST-19
天容　tiān róng　Celestial Countenance　SI-17

ròu 肉 flesh, meat, muscle; fleshy; pulp or flesh of fruit; as a radical it is pronounced rù.
This character is used as a radical and is found as a part of many characters that represent body parts. In its altered form it is the same as the moon radical （月） with the exception that it is found on the left or bottom of characters, and the moon radical is found on the right.

滑肉門　huá ròu mén　Slippery Flesh Gate　ST-24

rǔ 乳 milk; breast; nipple, teat; to suckle; triturate; give birth; brood over eggs; the young of animals.

乳中　rǔ zhōng　Breast Center　ST-17
乳根　rǔ gēn　Breast Root　ST-18

sān 三 three, third, threefold, triple, trinity.

三間　sān jiān　Third Space　LI-3
手三里　shǒu sān lǐ　Arm Three Li　LI-10
足三里　zú sān lǐ　Leg Three Li　ST-36
三陰交　sān yīn jiāo　Three Yin Intersection　SP-6
三焦俞　sān jiāo shū　Triple Burner Shu　BL-22
三陽絡　sān yáng luò　Three Yang Connection　TB-8

shān 山 mountain, hill.

承山　chéng shān　Mountain Support　BL-57

shāng 商 discuss, deliberate; trade, commerce; name of a dynasty; the second note in the ancient pentatonic scale. This character represents the sound associated with metal in five phase theory.

少商　shào shāng　Lesser Shang　LU-11
商陽　shāng yáng　Shang Yang　LI-1
商丘　shāng qiū　Shang Hill　SP-5
商曲　shāng qū　Shang Bend　KI-17

shàng 上 top, summit; up, upper; supreme, first, best; previous; on, above; to rise, offer up; to esteem, exalt. The line at the bottom of this character is simply a base of reference, while the vertical line represents something above the base.

上廉　shàng lián　Upper Ridge　LI-9
上巨虛　shàng jù xū　Upper Great Hollow　ST-37
上髎　shàng liáo　Upper Bone-Hole　BL-31
上關　shàng guān　Upper Gate　GB-3
上脘　shàng wǎn　Upper Venter　CV-13
上星　shàng xīng　Upper Star　GV-23

shào 少 lesser, minor. Pronounced *shǎo:* few, little.

The radical in this character is 小 *xiǎo,* which means small. The leftward slanting stroke is an abstract implication of the concept of diminishing. The meanings of the character are thus derived through the idea of diminishing something that is already small. This is the character used in the names of the shao yang (triple burner and gallbladder) and shao yin (heart and kidney) channels.

少商　shào shāng　Lesser Shang　LU-11
少海　shào hǎi　Lesser Sea　HT-3
少府　shào fǔ　Lesser Mansion　HT-8
少沖　shào chōng　Lesser Surge　HT-9
少澤　shào zé　Lesser Marsh　SI-1

shè 舍 hut, shed; to lodge, reside. Pronounced *shě:* to put away; release; set aside, omit.

氣舍　qì shè　Qi Abode　ST-11
府舍　fǔ shè　Bowel Abode　SP-13
意舍　yì shè　Mentation Abode　BL-49

shēn 身 body; the person, self.

身柱　shēn zhù　Body Pillar　GV-12

shēn 申 report to; apply to; give orders; extend; repeat; easy, relaxed; the ninth of the Twelve Earthly Branches.

申脈　shēn mài　Extending Vessel　BL-62

shén 神 spirit, spirits, gods.
This character has three commonly used meanings in Chinese medicine. In a general sense it refers to the whole of the psyche, including: the 志 *zhì,* disposition, the 意 *yì,* reflection, the 魂 *hún* and the 魄 *pò.* In this sense spirit also refers to the power of concentration or the quality of being present. A patient is described, for example, as having or not having spirit. Secondly, in a slightly more restricted way, the term spirit encompasses the Western concepts of mind and emotions. This is the spirit 神 *shén* that is stored in the heart, the yang counterpart of 靈 *líng,* the yin aspect of the spirit. Lastly, spirit is the driving force

within the body. This is illustrated by a quote from Zhang Jie Bin, the author of the *Differentiated Canon,* ''form is the body of the spirit and is used by the spirit. Without spirit the form cannot move, and without form the spirit cannot exist.''

神門　shén mén　Spirit Gate　HT-7
神堂　shén táng　Spirit Hall　BL-44
神封　shén fēng　Spirit Seal　KI-23
神藏　shén cáng　Spirit Storehouse　KI-25
本神　běn shén　Root Spirit　GB-13
神闕　shén què　Spirit Gate　CV-8
神道　shén dào　Spirit Path　GV-11
神庭　shén tíng　Spirit Court　GV-24

shèn 腎 kidney.

腎俞　shèn shū　kidney shu　BL-23

shí 食 eat; food; drink. Pronounced *sì* : food, rice; to feed.

食竇　shí dòu　Food Hole　SP-17

shí 石 rock, stone; stony, barren; mineral.

石關　shí guān　Stone Pass　KI-18
石門　shí mén　Stone Gate　CV-5

shì 使 employ, use; to send; to order; to cause, to allow; envoy, commissioner.

間使　jiān shǐ　Intermediary Courier　PC-5

shì 市 market, fair; city; trade.

陰市　yīn shì　Yin Market　ST-33
風市　fēng shì　Wind Market　GB-31

shì 室 chamber; mansion; home.

志室　zhì shì　Will Chamber　BL-52

shǒu 手 hand; arm.

手三里　shǒu sān lǐ　Arm Three Li　LI-10
手五里　shǒu wǔ lǐ　Arm Five Li　LI-13

shū 樞 pivot, axis, central point; indispensable, cardinal.
Note that all of the points that contain this character in their names are located in the central region of the body.

天樞　tiān shū　Celestial Pivot　ST-25
五樞　wǔ shū　Fifth Pivot　GB-27
懸樞　xuán shū　Suspended Pivot　GV-5
中樞　zhōng shū　Central Pivot　GV-7

shū 俞 an acupuncture point; to transport; pronounced *yú :* a surname.
Some sources say that the top part of 俞 is 八 *bā,* to divide, and that the bottom part is a mistranscription of the character 舟 *zhōu,* a boat. The character's meaning of to transport may be related to its being a pictograph of a boat made by hollowing out（八）a log.

In the medical context, the character 俞 may also be written 腧 and 輸 . The latter are formed by the addition of the vehicle 車 and flesh 肉 radicals, which emphasize the notions of transportation and connection with the body respectively. All three characters can refer specifically to the five transporting-shu points, stream-shu points, and the associated-shu points of the back, or they can refer to acupuncture points in general. The transporting-shu points have been so called in English because the character 輸 , preferred by most modern writers in this context, has the meaning of transport and because all three forms of the character suggest movement (i.e., a boat). The name "associated-shu" has been given to the "shu" points on the bladder channel to avoid confusion with the transporting-shu points and to highlight the points' associations with the organs. "Stream-shu" was chosen to preserve the metaphor of water flowing toward the sea. Neither "associated-shu" or "stream-shu" is a direct translation.

The character 俞 , according to modern-day authorities, should be pronounced *shū*, while *yú* should be reserved for the surname. The Japanese pronunciation of this character as *yú* suggests that this distinction may only be a modern one and may also explain why many Westerners have adopted the pronunciation *yú* .

臑俞 nào shū Upper Arm Shu SI-10
肩外俞 jiān wài shū Outer Shoulder Shu SI-14
肩中俞 jiān zhōng shū Central Shoulder Shu SI-15
肺俞 fèi shū Lung Shu BL-13
厥陰俞 jué yīn shū Jue Yin Shu BL-14
心俞 xīn shū Heart Shu BL-15
督俞 dū shū Governing Shu BL-16
膈俞 gé shū Diaphragm Shu BL-17
肝俞 gān shū Liver Shu BL-18
膽俞 dǎn shū Gallbladder Shu BL-19
脾俞 pí shū Spleen Shu BL-20
胃俞 wèi shū Stomach Shu BL-21
三焦俞 sān jiāo shū Triple Burner Shu BL-22
腎俞 shèn shū Kidney Shu BL-23
氣海俞 qì hǎi shū Sea-of-Qi Shu BL-24
大腸俞 dà cháng shū Large Intestine Shu BL-25
關元俞 guān yuán shū Origin Pass Shu BL-26
小腸俞 xiǎo cháng shū Small Intestine Shu BL-27
膀胱俞 páng guāng shū Bladder Shu BL-28
中膂俞 zhōng lǚ shū Central Backbone Shu BL-29
白環俞 bái huán shū White Ring Shu BL-30
膏肓俞 gāo huāng shū Gao Huang Shu BL-43
肓俞 huāng shū Huang Shu KI-16
俞府 shū fǔ Shu Mansion KI-27
腰俞 yāo shū Lumbar Shu GV-2

shù 束 bind, restrain, control, keep in order; bunch.

束骨 shù gǔ Bundle Bone BL-65

shuài 率 lead; follow, obey; universally; all.
Pronounced *lǜ* : rate.

率谷 shuài gǔ Valley Lead GB-8

shuǐ 水 water; fluid.
Though it is less distinct in the modern character than in the older script, the central line represents the flow of a river and the outer lines portray the ripples of flowing water.

水突 shuǐ tú Water Prominence ST-10
水道 shuǐ dào Waterway ST-28
水泉 shuǐ quán Water Spring KI-5
水分 shuǐ fēn Water Divide CV-9
水溝 shuǐ gōu Water Trough GV-26

sī 絲 silk; thread; strings of a musical instrument.

絲竹空 sī zhú kōng Silk Bamboo Hole TB-23

sì 四 four, fourth, fourfold, quadruple, quaternity.

四白 sì bái Four Whites ST-2
四滿 sì mǎn Fourfold Fullness KI-14
四瀆 sì dú Four Rivers TB-9

sù 素 plain, unornamented, ordinary, simple; vegetarian; white; original or normal constitution.

素髎 sù liáo White Bone-Hole GV-25

sūn 孫 grandchild; descendants; posterity; tertiary, minor.
The character is formed of 系 *xī,* to tie together, succession, and 子 *zǐ,* child. The meaning derives from the idea of a succession of children, i.e., descendants.

公孫 gōng sūn Yellow Emperor SP-4
角孫 jiǎo sūn Angle Vertex TB-20

suō 縮 contract, shrink.

筋縮 jīn suō Sinew Contraction GV-8

tái 台 lookout, tower; terrace, platform, stage.

靈台 líng tái Spirit Tower GV-10

tài 太 great, supreme; too, excessive; very.
This is the character used in the names of the tai yang (small intestine and bladder) and tai yin (lung and spleen) channels.

太淵　tài yuān　Great Abyss　LU-9
太乙　tài yǐ　Supreme Unity　ST-23
太白　tài bái　Supreme White　SP-3
太谿　tài xī　Great Ravine　KI-3
太沖　tài chōng　Supreme Surge　LV-3

táng 堂 hall, reception room; meeting place;
court of justice.
The character is composed of a roof, 尚 *shàng,* over earth, 土 *tǔ.* It represents a building with an earthen floor.

神堂　shén táng　Spirit Hall　BL-44
玉堂　yù táng　Jade Hall　CV-18

táo 陶 kiln; pottery; to be pleased.

陶道　táo dào　Kiln Path　GV-13

tiān 天 heaven, sky, celestial; a day; Nature, God, divine; the weather.
This character is composed of a picture of a person with arms and legs outstretched (大) and the sky above; hence the meanings sky, heaven, etc. It is found in many points that are located on the upper body, especially in the region of the heart or on the head. The relationship between the heavens and the heart is based on analogy; the heart rules the body as heaven rules the earth. The head's relation to the heavens is more direct;the head is the heaven (i.e., uppermost part) of the microcosmic universe of the body. Additionally, many points on the channels of the hollow organs bear the epithet celestial (天).This is most likely due to a line in *Essential Questions* that compares the qi of the hollow organs to that of heaven in that they both rule change and transformation.

天府　tiān fǔ　Celestial Storehouse　LU-3
天鼎　tiān dǐng　Celestial Tripod　LI-17

天樞　tiān shū　Celestial Pivot　ST-25
天溪　tiān xī　Celestial Ravine　SP-18
天宗　tiān zōng　Celestial Gathering　SI-11
天窗　tiān chuāng　Celestial Window　SI-16
天容　tiān róng　Celestial Countenance　SI-17
通天　tōng tiān　Celestial Connection　BL-7
天柱　tiān zhù　Celestial Pillar　BL-10
天池　tiān chí　Celestial Pool　PC-1
天泉　tiān quán　Celestial Spring　PC-2
天井　tiān jǐng　Celestial Well　TB-10
天髎　tiān liáo　Celestial Bone-Hole　TB-15
天牖　tiān yǒu　Celestial Window　TB-16
天衝　tiān chòng　Celestial Hub　GB-9
天突　tiān tú　Celestial Chimney　CV-22

tiáo 條 strip, band, section; measure word for long, thin objects.

條口　tiáo kǒu　Ribbon Opening　ST-38

tiào 跳 jump, leap; climb over; posture.
The foot radical 足 *zú* gives this character its meaning. 兆 *zhào* is a phonetic component.

環跳　huán tiào　Jumping Round　GB-30

tīng 聽 listen, hear; understand.

聽宮　tīng gōng　Auditory Palace　SI-19
聽會　tīng huì　Auditory Convergence　GB-2

tíng 庭 court, palace, courtyard; court of justice; hall, audience chamber.

內庭　nèi tíng　Inner Court　ST-44
中庭　zhōng tíng　Center Palace　CV-16
神庭　shén tíng　Spirit Court　GV-24

tōng 通 through, go through to, penetrate; understand, communicate; free, unblocked; succeed.
In Chinese medicine this character is used to express the

idea of unblocking or freeing the channels, the menses, the flow of milk, and the urine.

通里　tōng lǐ　Connecting Li　HT-5
通天　tōng tiān　Celestial Connection　BL-7
通谷　tōng gǔ　Valley Passage　BL-66
通谷　tōng gǔ　Open Valley　KI-20

tóng 瞳 pupil of the eye.

瞳子髎　tóng zǐ liáo　Pupil Bone-Hole　GB-1

tóu 頭 head; top; first, most important, best; end.

頭維　tóu wéi　Head Corner　ST-8
頭竅陰　tóu qiào yīn　Head Portal Yin　GB-11
頭臨泣　tóu lín qì　Head Overlooking Tears　GB-15

tú 突 abruptly, suddenly; rush out; stick out, protrude; offend; smooth; chimney.
This character's meaning derives from its depiction of a dog (犬 quǎn) rushing out of its den (穴 xuè, hole).

扶突　fú tú　Protuberance Assistant　LI-18
水突　shuǐ tú　Water Prominence　ST-10
天突　tiān tú　Celestial Chimney　CV-22

tù 兔 hare, rabbit.

伏兔　fú tù　Crouching Rabbit　ST-32

wài 外 out, outside; beyond; foreign; apart from.

外陵　wài líng　Outer Mound　ST-26
肩外俞　jiān wài shū　Outer Shoulder Shu　SI-14
外關　wài guān　Outer Pass　TB-5
外丘　wài qiū　Outer Hill　GB-36

wán 完 to complete, finish; completed; whole, unbroken.

完骨　wán gǔ　Completion Bone　GB-12

wǎn (guǎn) 脘 a duct in the body; core of a boil.
In Chinese medicine this character means one of two things,

depending on what source is consulted: 1) the stomach cavity and the adjacent parts of the esophagus and intestines; 2) the gastric organ itself, as opposed to the physiological properties attributed to that organ in Chinese medicine. This term is rendered in English as "venter."
Some older books replace this character with 管 *guǎn,* meaning pipe or duct.

下脘   xià wǎn   Lower Venter   CV-10
中脘   zhōng wǎn   Central Venter   CV-12
上脘   shàng wǎn   Upper Venter   CV-13

wàn 腕 wrist; flexible joint.

腕骨   wàn gǔ   Wrist Bone   SI-4

wéi 維 tie, hold together; hold fast.
This character originally represented the four corners of a net, and by extension came to mean the four limbs and the four directions.   This older meaning is reflected in the first of the two point names below.

頭維   tóu wéi   Head Corner   ST-8
維道   wéi dào   Linking Path   GB-28

wěi 委 entrust; appoint; to give up, to bow under a burden; indirect, roundabout, tortuous, crooked, bent; to be or feel wronged; a grievance.
This character's meaning of entrust is said to come from the fact that the grain (禾 *hé*) was entrusted to women (女 *nǚ*) when men had to leave home on other business.   The idea of a curved stalk heavy with grain or a woman bent over with her burden may be responsible for the extended meanings of curved, tortuous or bent.

委陽   wěi yáng   Bend Yang   BL-39
委中   wěi zhōng   Bend Middle   BL-40

wěi 尾 tail; end; rear.

鳩尾   jiū wěi   Turtledove Tail   CV-15

wèi 胃 stomach.

胃俞 wèi shū Stomach Shu BL-21
胃倉 wèi cāng Stomach Granary BL-50

wēn 溫 warm; mild, genial; review.

溫溜 wēn liù Warm Dwelling LI-7

wū 屋 house, building.

屋翳 wū yì Roof ST-15

wǔ 五 five, fifth, fivefold.
中 *zhōng,* center, is often implied when this character is used in point names. This is because in Chinese numerology the central position is associated with the number five. The ancient form of the character was an X, an obvious reference to the center. Later lines were added at the top and bottom of the character indicating yin below and yang above, demonstrating that the five phases result from the interplay of yin and yang.

手五里 shǒu wǔ lǐ Arm Five Li LI-13
五處 wǔ chù Fifth Place BL-5
五樞 wǔ shū Fifth Pivot GB-27
地五會 dì wǔ huì Earth Fivefold Convergence GB-42
足五里 zú wǔ lǐ Foot Five Li LV-10

xī 膝 knee.

膝陽關 xī yáng guān Knee Yang Joint GB-33
膝關 xī guān Knee Joint LV-7

xī 谿 or 溪 ravine, stream gully, gully stream.
This character has two forms, as shown above. The character 溪 is a more recent invention, and though it is now used in the point names it did not exist at the time that the names were created. Both characters indicate a mountain ravine through which mountain streams can run, but 溪 contains a water radical and is thus associated more with the stream than the ravine it runs through. In the acupunc-

ture point names the word ravine is almost always locational in nature. According to *Essential Questions* a "large union of the flesh" is called a valley (谷 *gǔ*) and a "small union of the flesh" is called a ravine（谿）.

解谿　jiě xī　Ravine Divide　ST-41
天谿　tiān xī　Celestial Ravine　SP-18
後谿　hòu xī　Back Ravine　SI-3
陽谿　yáng xī　Yang Ravine　LI-5
太谿　tài xī　Great Ravine　KI-3
俠谿　xiá xī　Pinched Ravine　GB-43

xī 郄 cleft.

陰郄　yīn xī　Yin Cleft　HT-6
浮郄　fú xī　Superficial Cleft　BL-38
郄門　xī mén　Cleft Gate　PC-4

xí 息 a full breath, a gasp, a respiration; to produce interest; to stop, repose, quiet.

顱息　lú xí　Skull Rest　TB-19

xī 譆 an exclamatory sound, "shee."

譩譆　yī xǐ　Yi Xi　BL-45

xià 俠 generous; bold, as a knight-errant.
This character is often used to express the meaning of the character 夾 *jiā,* to pinch from two sides.

俠白　xiá bái　Guarding White　LU-4
俠谿　xiá xī　Pinched Ravine　GB-43

xià 下 below, under; to descend; lower, inferior; to deposit, lay; to set to (work); a time.
The upper line of this character denotes the horizon or the ground, and the perpendicular line implies something below or inferior to it.

下廉　xià lián　Lower Ridge　LI-8
下關　xià guān　Below the Joint　ST-7
下巨虛　xià jù xū　Lower Great Hollow　ST-39

下髎 xià liáo Lower Bone-Hole BL-34
下脘 xià wǎn Lower Venter CV-10

xiàn 陷 to sink, fall; involve; to beguile, betray.

陷谷 xiàn gǔ Sunken Valley ST-43

xiāng 鄉 countryside; village; district.

胸鄉 xiōng xiāng Chest Village SP-19

xiāng 香 fragrant, aromatic.

迎香 yíng xiāng Welcome Fragrance LI-20

xiāo 消 to melt, thaw; to disperse; to disappear; to cancel, annul.

消濼 xiāo luò Dispersing Riverbed TB-12

xiǎo 小 small; petty, mean; a concubine.
This character is made up of 八 bā, meaning to divide, and a vertical line representing the thing divided. It thus implies the idea of making a thing smaller by splitting it up.

小海 xiǎo hǎi Small Sea SI-8
小腸俞 xiǎo cháng shū Small Intestine Shu BL-27

xīn 心 heart; mind; affections.
This character is a stylized pictograph of the heart. In Chinese 心 refers as much to the emotions and the psyche as it does to the actual organ of the heart.

心俞 xīn shū Heart Shu BL-15

xìn 囟 top of the head; skull; frontal region of the head; the fontanels.

囟會 xìn huì Fontanel Meeting GV-22

xìn 信 to believe in, trust; truth, sincerity; confidence; a letter, a token of confidence; an envoy; news; sign, signal.
The image of a man (人 rén) and his word (言 yán) led to the many meanings of this character.

交信　jiāo xìn　Intersection Reach　KI-8

xīng 星 star, heavenly body; point of light, spark.

上星　shàng xīng　Upper Star　GV-23

xíng 行 to walk, to travel; to do, act. Pronounced *háng*: row, line; business.

The left three strokes of 行 *xíng* (i.e., 彳 *chì*) mean walk to the left, and the right three strokes (亍 *chú*) mean walk to the right. In Chinese medicine this character is used to express the function of moving qi, blood or fluids. It is also the character that is translated as phase in the term five phases (五行 *wǔ xíng*), which are five movements (steps) in a cycle.

行間　xíng jiān　Moving Between　LV-2

xiōng 胸 chest; breast, bosom; mind, intelligence.

胸鄉　xiōng xiāng　Chest Village　SP-19

xū 虚 false, untrue, unreal, vain; hollow, empty, vacuous, insubstantial; pure, unprejudiced, humble.

This character is employed in Chinese medicine to express the parameter of vacuity in the eight parameters. It is the opposite of repletion (實 *shí*).

上巨虚　shàng jù xū　Upper Great Hollow　ST-37
下巨虚　xià jù xū　Lower Great Hollow　ST-39

xū 墟 old burial grounds; wild waste land; a fair, market.

靈墟　líng xū　Spirit Ruins　KI-24
丘墟　qiū xū　Hill Ruins　GB-40

xuán 懸 to hang, suspend; in suspense, anxious; distant from, separated.

懸顱　xuán lú　Suspended Skull　GB-5
懸厘　xuán lí　Suspended Tuft　GB-6
懸鐘　xuán zhōng　Suspended Bell　GB-39
懸樞　xuán shū　Suspended Pivot　GV-5

xuán 璇 a fine kind of jade.

璇璣 xuán jī Jade Pivot CV-21

xuè 穴 cave, den, hole; underground dwelling; to bore a hole.
This is the character used in Chinese to represent the acupuncture points. The top part of the character represents a roof, while the bottom portion, 八, means to divide. Its meaning is thus derived from the idea of a space which is obtained through the removal of rocks or dirt, i.e., a cave or den.

氣穴 qì xuè Qi Point KI-13

xuè 血 blood.
The radical 皿 min, meaning a vessel for catching sacrificial blood, gives this character its meaning. The additional line on top represents the blood as it pours into the vessel.

血海 xuè hǎi Sea of Blood SP-10

yǎ 啞 dumb, mute.
The right hand portion of the character （亞） is said to picture two persons whose physical structure deviates from the norm, i.e., hunchbacks. Muteness is a deviation from the norm that affects the speech, here represented by the mouth （口） on the left.

啞門 yǎ mén Mute's Gate GV-15

yàn 厭 dislike, detest; reject; be tired of, bored with.

頷厭 hàn yàn Forehead Fullness GB-4

yáng 揚 to scatter, spread; to raise; to winnow; to publish abroad; to praise.

飛揚 fēi yáng Taking Flight BL-58

yáng 陽 yang, the complement of yin.
The left part of this character is the radical form of 阜 fù, which represents a mound. The right hand part of the

which represents a mound. The right hand part of the character pictures the sun above the horizon (旦) and rays of light shining down (勿), 陽 *yáng,* therefore, was originally a pictograph representing the sunny side of a hill. (Compare 陰 *yīn.*)

商陽　shāng yáng　Shang Yang　LI-1
陽谿　yáng xī　Yang Ravine　LI-5
沖陽　chōng yáng　Surging Yang　ST-42
陽谷　yáng gǔ　Yang Valley　SI-5
會陽　huì yáng　Meeting of Yang　BL-35
委陽　wěi yáng　Bend Yang　BL-39
陽綱　yáng gāng　Yang Headrope　BL-48
合陽　hé yáng　Yang Union　BL-55
跗陽　fū yáng　Instep Yang　BL-59
陽池　yáng chí　Yang Pool　TB-4
三陽絡　sān yáng luò　Three Yang Connection　TB-8
陽白　yáng bái　Yang White　GB-14
膝陽關　xī yáng guān　Knee Yang Joint　GB-33
陽陵泉　yáng líng quán　Yang Mound Spring　GB-34
陽交　yáng jiāo　Yang Intersection　GB-35
陽輔　yáng fǔ　Yang Assistance　GB-38
腰陽關　yāo yáng guān　Lumbar Yang Pass　GV-3
至陽　zhì yáng　Extremity of Yang　GV-9

yǎng 養 to nourish; to rear, bring up, care for; support, maintain.

Note the food radical, 食 *shí ,* that gives this character its meaning. The upper portion is 羊 *yáng,* meaning goat, and functioning here as a phonetic element. It may also be said to lend meaning to the character in the sense that one can obtain nourishment from eating mutton, or in the sense that one can rear goats.

養老　yǎng lǎo　Nursing the Aged　SI-6

yāo 腰 low back, loins, waist; kidney (of animals).

腰俞　yāo shū　Lumbar Shu　GV-2
腰陽關　yāo yáng guān　Lumbar Yang Pass　GV-3

yè 腋 armpit.

淵腋　yuān yè　Armpit Abyss　GB-22

yè 液 fluid, humor; juice, sap.

液門　yè mén　Humor Gate　TB-2

yì 譩 an exclamatory sound, "ee."

譩譆　yī xǐ　Yi Xi　BL-45

yǐ 乙 one; the second of the ten celestial branches, hence second in a series, as the letter b in English; crooked, bent.

太乙　tài yǐ　Supreme Unity　ST-23

yì 意 reflection, an idea, a thought, a wish; intention, purpose, will.
Meaning is derived from two parts: 音 *yīn,* meaning sound or voice, and 心 *xīn,* heart and mind. A person's heartfelt (心) thoughts and intentions are deduced from the words (音) he speaks. The *Spiritual Axis* states in one passage that reflection is stored in the spleen, and elsewhere defines reflection as the ability of the heart (mind) to recall or reflect. (心有所憶謂之意 .)

意舍　yì shè　Mentation Abode　BL-49

yì 翳 a feather screen; a shade, screen; to shade, screen.

屋翳　wū yì　Roof　ST-15
翳風　yì fēng　Wind Screen　TB-17

yīn 殷 abundant; flourishing; great; many; highest degree of; to determine exactly; to regulate; the name of a Chinese imperial dynasty.

殷門　yīn mén　Gate of Abundance　BL-37

yīn 陰 yin, the complement of yang.
The left part of this character is the radical form of 阜 *fù,* which represents a mound. The right part pictures the

presence （今） of clouds （云） , and by extension, shade. The character 陰 is thus a representation of the shady side of a hill. Its extended meanings are derived from this fact. (Compare 陽 *yáng*.)

陰市　yīn shì　Yin Market　ST-33
三陰交　sān yīn jiāo　Three Yin Intersection　SP-6
陰陵泉　yīn líng quán　Yin Mound Spring　SP-9
陰郄　yīn xī　Yin Cleft　HT-6
厥陰俞　jué yīn shū　Jue Yin Shu　BL-14
至陰　zhì yīn　Reaching Yin　BL-67
陰谷　yīn gǔ　Yin Valley　KI-10
陰都　yīn dū　Yin Metropolis　KI-19
頭竅陰　tóu qiào yīn　Head Portal Yin　GB-11
足竅陰　zú qiào yīn　Foot Portal Yin　GB-44
陰包　yīn bāo　Yin Bladder　LV-9
陰廉　yīn lián　Yin Corner　LV-11
會陰　huì yīn　Meeting of Yin　CV-1
陰交　yīn jiāo　Yin Intersection　CV-7

yín 齦 gum, gingiva.

齦交　yín jiāo　Gum Intersection　GV-28

yǐn 隱 hidden, mysterious, secret; to conceal; small, minute.

隱白　yǐn bái　Hidden White　SP-1

yīng 膺 the breast.
This character is used both in the concrete anatomical sense of the anterior chest, and in the more abstract sense of the seat of the emotions.

膺窗　yīng chuāng　Breast Window　ST-16

yíng 迎 meet, greet, welcome, receive; move toward, meet face to face; coming in the opposite direction.

迎香　yíng xiāng　Welcome Fragrance　LI-20
大迎　dà yíng　Great Reception　ST-5
人迎　rén yíng　Man's Prognosis　ST-9

yíng 營 camp, barracks; operate, run; plan, build; circulate; seek.

正營 zhèng yíng Upright Construction GB-17

yŏng 涌 to well up, bubble up, gush; flow rapidly.

涌泉 yŏng quăn Gushing Spring KI-1

yōu 幽 dark, gloomy; secret, retired; lonely; subtle.
This character originally implied the deep, shady reaches of a mountain （山） where only slender threads （么） of light penetrate.

幽門 yōu mén Dark Gate KI-21

yŏu 牖 window; lattice window; to teach, enlighten.

天牖 tiān yŏu Celestial Window TB-16

yú 髃 collarbone, clavicle.

肩髃 jiān yú Shoulder Bone LI-15

yú 魚 fish.

魚際 yú jì Fish Border LU-10

yù 玉 jade; gem, precious stone; valuable.

玉枕 yù zhĕn Jade Pillow BL-9
玉堂 yù táng Jade Hall CV-18

yù 彧 elegant; accomplished.

彧中 yù zhōng Lively Center KI-26

yuān 淵 gulf, abyss, deep water source; profound.

太淵 tài yuān Great Abyss LU-9
清冷淵 qīng lĕng yuān Clear Cold Abyss TB-11
淵腋 yuān yè Armpit Abyss GB-22

yuán 元 first, primary; basic, fundamental; unit, component.

The two lines （二） on the top of this character are the ancient character meaning above or top (now written as 上 shàng). The bottom part of the character is a drawing of two legs. The implication is that the head is at the very top. The meanings of origin, staring point, etc., are derived through extension of this idea.

關元俞 guān yuán shū Origin Pass Shu BL-26
關元 guān yuán Origin Pass CV-4

yuán 垣 wall, city wall; the space enclosed by a constellation.

曲垣 qū yuán Crooked Wall SI-13
神庭 shén tíng Spirit Court GV-24

yuè 月 moon; month; full-moon shaped, round.

日月 rì yuè Sun and Moon GB-24

yún 雲 cloud.

The original form of this character was simply 云, the two lines （二） at the top being the ancient character meaning above or top and thus implying the skies, while the angular line at the bottom depicts the vapors rising up from the earth to form clouds. Over time the ancient character was borrowed to mean to speak or to say, and the rain radical （雨） was added at the top to reinforce the original meaning of clouds.

雲門 yún mén Cloud Gate LU-2

zǎn (cuán) 攢 save, accumulate; hoard.

攢竹 zǎn zhú Bamboo Gathering BL-2

zé 澤 pond, pool; marsh, swamp; damp, moist; sheen, luster; favor, beneficence.

尺澤 chǐ zé Cubit Marsh LU-5

少澤　shào zé　Lesser Marsh　SI-1
曲澤　qū zé　Marsh at the Bend　PC-3

zhāng 章 a strain of music; a chapter; the camphor laurel.

章門　zhāng mén　Camphorwood Gate　LV-13

zhào 照 to shine, illuminate; to reflect; to look after; license; according to; understand; contrast; photograph.

照海　zhào hǎi　Shining Sea　KI-6

zhé 輒 the sides of a chariot where the arms were carried; abruptly, suddenly, at once; then.

輒筋　zhé jīn　Sinew Seat　GB-23

zhēn 眞 true, real.

肩眞　jiān zhēn　True Shoulder　SI-9

zhěn 枕 pillow; rest the head on.

玉枕　yù zhěn　Jade Pillow　BL-9

zhèng 正 correct, right; straight, upright; situated in the middle; honest, upright; sharp (of time); positive; precisely correct, from.
To stop (止 *zhǐ*) at the appointed limit explains the meaning from which the other meanings are derived.

支正　zhī zhèng　Branch to the Correct　SI-7
正營　zhèng yíng　Upright Construction　GB-17

zhī 支 branch; descendants; pay out; support, prop up; manage; withstand; measure word for stick-like objects such as pens.
In the old script the character was more clearly a picture of hand grasping a branch. This is the character used to indicate the twelve earthly branches.

支正　zhī zhèng　Branch to the Correct　SI-7
支溝　zhī gōu　Branch Ditch　TB-6

zhì 志 will, ambition, disposition, determination.
This character indicates resoluteness of intent. In the *Spiritual Axis* the kidney is said to store the will (disposition, 志). This is usually thought to be a reference to the kidney's contribution to a person's ability to focus and reflect or recall (意 *yì*).

志室 zhì shì Will Chamber BL-52

zhì 秩 order; sequence.

秩邊 zhì biān Sequential Limit BL-54

zhì 至 arrive; to, until; consummate; extremely, most.

至陽 zhì yáng Extremity of Yang GV-9
至陰 zhì yīn Reaching Yin BL-67

zhōng 中 center, middle; central; within, in.
This is a pictograph of an arrow piercing the center of a target.

中府 zhōng fǔ Central Treasury LU-1
乳中 rǔ zhōng Breast Center ST-17
肩中俞 jiān zhōng shū Central Shoulder Shu SI-15
中膂俞 zhōng lǚ shū Central Backbone Shu BL-29
中髎 zhōng liáo Central Bone-Hole BL-33
委中 wěi zhōng Bend Middle BL-40
中注 zhōng zhù Central Flow KI-15
彧中 yù zhōng Lively Center KI-26
中衝 zhōng chōng Central Hub PC-9
中渚 zhōng zhǔ Central Islet TB-3
中瀆 zhōng dú Central River GB-32
中封 zhōng fēng Mound Center LV-4
中都 zhōng dū Central Metropolis LV-6
中極 zhōng jí Central Pole CV-3
中脘 zhōng wǎn Central Venter CV-12
中庭 zhōng tíng Center Palace CV-16
膻中 dàn zhōng Chest Center CV-17
脊中 jǐ zhōng Spinal Center GV-6
中樞 zhōng shū Central Pivot GV-7
人中 rén zhōng Human Center GV-26

zhōng 鐘 cup, goblet; bell.

大鐘　dà zhōng　Large Goblet　KI-4
懸鐘　xuán zhōng　Suspended Bell　GB-39

zhōu 周 encircle; all round, everywhere; complete, entire, the whole; comprehensive, catholic; to relieve, to assist; near, as relative; the name of a Chinese imperial dynasty.

周榮　zhōu róng　All-Round Flourishing　SP-20

zhǒu 肘 elbow.

肘髎　zhǒu liáo　Elbow Bone-Hole　LI-12

zhú 築 build; to beat down hard; to ram earth (i.e., to make mud walls).

築賓　zhú bīn　Guest House　KI-9

zhú 竹 bamboo.

攢竹　zǎn zhú　Bamboo Gathering　BL-2
絲竹空　sī zhú kōng　Silk Bamboo Hole　TB-23

zhǔ 渚 islet; bank.

中渚　zhōng zhǔ　Central Islet　TB-3

zhù 柱 pillar, column, post; cylinder.

天柱　tiān zhù　Celestial Pillar　BL-10
身柱　shēn zhù　Body Pillar　GV-12

zhù 注 pour; flow; explanatory notes.

中注　zhōng zhù　Central Flow　KI-15

zhù 杼 reed; shuttle.

大杼　dà zhù　Great Shuttle　BL-11

zhuī 椎 mallet, bludgeon (now written 槌 *chuí*); vertebra.

大椎　dà zhuī　Great Hammer　GV-14

zǐ 紫 purple, violet.

紫宮　zǐ gōng　Purple Palace　CV-19

zǐ 子 offspring; son; noun suffix.

瞳子髎　tóng zǐ liáo　Pupil Bone-Hole　GB-1

zōng 宗 ancestor; clans descended from a common ancestor; sect, faction, school; principal.
In Chinese medicine the character 宗 zong usually implies gathering (which in modern writing is represented by the character 綜). For example, 宗筋 *zōng jīn,* is the sinew gathering (the genitals, where the sinews gather), and 宗氣 *zōng qì* is the qi that gathers in the chest (generally translated as ancestral qi).

天宗　tiān zōng　Celestial Gathering　SI-11
會宗　huì zōng　Convergence and Gathering　TB-7

zú 足 foot, leg; sufficient, ample; full, as much as.

足三里　zú sān lǐ　Leg Three Li　ST-36
足臨泣　zú lín qì　Foot Overlooking Tears　GB-41
足竅陰　zú qiào yīn　Foot Portal Yin　GB-44
足五里　zú wǔ lǐ　Foot Five Li　LV-10

zuì 最 most; assemble, collect.

孔最　kǒng zuì　Collection Hole　LU-6

Appendix B

The Names of the Special Point Groupings

A book about the Chinese names for acupuncture points would not be complete without a discussion of the Chinese names for the special point groupings. The names of these groupings, like the names of the points themselves, can guide us to a deeper understanding of the points and their functions. A different challenge exists here, however. Where the names of points have simply been replaced by the alphanumeric code in the West, the names of the special point groupings have, of necessity, been given English renderings. Although these titles serve a useful purpose, in several cases the English name for the point group is not an actual translation of the original Chinese, but a name chosen to fit descriptions of the nature or function of the group. The following discussion aims to help students to gain a clearer understanding of both the Chinese and English names of the special point groupings. Most of the characters discussed here can be found, along with further information concerning their origins and meanings, in the *Glossary of Single Characters*.

Five transporting-shu points (五輸穴 *wǔ shū xuè*):

The five transporting-shu points are the special sets of five points located below the elbow or knee on each of the twelve primary channels. They include well-jing points (井穴 *jǐng xuè*), spring-ying points (滎穴 *yíng xuè*), stream-shu points (俞穴 *shū xuè*), river-jing points (經穴 *jīng xuè*) and uniting-he points (合穴 *hé xuè*). Their Chinese and English names largely reflect an analogy that likens the nature of qi at these points to the flow of water from its source in the mountains to its home in the sea.

Although the English generic name transporting-shu points would appear to be, at least tenuously, in keeping with the image of flowing water, its directness belies a certain vagueness inherent in the Chinese. This vagueness is rooted in the fact that there are three characters (輸, 俞 and 腧, all pronounced *shū*) that are used interchangeably to refer to this point group. Of these three characters, only 輸, which is distinguished by the vehicle radical 車 has the unequivocal meaning of to transport in current use. The character 俞, which represents a boat made from a hollowed log, is also said in some old dictionaries to have the meaning of transportation. The character 腧 is derived from 俞 by the addition of the flesh radical 月 (a simplification of 肉 *rù*), implying a connection with the body.

Vagueness of the meanings of these characters is compounded rather than resolved by their usage. 俞 and its two derivates can be used to denote the five transporting-shu points as a group and, within that group, the stream-shu points. They can also refer to the associated-shu points of the back and to acupuncture points in general. The notion of transportation can be said to apply in all these cases, and could be related to the idea of acupuncture points in general as points on the body where qi is "transported." Although this reasoning explains the English name for this group of points, it is somewhat forced. The authors of the *Inner Canon* spoke of transporting-shu points in such a way as to suggest that they simply meant "(the) five acupuncture points." They were inconsistent in the usage of characters, and did not give these points a specific label that unequivocally attached to them a notion of transportation different from that other points. Nor did they define them in terms of a metaphor of transportation. The notion of transportation and its connection with the water metaphor is only implied and was developed by later writers.

Well-jing points (井穴 *jǐng xuè*): 井 *jǐng*, which means a well, is used to denote the well-jing points because the nature of the qi at these points is said to be small and still like water in a well.

Spring-ying points (滎穴 *yíng xuè*):   The character 滎 *yíng* can mean the dashing of waves, the streaming of water, a brook, or the rising of water as at a spring. It is used in acupuncture to represent the nature of the qi at the spring-ying points, which is likened to the flow of water from a spring.

Stream-shu points (俞穴 *shū xuè*):   Qi at the stream-shu points is said to resemble water pouring downward, as from a shallow place to a deeper one. This describes the qi as it flows from the shallow flesh of the wrist or ankle to the deep flesh of the forearm or calf. The English rendering of the name of this point category as "stream" is not a direct translation, but is based on classical Chinese descriptions likening the nature of the qi flow at these points to a stream which is flowing toward a river.   As mentioned above, the characters 腧 and 輸 are also sometimes used to represent the stream-shu points.

River-jing points (經穴 *jīng xuè*):   Although the character 經 *jīng* is not defined to mean river, the construction of the character does allow for this interpretation (see: *Glossary of Single Characters*).   The rendering of the name of this point grouping as "river-jing points" is based primarily on descriptions in the classics that describe the nature of the qi at these points to be like a flowing river.

Uniting-he points (合穴 *hé xuè*):   The character 合 *hé* means to unite, and in the name for the uniting-he points it represents the nature of the qi as it enters deeply into the body and unites with the organ to which the channel relates. The classical metaphor likens the nature of the qi at these points to the water of a river as it unites with the sea.

Lower uniting-he points (下合穴 *xià hé xuè*):   These are the six points located on the lower limbs where the qi of the six bowels gathers. The character 下 *xià*, meaning lower, is indicative of the location of these points.   The meaning of 合 *hé* is the same as that explained under uniting-he points above.

Alarm-mu points (募穴 *mù xuè*): 募 *mù* means to collect, to gather or to muster, and is used in phrases meaning
the enlistment of troops or the gathering of taxes. It is
used in Chinese medicine to refer to the alarm-mu points
because these are points where the qi of a specific viscus or
bowel gathers. The English designation of this point grouping as "alarm" points is a reflection of their function as
diagnostic indicators, and does not reflect the meaning of
the Chinese name.

Associated-shu points (俞穴 *shū xuè*): These points
are called associated-shu points in English in reference to
their association with a particular viscus or bowel. This
name is again not a translation of the Chinese name for the
special grouping, but is based rather on the nature of the
points. Though the logic of the Chinese name is not entirely clear, the character 俞 *shū* (or 腧 or 輸 - see above),
meaning to transport, may be an indication that the qi of
the related organs is transported to these points. Because of
the interchangability of the characters 俞, 腧 and 輸, the
Chinese differentiate references to transporting-shu points,
stream-shu points and associated-shu points mainly by context. In English we have three distinctly different names.

Source-yuan points (原穴 *yuán xuè*): The character 原
yuán is a highly altered version of what was originally a
pictograph of water flowing out of the side of a cliff, and
thus stands for the concept of a source. This character is
used to denote both source qi and source-yuan points, as
the source qi of an organ is said to reside at the source-
yuan point of its associated channel.

It is interesting to note that the clinical importance of the
source-yuan points is reflected in their names. The original
five pairs of source-yuan points for the five viscera all contain the characters 大 *dà* or 太 *tài* (great or supreme).
The source-yuan points listed in the *Spiritual Axis* are as
follows: Great Abyss (LU-9) for the lung; Great Mound
(PC-7) for the heart; Supreme Surge (LV-3) for the liver;

Supreme White (SP-3) for the spleen and Great Ravine (KI-3) for the kidney. The *gāo* and *huāng* also had source-yuan points assigned to them. Note that the source-yuan point of the heart was Great Mound (PC-7), which differs from the present-day assignation of Spirit Gate (HT-7).

Cleft-xi points (郄穴 *xī xuè*): 郄 *xī* means a cleft or fissure and refers to one point on each of the twelve channels and four of the extraordinary vessels where qi and blood collect in a cleft-like depression. In this case the English rendering reflects the original Chinese.

Connecting-luo points (絡穴 *luò xuè*): The character 絡 *luò* is used to describe the quality of hemp and silk fibers, and by extension means to enmesh and to connect. The connecting vessels (絡脈 *luò mài*) enmesh and at the same time connect the tissues of the body. The connecting-luo points are so named because the connecting vessels connect at these points to join the primary channel and its interior-exterior counterpart.

Meeting-hui points (會穴 *huì xuè*): The character 會 *huì* means to meet or assemble. In acupuncture, meeting-hui points are points that influence a specific aspect of the body such as the sinews, bones, blood, etc. The name of this point grouping most probably implies that the essence of the sinews, bones, blood, etc., in an abstract way, collects or meets at these points, thus accounting for their effectiveness in treating disorders of those particular aspects.

Intersection-jiaohui points (交會穴 *jiāo huì xuè*): The two characters in the term 交會 *jiāo huì* mean to intersect and to meet, respectively. This term is usually used in acupuncture to refer to points where two or more channels intersect, although it is also used in referring to the confluence-jiaohui points of the eight extraordinary vessels. In English we have different renderings in order to draw a distinction between the two, where the Chinese rely mostly on context for differentiation.

Index One

English Order List of Main Point Names

Branch Ditch TB-6   支溝 *zhī gōu*
Branch to the Correct SI-7   支正 *zhī zhèng*
Breast Center ST-17   乳中 *rǔ zhōng*
Breast Root ST-18   乳根 *rǔ gēn*
Breast Window ST-16   膺窗 *yīng chuāng*
Bright Eyes BL-1   睛明 *jīng míng*
Bright Light GB-37   光明 *guāng míng*
Broken Sequence LU-7   列缺 *liè quē*
Bundle Bone BL-65   束骨 *shù gǔ*
Calf's Nose ST-35   犢鼻 *dú bí*
Camphorwood Gate LV-13 章門 *zhāng mén*
Capital Bone BL-64   京骨 *jīng gǔ*
Capital Gate GB-25   京門 *jīng mén*
Celestial Bone-Hole TB-15   天髎 *tiān liáo*
Celestial Chimney CV-22   天突 *tiān tú*
Celestial Connection BL-7   通天 *tōng tiān*
Celestial Countenance SI-17   天容 *tiān róng*
Celestial Gathering SI-11   天宗 *tiān zōng*
Celestial Hub GB-9   天衝 *tiān chòng*
Celestial Pillar BL-10   天柱 *tiān zhù*
Celestial Pivot ST-25   天樞 *tiān shū*
Celestial Pool PC-1   天池 *tiān chí*
Celestial Ravine SP-18   天谿 *tiān xī*
Celestial Spring PC-2   天泉 *tiān quán*
Celestial Storehouse LU-3   天府 *tiān fǔ*
Celestial Tripod LI-17   天鼎 *tiān dǐng*
Celestial Well TB-10   天井 *tiān jǐng*
Celestial Window SI-16   天窗 *tiān chuāng*
Celestial Window TB-16   天牖 *tiān yǒu*
Center Palace CV-16   中庭 *zhōng tíng*
Central Backbone Shu BL-29   中膂俞 *zhōng lǔ shū*
Central Bone-Hole BL-33   中髎 *zhōng liáo*
Central Flow KI-15   中注 *zhōng zhù*
Central Hub PC-9   中衝 *zhōng chōng*
Central Islet TB-3   中渚 *zhōng zhǔ*
Central Metropolis LV-6   中都 *zhōng dū*
Central Pivot GV-7   中樞 *zhōng shū*
Central Pole CV-3   中極 *zhōng jí*
Central River GB-32   中瀆 *zhōng dú*
Central Shoulder Shu SI-15   肩中俞 *jiān zhōng shū*

Central Treasury LU-1 中府 *zhōng fǔ*
Central Venter CV-12 中脘 *zhōng wǎn*
Channel Ditch LU-8 經渠 *jīng qú*
Cheek Bone-Hole SI-18 顴髎 *quán liáo*
Chest Center CV-17 膻中 *dàn zhōng*
Chest Village SP-19 胸鄉 *xiōng xiāng*
Clear Cold Abyss TB-11 清冷淵 *qīng lěng yuān*
Cleft Gate PC-4 郄門 *xī mén*
Cloud Gate LU-2 雲門 *yún mén*
Collection Hole LU-6 孔最 *kǒng zuì*
Completion Bone GB-12 完骨 *wán gǔ*
Connecting Li HT-5 通里 *tōng lǐ*
Convergence and Gathering TB-7 會宗 *huì zōng*
Corridor Walk KI-22 步廊 *bù láng*
Crooked Wall SI-13 曲垣 *qū yuán*
Crouching Rabbit ST-32 伏兔 *fú tù*
Cubit Marsh LU-5 尺澤 *chǐ zé*
Curved Bone CV-2 曲骨 *qū gǔ*
Cyan Spirit HT-2 青靈 *qīng líng*
Cycle Gate LV-14 期門 *qí mén*
Dark Gate KI-21 幽門 *yōu mén*
Declining Connection BL-8 絡卻 *luò què*
Deviating Turn BL-4 曲差 *qū chā*
Diaphragm Pass BL-46 膈關 *gé guān*
Diaphragm Shu BL-17 膈俞 *gé shū*
Dispersing Riverbed TB-12 消濼 *xiāo luò*
Ear Gate TB-21 耳門 *ěr mén*
Earth Fivefold Convergence GB-42 地五會 *dì wǔ huì*
Earth Granary ST-4 地倉 *dì cāng*
Earth's Crux SP-8 地機 *dì jī*
Elbow Bone-Hole LI-12 肘髎 *zhǒu liáo*
Empty Basin ST-12 缺盆 *quē pén*
Extending Vessel BL-62 申脈 *shēn mài*
Extremity of Yang GV-9 至陽 *zhì yáng*
Extremity of the Mouth GV-27 兌端 *duì duān*
Eye Window GB-16 目窗 *mù chuāng*
Eyebrow Ascension BL-3 眉衝 *méi chōng*
Fifth Pivot GB-27 五樞 *wǔ shū*
Fifth Place BL-5 五處 *wǔ chù*
Fish Border LU-10 魚際 *yú jì*

Floating White GB-10   浮白 *fú bái*
Florid Canopy CV-20   華蓋 *huá gài*
Fontanel Meeting GV-22   囟會 *xìn huì*
Food Hole SP-17   食竇 *shí dòu*
Foot Five Li LV-10   足五里 *zú wǔ lǐ*
Foot Overlooking Tears GB-41   足臨泣 *zú lín qì*
Foot Portal Yin GB-44   足竅陰 *zú qiào yīn*
Forehead Fullness GB-4   頷厭 *hàn yàn*
Four Rivers TB-9   四瀆 *sì dú*
Four Whites ST-2   四白 *sì bái*
Fourfold Fullness KI-14   四滿 *sì mǎn*
Front Valley SI-2   前谷 *qián gǔ*
Gallbladder Shu BL-19   膽俞 *dǎn shū*
Gao Huang Shu BL-43   膏肓俞 *gāo huāng shū*
Gate of Abundance BL-37   殷門 *yīn mén*
Girdling Vessel GB-26   帶脈 *dài mài*
Governing Shu BL-16   督俞 *dū shū*
Grain Bone-Hole LI-19   禾髎 *hé liáo*
Grasping the Wind SI-12   秉風 *bǐng fēng*
Great Abyss LU-9   太淵 *tài yuān*
Great Bone LI-16   巨骨 *jù gǔ*
Great Bone-Hole ST-3   巨髎 *jù liáo*
Great Embracement SP-21   大包 *dà bāo*
Great Gigantic ST-27   大巨 *dà jù*
Great Hammer GV-14 大椎 *dà zhuī*
Great Horizontal SP-15   大橫 *dà hèng*
Great Manifestation KI-12   大赫 *dà hè*
Great Metropolis SP-2   大都 *dà dū*
Great Mound PC-7 大陵 *dà líng*
Great Ravine KI-3   太谿 *tài xī*
Great Reception ST-5   大迎 *dà yíng*
Great Shuttle BL-11   大杼 *dà zhù*
Great Tower Gate CV-14   巨闕 *jù què*
Guarding White LU-4   俠白 *xiá bái*
Guest House KI-9   築賓 *zhú bīn*
Gum Intersection GV-28   齦交 *yín jiāo*
Gushing Spring KI-1   涌泉 *yǒng quǎn*
Harmony Bone-Hole TB-22 和髎 *hé liáo*
Head Corner ST-8 頭維 *tóu wéi*
Head Overlooking Tears GB-15   頭臨泣 *tóu lín qì*

Head Portal Yin GB-11   頭竅陰 *tóu qiào yīn*
Heart Shu BL-15   心俞 *xīn shū*
Hidden White SP-1   隱白 *yǐn bái*
Highest Spring HT-1   極泉 *jí quán*
Hill Ruins GB-40   丘墟 *qiū xū*
Huang Gate BL-51   肓門 *huāng mén*
Huang Shu KI-16   肓俞 *huāng shū*
Humor Gate TB-2   液門 *yè mén*
Hun Gate BL-47   魂門 *hún mén*
Hundred Convergences GV-20   百會 *bǎi huì*
Inner Court ST-44   內庭 *nèi tíng*
Inner Pass PC-6   內關 *nèi guān*
Instep Yang BL-59   跗陽 *fū yáng*
Interior Strengthening CV-11   建里 *jiàn lǐ*
Intermediary Courier PC-5   間使 *jiān shǐ*
Intersection Reach KI-8   交信 *jiāo xìn*
Jade Hall CV-18   玉堂 *yù táng*
Jade Pillow BL-9   玉枕 *yù zhěn*
Jade Pivot CV-21   璇璣 *xuán jī*
Jawbone ST-6 頰車 *jiá chē*
Jue Yin Shu BL-14   厥陰俞 *jué yīn shū*
Jumping Round GB-30   環跳 *huán tiào*
Kidney Shu BL-23   腎俞 *shèn shū*
Kiln Path GV-13   陶道 *táo dào*
Knee Joint LV-7   膝關 *xī guān*
Knee Yang Joint GB-33   膝陽關 *xī yáng guān*
Kunlun Mountains BL-60   昆侖 *kūn lún*
Large Goblet KI-4   大鐘 *dà zhōng*
Large Intestine Shu BL-25   大腸俞 *dà cháng shū*
Large Pile LV-1   大敦 *dà dūn*
Leaking Valley SP-7   漏谷 *lòu gǔ*
Leg Three Li ST-36   足三里 *zú sān lǐ*
Lesser Mansion HT-8   少府 *shào fǔ*
Lesser Marsh SI-1   少澤 *shào zé*
Lesser Sea HT-3   少海 *shào hǎi*
Lesser Shang LU-11   少商 *shào shāng*
Lesser Surge HT-9   少沖 *shào chōng*
Life Gate GV-4   命門 *mìng mén*
Light Guard BL-6   承光 *chéng guāng*
Linking Path GB-28   維道 *wéi dào*

Lively Center KI-26 彧中 *yù zhōng*
Liver Shu BL-18 肝俞 *gān shū*
Long Strong GV-1 長強 *cháng qiáng*
Lower Bone-Hole BL-34 下髎 *xià liáo*
Lower Great Hollow ST-39 下巨虛 *xià jù xū*
Lower Ridge LI-8 下廉 *xià lián*
Lower Venter CV-10 下脘 *xià wǎn*
Lumbar Shu GV-2 腰俞 *yāo shū*
Lumbar Yang Pass GV-3 腰陽關 *yāo yáng guān*
Lung Shu BL-13 肺俞 *fèi shū*
Man's Prognosis ST-9 人迎 *rén yíng*
Marsh at the Bend PC-3 曲澤 *qū zé*
Meeting of Yang BL-35 會陽 *huì yáng*
Meeting of Yin CV-1 會陰 *huì yīn*
Metal Gate BL-63 金門 *jīn mén*
Mound Center LV-4 中封 *zhōng fēng*
Mountain Support BL-57 承山 *chéng shān*
Moving Between LV-2 行間 *xíng jiān*
Mute's Gate GV-15 啞門 *yǎ mén*
Not Contained ST-19 不容 *bù róng*
Nursing the Aged SI-6 養老 *yǎng lǎo*
Open Valley KI-20 通谷(腹) *tōng gǔ (fù)*
Origin Pass CV-4 關元 *guān yuán*
Origin Pass Shu BL-26 關元俞 *guān yuán shū*
Outer Hill GB-36 外丘 *wài qiū*
Outer Mound ST-26 外陵 *wài líng*
Outer Pass TB-5 外關 *wài guān*
Outer Shoulder Shu SI-14 肩外俞 *jiān wài shū*
Palace of Toil PC-8 勞宮 *láo gōng*
Pass Gate ST-22 關門 *guān mén*
Passage Hub TB-1 關衝 *guān chōng*
Pinched Ravine GB-43 俠谿 *xiá xī*
Po Door BL-42 魄戶 *pò hù*
Pool at the Bend LI-11 曲池 *qū chí*
Protuberance Assistant LI-18 扶突 *fú tú*
Pubic Bone KI-11 橫骨 *héng gǔ*
Pupil Bone-Hole GB-1 瞳子髎 *tóng zǐ liáo*
Purple Palace CV-19 紫宮 *zǐ gōng*
Qi Abode ST-11 氣舍 *qì shè*
Qi Door ST-13 氣戶 *qì hù*

Qi Point   KI-13   氣穴   *qì xuè*
Ravine Divide   ST-41   解谿   *jiě xī*
Reaching Yin   BL-67   至陰   *zhì yīn*
Recover Flow   KI-7   復溜   *fù liū*
Reflection Abode   BL-49   意舍   *yì shè*
Return   ST-29   歸來   *guī lái*
Ribbon Opening   ST-38   條口   *tiáo kǒu*
Ridge Spring   CV-23   廉泉   *lián quán*
Roof   ST-15   屋翳   *wū yì*
Root Spirit   GB-13   本神   *běn shén*
Sauce Receptacle   CV-24   承漿   *chéng jiāng*
Sea of Blood   SP-10   血海   *xuè hǎi*
Sea of Qi   CV-6   氣海   *qì hǎi*
Sea-of-Qi Shu   BL-24   氣海俞   *qì hǎi shū*
Second Bone-Hole   BL-32   次髎   *cì liáo*
Second Space   LI-2   二間   *èr jiān*
Sequential Limit   BL-54   秩邊   *zhì biān*
Severe Mouth   ST-45   厲兌   *lì duì*
Shang Bend   KI-17   商曲   *shāng qū*
Shang Hill   SP-5   商丘   *shāng qiū*
Shang Yang   LI-1   商陽   *shāng yáng*
Shining Sea   KI-6   照海   *zhào hǎi*
Shoulder Bone   LI-15   肩髃   *jiān yú*
Shoulder Bone-Hole   TB-14   肩髎   *jiān liáo*
Shoulder Well   GB-21   肩井   *jiān jǐng*
Shu Mansion   KI-27   俞府   *shū fǔ*
Silk Bamboo Hole   TB-23   絲竹空   *sī zhú kōng*
Sinew Contraction   GV-8   筋縮   *jīn suō*
Sinew Seat   GB-23   輒筋   *zhé jīn*
Sinew Support   BL-56   承筋   *chéng jīn*
Skull Rest   TB-19   顱息   *lú xí*
Slippery Flesh Gate   ST-24   滑肉門   *huá ròu mén*
Small Intestine Shu   BL-27   小腸俞   *xiǎo cháng shū*
Small Sea   SI-8   小海   *xiǎo hǎi*
Spasm Vessel   TB-18   瘈脈   *chì mài*
Spinal Center   GV-6   脊中   *jǐ zhōng*
Spirit Court   GV-24   神庭   *shén tíng*
Spirit Gate   HT-7   神門   *shén mén*
Spirit Gate   CV-8   神闕   *shén què*
Spirit Hall   BL-44   神堂   *shén táng*

Spirit Path GV-11   神道 *shén dào*
Spirit Pathway HT-4   靈道 *líng dào*
Spirit Ruins KI-24   靈墟 *líng xū*
Spirit Seal KI-23   神封 *shén fēng*
Spirit Storehouse KI-25   神藏 *shén cáng*
Spirit Support GB-18   承靈 *chéng líng*
Spirit Tower GV-10   靈台 *líng tái*
Spleen Shu BL-20   脾俞 *pí shū*
Spring at the Bend LV-8   曲泉 *qū quán*
Squatting Bone-Hole GB-29   居髎 *jū liáo*
Stomach Granary BL-50   胃倉 *wèi cāng*
Stomach Shu BL-21   胃俞 *wèi shū*
Stone Gate CV-5   石門 *shí mén*
Stone Pass KI-18   石關 *shí guān*
Storeroom ST-14   庫房 *kù fáng*
Subservient Visitor BL-61   僕參 *pú cān*
Sun and Moon GB-24   日月 *rì yuè*
Sunken Valley ST-43   陷谷 *xiàn gǔ*
Superficial Cleft BL-38   浮郄 *fú xī*
Support BL-36   承扶 *chéng fú*
Supreme Surge LV-3   太沖 *tài chōng*
Supreme Unity ST-23   太乙 *tài yǐ*
Supreme White SP-3   太白 *tài bái*
Surging Gate SP-12   沖門 *chōng mén*
Surging Qi ST-30   氣沖 *qì chōng*
Surging Yang ST-42   沖陽 *chōng yáng*
Suspended Bell GB-39   懸鐘 *xuán zhōng*
Suspended Pivot GV-5   懸樞 *xuán shū*
Suspended Skull GB-5   懸顱 *xuán lú*
Suspended Tuft GB-6   懸厘 *xuán lí*
Taking Flight BL-58   飛揚 *fēi yáng*
Tear Container ST-1   承泣 *chéng qì*
Temporal Hairline Curve GB-7   曲鬢 *qū bìn*
Thigh Joint ST-31   髀關 *bì guān*
Third Space LI-3   三間 *sān jiān*
Three Yang Connection TB-8   三陽絡 *sān yáng luò*
Three Yin Intersection SP-6   三陰交 *sān yīn jiāo*
Triple Burner Shu BL-22   三焦俞 *sān jiāo shū*
True Shoulder SI-9   肩眞 *jiān zhēn*
Turtledove Tail CV-15   鳩尾 *jiū wěi*

Union Valley LI-4 合谷 *hé gǔ*
Unyielding Space GV-18 強間 *qiáng jiān*
Upper Arm LI-14 臂臑 *bì nào*
Upper Arm Convergence TB-13 臑會 *nào huì*
Upper Arm Shu SI-10 臑俞 *nào shū*
Upper Bone-Hole BL-31 上髎 *shàng liáo*
Upper Gate GB-3 上關 *shàng guān*
Upper Great Hollow ST-37 上巨虛 *shàng jù xū*
Upper Ridge LI-9 上廉 *shàng lián*
Upper Star GV-23 上星 *shàng xīng*
Upper Venter CV-13 上脘 *shàng wǎn*
Upright Construction GB-17 正營 *zhèng yíng*
Urgent Pulse LV-12 急脈 *jí mài*
Valley Lead GB-8 率谷 *shuài gǔ*
Valley Passage BL-66 通谷 *tōng gǔ*
Veering Passageway LI-6 偏歷 *piān lì*
Warm Dwelling LI-7 溫溜 *wēn liù*
Water Divide CV-9 水分 *shuǐ fēn*
Water Prominence ST-10 水突 *shuǐ tú*
Water Spring KI-5 水泉 *shuǐ quán*
Water Trough GV-26 水溝 *shuǐ gōu*
Waterway ST-28 水道 *shuǐ dào*
Welcome Fragrance LI-20 迎香 *yíng xiāng*
White Bone-Hole GV-25 素髎 *sù liáo*
White Ring Shu BL-30 白環俞 *bái huán shū*
Will Chamber BL-52 志室 *zhì shì*
Wind Gate BL-12 風門 *fēng mén*
Wind Mansion GV-16 風府 *fēng fǔ*
Wind Market GB-31 風市 *fēng shì*
Wind Pool GB-20 風池 *fēng chí*
Wind Screen TB-17 翳風 *yì fēng*
Winnower Gate SP-11 箕門 *jī mén*
Woodworm Canal LV-5 蠡溝 *lǐ gōu*
Wrist Bone SI-4 腕骨 *wàn gǔ*
Yang Assistance GB-38 陽輔 *yáng fǔ*
Yang Headrope BL-48 陽綱 *yáng gāng*
Yang Intersection GB-35 陽交 *yáng jiāo*
Yang Mound Spring GB-34 陽陵泉 *yáng líng quán*
Yang Pool TB-4 陽池 *yáng chí*
Yang Ravine LI-5 陽谿 *yáng xī*

Yang Union   BL-55   合陽   *hé yáng*
Yang Valley   SI-5   陽谷   *yáng gǔ*
Yang White   GB-14   陽白   *yáng bái*
Yellow Emperor   SP-4   公孫   *gōng sūn*
Yi Xi   BL-45   譩譆   *yì xī*
Yin Bladder   LV-9   陰包   *yīn bāo*
Yin Cleft   HT-6   陰郄   *yīn xī*
Yin Corner   LV-11   陰廉   *yīn lián*
Yin Intersection   CV-7   陰交   *yīn jiāo*
Yin Market   ST-33   陰市   *yīn shì*
Yin Metropolis   KI-19   陰都   *yīn dū*
Yin Mound Spring   SP-9   陰陵泉   *yīn líng quán*
Yin Valley   KI-10   陰谷   *yīn gǔ*

Index Two

Pinyin List of Primary and Alternate Acupoint Names

Alternate names are marked with an asterisk.

bié yáng 別陽 TB-4   *Divergent Yang**
bìn bǔ 髕骨 GB-30   *Kneecap**
bìn gǔ 臏骨 GB-30   *Kneecap**
bǐng fēng 秉風 SI-12   *Grasping the Wind*
bó jǐng 膊井 GB-21   *Shoulder Well**
bó yāng 脖胦 CV-6   *Navel**
bó yāng 脖胦 CV-4   *Navel**
bǔ yuán 補元 ST-25   *Origin Supplementer**
bù láng 步郎 KI-22   *Walking Gentleman**
bù láng 步廊 KI-22   *Corridor Walk*
bù róng 不容 ST-19   *Not Contained*
cáo xī 曹谿 GV-16   *Cao's Ravine**
cáo xī lù 曹溪路 GV-1   *Cao's Ravine Road**
chǎn mén 產門 CV-4   *Delivery Gate**
chāng yáng 昌陽 KI-7   *Glorious Yang**
cháng āi 腸哀 SP-16   *Intestinal Lament**
cháng gǔ 長穀 ST-25   *Long Grain**
cháng huì 長顀 LI-19   *Long Plate**
cháng jī 長雞 ST-25   *Long Chicken**
cháng jiá 長頰 LI-19   *Long Cheek**
cháng jié 腸結 SP-14   *Intestinal Bind**
cháng liáo 長窌 LI-19   *Long Bone-Hole**
cháng liáo 長膠 LI-19   *Long Bone-Hole**
cháng pín 長頻 LI-19   *Long Shore**
cháng píng 長平 LV-13   *Long Level**
cháng qiáng 長強 GV-1   *Long Strong*
cháng qū 腸屈 SP-16   *Intestinal Bend**
cháng shān 腸山 BL-57   *Intestine Mountain**
cháng wéi 長維 ST-25   *Long Link**
cháng xī 長谿 ST-25   *Long Ravine**
cháng zhuŏ 長頵 LI-19   *Long Cheek**
cháo tiān diān 朝天巔 GV-1
             *Heavenward Looking Summit**
chén qì 塵氣 GV-12   *Dust Qi**
chéng fú 承扶 BL-36   *Support*
chéng fú pí bù 承扶皮部 BL-36   *Skin Region Support**
chéng guāng 承光 BL-6   *Light Guard*
chéng jiāng 承漿 CV-24   *Sauce Receptacle*
chéng jīn 承筋 BL-56   *Sinew Support*
chéng líng 承靈 GB-18   *Spirit Support*

chéng mǎn 承滿 ST-20   *Assuming Fullness*
chéng mìng 承命 SP-6   *Life Support**
chéng qì 承泣 ST-1   *Tear Container*
chéng shān 承山 BL-57   *Mountain Support*
chí shū 持樞 CV-4   *Junior Pivot**
chí tóu 池頭 LI-7   *Pool's Head**
chǐ gài 尺蓋 ST-12   *Cubit Cover**
chǐ zé 尺澤 LU-5   *Cubit Marsh*
chì mài 瘈脈 TB-18   *Spasm Vessel*
chōng mén 沖門 SP-12   *Surging Gate*
chōng yáng 沖陽 LI-20   *Surging Yang**
chōng yáng 沖陽 ST-42   *Surging Yang*
chōng yáng 衝陽 LI-20   *Thoroughfare Yang**
chuài cháng 腨腸 BL-56   *Calf Intestine**
chuài cháng 腨腸 KI-9   *Calf Intestine**
chuāng lóng 窗龍 SI-16   *Window Dragon**
chuāng lóng 窗籠 SI-16   *Window Basket**
chuāng sǒng 窗聳 SI-16   *Lofty Window**
chuí jiāng 垂漿 CV-4   *Fallen Sauce**
chún shàng duān 唇上端 GV-27
     Upper Extremity of the Lip*
cī gōng 慈宮 SP-12   *Palace of Charity**
cì liáo 次髎 BL-32   *Second Bone-Hole*
cì mén 次門 CV-4   *Second Gate**
dà bāo 大包 SP-21   *Great Embracement*
dà bāo 大胞 SP-21   *Great Bladder**
dà cháng mù 大腸募 ST-25   *Large Intestine Mu**
dà cháng shū 大腸俞 BL-25   *Large Intestine Shu*
dà chōng 大沖 LV-3   *Large Surge**
dà dū 大都 SP-2   *Great Metropolis*
dà dūn 大敦 LV-1   *Large Pile*
dà gǔ 大骨 BL-64   *Large Bone**
dà hǎi 大海 CV-4   *Great Sea**
dà hè 大赫 KI-12   *Great Manifestation*
dà héng 大橫 SP-15   *Great Horizontal*
dà jìn 大禁 LI-13   *Great Prohibition**
dà jù 大巨 ST-27   *Great Gigantic*
dà kùn 大涃 CV-4   *Great Reservoir**
dà líng 大陵 PC-7   *Great Mound*
dà shùn 大順 LV-1   *Great Favorableness**

dà yīn 大陰 LV-6　*Great Yin**
dà yīn 大陰 SP-6　*Great Yin**
dà yíng 大迎 ST-5　*Great Reception*
dà yǔ 大羽 GV-18　*Great Feather**
dà zhōng 大鐘 KI-4　*Large Goblet*
dà zhōng jí 大中極 CV-4　*Great Central Pole**
dà zhù 大杼 BL-11　*Great Shuttle**
dà zhuī 大椎 GV-14　*Great Hammer*
dài mài 帶脈 GB-26　*Girdling Vessel*
dān tiān 丹田 CV-7　*Cinnabar Field**
dān tián 丹田 CV-4　*Cinnabar Field**
dān tián 丹田 CV-5　*Cinnabar Field**
dǎn mù 膽募 GB-23　*Gallbladder Mu**
dǎn mù 膽募 GB-24　*Gallbladder Mu**
dǎn shū 膽俞 BL-19　*Gallbladder Shu*
dàn zhōng 膻中 CV-17　*Chest Center*
dāng rǔ 當乳 ST-17　*On the Nipple**
dǐ gǔ 骶骨 GV-1　*Sacral Bone**
dǐ shàng 骶上 GV-1　*Sacrum Above**
dì cāng 地倉 ST-4　*Earth Granary*
dì chōng 地沖 KI-1　*Earth Surge**
dì chōng 地衝 KI-1　*Earth Thoroughfare**
dì jī 地箕 SP-8　*Earth Winnower**
dì jī 地機 SP-8　*Earth's Crux*
dì wǔ 地五 GB-42　*Earth Five**
dì wǔ huì 地五會 GB-42　*Earth Fivefold Convergence*
diān shàng 巔上 GV-20　*Mountain Top**
dié yáng 跌陽 ST-42　*Unrestrained Yang**
dǐng mén 頂門 GV-22　*Vertex Gate**
dū shū 督俞 BL-16　*Governing Shu*
dú bí 犢鼻 ST-35　*Calf's Nose*
duàn jiāo 斷交 GV-28　*Extremity Intersection**
duì chōng 兌衝 HT-7　*Protuberant Hub**
duì duān 兌端 GV-27　*Extremity of the Mouth*
duì gǔ 兌骨 HT-7　*Protuberant Bone**
duì gǔ 兌骨 HT-8　*Protuberant Bone**
duì gǔ 兌骨 SI-18　*Mouth Bone**
duì tōng duì 兌通兌 GV-27　*Mouth Means Edge**
duì zhōng 兌中 HT-7　*Protuberance**
duō suǒ wén 多所聞 SI-19　*More Heard**

ěr hé liǎo 耳和髎 TB-22 *Ear Harmony Bone-Hole**
ěr mén 耳門 TB-21 *Ear Gate*
èr jiān 二間 LI-2 *Second Space*
fǎ jì 髮際 GV-24 *Hairline**
fáng liáo 肪髎 LV-13 *Lard Bone-Hole**
fēi hǔ 飛虎 TB-6 *Flying Tiger**
fēi yáng 飛揚 BL-58 *Taking Flight*
fēi yáng 飛陽 BL-58 *Flying Yang**
fèi dǐ 肺底 GV-9 *Bottom of the Lung**
fèi mù 肺募 LU-1 *Lung Mu**
fèi shū 肺俞 BL-13 *Lung Shu*
fēn jiān 分間 GB-38 *Parting Space**
fēn ròu 分肉 GB-38 *Parting of the Flesh**
fēn shuǐ 分水 CV-9 *Divided Waters**
fēn zhōng 分中 GB-30 *Divided Center**
fēng chí 風池 GB-20 *Wind Pool*
fēng fǔ 風府 BL-12 *Wind Mansion**
fēng fǔ 風府 GV-16 *Wind Mansion*
fēng lóng 豐隆 ST-40 *Bountiful Bulge*
fēng mén 風門 BL-12 *Wind Gate*
fēng shì 風市 GB-31 *Wind Market*
fū yáng 跗陽 BL-59 *Instep Yang*
fú bái 伏白 KI-7 *Deep-Lying White**
fú bái 浮白 GB-10 *Floating White*
fú jiù 伏臼 KI-7 *Deep-Lying Mortar**
fú tú 扶突 LI-18 *Protuberance Assistant*
fú tù 伏兔 ST-32 *Crouching Rabbit*
fú xī 浮郄 BL-38 *Superficial Cleft*
fǔ shè 府舍 SP-13 *Bowel Abode*
fǔ zhōng shū 府中俞 LU-1 *Treasury Center Shu**
fùāi 腹哀 SP-16 *Abdominal Lament*
fù bái 復白 KI-7 *Returning White**
fù chū 腹出 SP-14 *Abdominal Exit**
fù fēn 附分 BL-41 *Attached Branch*
fù jié 腹結 SP-14 *Abdominal Bind*
fù kū 腹窟 SP-14 *Abdominal Hole**
fù liū 復溜 KI-7 *Recover Flow*
fù qū 腹屈 SP-14 *Abdominal Bend**
fù yáng 付陽 BL-59 *Give Yang**
fù yáng 附陽 BL-59 *Yang Attachment**

gān mù 肝募 LV-14   *Liver Mu**
gān shū 肝俞 BL-18   *Liver Shu*
gāo gài 高蓋 BL-16   *High Cover**
gāo gài 高蓋 BL-23   *High Cover**
gāo huāng shū 膏肓俞 BL-43   *Gao Huang Shu*
gāo qū 高曲 KI-17   *High Bend**
gāo yì 高益 BL-16   *High Boost**
gé guān 膈關 BL-46 (B-41)   *Diaphragm Pass*
gé shū 膈俞 BL-17   *Diaphragm Shu*
gōng sūn 公孫 SP-4   *Yellow Emperor*
gǔ dǐ 骨骶 GV-1   *Sacral Bone**
gǔ mén 谷門 ST-25   *Valley Gate**
gǔ mén 穀門 ST-2   *Grain Gate**
guān chōng 關衝 TB-1   *Passage Hub*
guān liáng 關梁 BL-63   *Gate Beam**
guān líng 關陵 GB-33   *Joint Mound**
guān mén 關門 ST-22   *Pass Gate*
guān yáng 關陽 GB-33   *Joint Yang**
guān yuán 關元 CV-4   *Origin Pass*
guān yuán 關原 CV-4   *Source Pass**
guān yuán shū 關元俞 BL-26   *Origin Pass Shu*
guāng míng 光明 GB-37   *Bright Light*
guī lái 歸來 ST-29   *Return*
guī wěi 龜尾 GV-1   *Tortoise Tail**
guī wěi cháng jiāng 龜尾長彊 GV-1
         *Tortoise Tail Long Border**
guǐ cáng 鬼藏 CV-1   *Ghost Store**
guǐ chén 鬼臣 LI-11   *Ghost Minister**
guǐ chuáng 鬼床 ST-4   *Ghost Bed**
guǐ chuáng 鬼床 ST-6   *Ghost Bed**
guǐ gōng 鬼宮 GV-26   *Ghost Palace**
guǐ kè tīng 鬼客廳 GV-26   *Ghost Reception Room**
guǐ kū 鬼窟 PC-8   *Ghost Cave**
guǐ lěi 鬼壘 SP-1   *Ghost Pile**
guǐ lín 鬼林 GV-16   *Ghost Forest**
guǐ lín 鬼林 ST-6   *Ghost Forest**
guǐ lù 鬼路 BL-62   *Ghost Road**
guǐ lù 鬼路 PC-5   *Ghost Road**
guǐ lù 鬼路 PC-8   *Ghost Road**
guǐ mén 鬼門 GV-22   *Ghost Gate**

guǐ shì	鬼市	CV-24	*Ghost Market* *
guǐ shì	鬼市	GV-26	*Ghost Market* *
guǐ shòu	鬼受	LU-5	*Ghost Endurance* *
guǐ táng	鬼堂	GV-23	*Ghost Hall* *
guǐ táng	鬼堂	LU-5	*Ghost Hall* *
guǐ tuǐ	鬼腿	LI-11	*Ghost Leg* *
guǐ xié	鬼邪	LI-10	*Ghost Evil* *
guǐ xié	鬼邪	ST-36	*Ghost Evil* *
guǐ xīn	鬼心	LU-10	*Ghost Heart* *
guǐ xīn	鬼心	PC-7	*Ghost Heart* *
guǐ xìn	鬼信	LU-11	*Ghost Sincerity* *
guǐ xuè	鬼穴	GV-16	*Ghost Hole* *
guǐ yǎn	鬼眼	SP-1	*Ghost Eye* *
guǐ zhěn	鬼枕	GV-16	*Ghost Pillow* *
hǎi dǐ*	海底	CV-1	*Seabed* *
hán fǔ	寒府	GB-33	*Cold Mansion* *
hán kǒu	含口	LI-4	*Holding Mouth* *
hàn yàn	頷厭	GB-4	*Forehead Fullness*
hé chē lù	河車路	GV-1	*River Cart Road* *
hé gān	髑骭	CV-15	*Breast Bone* *
hé gǔ	合谷	LI-4	*Union Valley*
hé gǔ	合骨	LI-4	*Uniting Bones* *
hé hé	髑髑	CV-15	*Breast Bone* *
hé kōng	和空	TB-22	*Harmony Hollow* *
hé liáo	禾髎	TB-22	*Grain Bone-Hole* *
hé liáo	禾髎	LI-19	*Grain Bone-Hole*
hé liáo	和髎	TB-22	*Harmony Bone-Hole*
hé lú	合顱	GV-17	*Skull Union* *
hé yáng	合陽	BL-55	*Yang Union*
hè dǐng	鶴頂	ST-34	*Crane Top* *
héng gǔ	橫骨	KI-11	*Pubic Bone*
héng hù	橫戶	CV-7	*Horizontal Door* *
héng shé	橫舌	GV-15	*Opposite the Tongue* *
hóu zhōng	喉中	CV-23	*Larynx Center* *
hòu dǐng	後頂	GV-19	*Behind the Vertex*
hòu guān	後關	GB-2	*Hind Gate* *
hòu qū	後曲	GB-1	*Hind Curve* *
hòu xī	後谿	SI-3	*Back Ravine*
hòu zhāng mén	後章門	LV-13	*Rear Camphorwood Gate* *

hǔ kǒu 虎口 LI-4　　*Tiger's Mouth**
huá gài 華蓋 CV-20　*Florid Canopy*
huá ròu mén 滑肉門 ST-24　*Slippery Flesh Gate*
huá yōu mén 滑幽門 ST-24　*Slippery Dark Gate**
huán gǔ 環谷 GB-30　*Round Valley**
huán tiào 環跳 GB-30　*Jumping Round*
huāng mén 肓門 BL-51 (B-46)　*Huang Gate*
huāng shū 肓俞 KI-16　*Huang Shu*
huāng zhī yuán 肓之原 CV-4　*Huang Origin**
huāng zhī yuán 肓之原 CV-6　*Huang Origin**
huí gǔ 回骨 CV-2　*Return Bone**
huì é 會額 GV-17　*Meeting of the Forehead**
huì gǔ 會骨 ST-42　*Meeting Bones**
huì qū 會屈 ST-42　*Meeting Bend**
huì wéi 會維 ST-4　*Linking Confluence**
huì yáng 會陽 BL-35　*Meeting of Yang*
huì yīn 會陰 CV-1　*Meeting of Yin*
huì yǒng 會湧 ST-42　*Meeting Gush**
huì yuán 會原 ST-42　*Meeting Source**
huì zōng 會宗 TB-7　*Convergence and Gathering*
hún mén 魂門 BL-47 (B-42)　*Hun Gate*
huò zhōng 或中 KI-26　*Possible Center**
jī dǐng 雞頂 ST-34　*Chicken Top**
jī guān 機關 GB-2　*Hinge**
jī guān 機關 ST-6　*Hinge**
jī mén 箕門 SP-11　*Winnower Gate*
jí mài 急脈 LV-12　*Urgent Pulse*
jí quán 極泉 HT-1　*Highest Spring*
jǐ dǐ duān 脊骶端 GV-1
　　　　　*End of the Sacral Spine**
jǐ nèi shū 脊內俞 BL-29　*Spine Inner Shu**
jǐ shū 脊俞 GV-6　*Spine Shu**
jǐ zhōng 脊中 GV-6　*Spinal Center*
jǐ zhù 脊柱 GV-6　*Spine Pillar**
jì lè 季肋 LV-13　*Free Ribs**
jì xié 季脅 LV-13　*Free Ribs**
jì yāng 季胦 CV-6　*Small Navel**
jiā bái 夾白 LU-4　*Pinching White**
jiā xī 夾谿 GB-42　*Pinched Ravine**
jiá chē 頰車 ST-6　*Jawbone*

jiān gǔ 間谷 LI-2 *Space Valley**
jiān jiān 肩尖 LI-15 *Shoulder Tip**
jiān jǐng 肩井 GB-21 *Shoulder Well*
jiān liáo 肩髎 TB-14 *Shoulder Bone-Hole*
jiān shǐ 間使 PC-5 *Intermediary Courier*
jiān wài shū 肩外俞 SI-14 *Outer Shoulder Shu*
jiān yú 肩髃 LI-15 *Shoulder Bone*
jiān zhēn 肩眞 SI-9 *True Shoulder*
jiān zhōng shū 肩中俞 SI-15
        Central Shoulder Shu
jiàn lǐ 建里 CV-11 *Interior Strengthening*
jiāo chōng 交沖 GV-19 *Intersection Surge**
jiāo chōng 交衝 GV-19 *Intersection Hub**
jiāo xìn 交信 KI-8 *Intersection Reach*
jiāo yí 交儀 LV-5 *Intersection Apparatus**
jiǎo sūn 角孫 TB-20 *Angle Vertex*
jiě xī 解谿 ST-41 *Ravine Divide*
jīn huì 筋會 GB-34 *Sinew Convergence**
jīn mén 金門 CV-1 *Metal Gate**
jīn mén 金門 BL-63 *Metal Gate*
jīn shù 筋束 GV-8 *Sinew Binder**
jīn suō 筋縮 GV-8 *Sinew Contraction*
jīng gōng 精宮 BL-52 *Palace of Essence**
jīng gōng 精宮 GV-4 *Palace of Essence**
jīng gǔ 京骨 BL-64 *Capital Bone*
jīng lù 精露 CV-4 *Essential Dew**
jīng lù 精露 CV-5 *Essential Dew**
jīng mén 京門 GB-25 *Capital Gate*
jīng míng 睛明 BL-1 *Bright Eyes*
jīng míng 精明 BL-1 *Bright Essence**
jīng qú 經渠 LU-8 *Channel Ditch*
jīng shǐ 經始 HT-9 *Channel Start**
jǐng chōng 頸沖 LI-14 *Neck Surge**
jǐng chōng 頸衝 LI-14 *Neck Thoroughfare**
jiū wěi 鳩尾 CV-15 *Turtledove Tail*
jū liáo 居髎 GB-29 *Squatting Bone-Hole*
jù chù 巨處 BL-5 *Great Place**
jù gǔ 巨骨 LI-16 *Great Bone*
jù liáo 巨髎 TB-23 *Giant Bone-Hole**
jù liáo 巨髎 ST-3 *Great Bone-Hole*

jù què 巨闕 CV-14　***Great Tower Gate***
jù xū 巨虛 ST-37　***Great Hollow****
jù xū shàng lián 巨虛上廉 ST-37
　　　Upper Ridge of Great Hollow*
jù xū xià lián 巨虛下廉 ST-39
　　　Lower Ridge of Great Hollow*
jué gǔ 厥骨 GV-1　***Jue Bone****
jué gǔ 絶骨 GB-38　***Severed Bone****
jué gǔ 絶骨 GB-39　***Severed Bone***
jué gǔ 橛骨 GV-1　***Peg Bone****
jué shū 厥俞 BL-14　***Jue Shu****
jué xīn 蹶心 KI-1　***Stumbling Heart****
jué yáng 厥陽 BL-58　***Jue Yang****
jué yáng 厥楊 BL-58　***Jue Poplar****
jué yáng 絶陽 LI-1　***Yang Extremity****
jué yīn shū 厥陰俞 BL-14　***Jue Yin Shu***
jué yùn 絶孕 CV-5　***Infertility****
kè wáng 客王 GB-3　***Guest King****
kè zhǔ 客主 GB-3　***Guest-Host****
kè zhǔ rén 客主人 GB-3　***Guest-Host-Person****
kǒng zuì 孔最 LU-6　***Collection Hole***
kù fáng 庫房 ST-14　***Storeroom***
kuà gǔ 骻骨 ST-34　***Hip Bone****
kuān gǔ 髖骨 GB-30　***Hip Bone****
kūn lún 昆侖 CV-4　***Kunlun Mountains****
kūn lún 昆侖 BL-60　***Kunlun Mountains***
láo gōng 勞宮 PC-8　***Palace of Toil***
lè liáo 肋髎 GB-13　***Rib Bone-Hole****
lèi kōng 淚空 BL-2　***Tear Hole****
lèi kǒng 淚孔 BL-1　***Tear Hole****
lèi qiāng 淚腔 BL-1　***Tear Cavity****
lǐ gōu 蠡溝 LV-5　***Woodworm Canal***
lì duì 厲兌 ST-45　***Severe Mouth***
lì jī 利機 BL-35　***Crux Disinhibitor****
lì jī 利機 CV-4　***Crux Disinhibitor****
lì jī 利機 CV-5　***Crux Disinhibitor****
lián quán 廉泉 CV-23　***Ridge Spring***
liáng guān 梁關 BL-63　***Beam Gate****
liáng mén 梁門 ST-21　***Beam Gate***
liáng qiū 梁丘 ST-34　***Beam Hill***

liè quē 列缺 LU-7   ***Broken Sequence***

lín qī (tóu) 臨泣 (頭) GB-15

        Overlooking Tears (head)*

lín qì (zú) 臨泣(足) GB-41   ***Overlooking Tears (Leg)****

líng dào 靈道 HT-4   ***Spirit Pathway***

líng qiáng 靈墙 KI-24   ***Spirit Wall****

líng tái 靈台 GV-10   ***Spirit Tower***

líng xū 靈墟 KI-24   ***Spirit Ruins***

lǐng shàng 嶺上 GV-20   ***Ridge Top****

lǐng shàng tiān mǎn 嶺上天滿 GV-20

        Ridge Top Celestial Fullness*

lóng hǔ 龍虎 GV-1   ***Dragon Tiger****

lóng hǔ xuè 龍虎穴 GV-1   ***Dragon and Tiger Point****

lóng quán 龍泉 KI-2   ***Dragon in the Spring****

lóng yuān 龍淵 KI-2   ***Dragon in the Abyss****

lòu gǔ 漏谷 SP-7   ***Leaking Valley***

lòu yīn 漏陰 KI-6   ***Leaky Yin****

lú xí 顱息 TB-19   ***Skull Rest***

lú xìn 顱囟 TB-19   ***Skull****

lǚ gōng 呂宮 KI-3   ***Lu Palace****

lǚ xì 呂細 KI-3   ***Small Lu****

luò què 絡卻 BL-8   ***Declining Connection***

luò xī 絡郄 BL-8   ***Connecting Cleft****

méi běn 眉本 BL-2   ***Root of the Eyebrow****

méi chōng 眉衝 BL-3   ***Eyebrow Ascension***

méi tóu 眉頭 BL-2   ***Eyebrow****

méi zhōng 眉中 BL-2   ***At the Eyebrow****

mǐ niè 米嚙 GB-5   ***Rice Bite****

mǐ niè 米嚙 GB-5   ***Rice Bite****

miàn liáo 面節 ST-1   ***Face Bone-Hole****

miàn liáo 面髎 ST-1   ***Face Bone-Hole****

miàn wáng 面王 GV-25   ***King of Face****

miàn zhèng 面正 GV-25   ***Face Center****

míng guāng 明光 BL-2   ***Bright Light****

míng táng 名堂 GV-23   ***Hall of Fame****

míng táng 明堂 GV-23   ***Bright Hall****

mìng dì 命蒂 CV-8   ***Life Stem****

mìng guān 命關 SP-17   ***Life Pass****

mìng mén 命門 CV-4   ***Life Gate****

mìng mén 命門 CV-5   ***Life Gate****

mìng mén 命門 GV-4   *Life Gate*

mù chuāng 目窗 GB-16   *Eye Window*

mù liáo 目髎 TB-23   *Eye Bone-Hole**

mù nèi zì 目内眥 BL-1   *Inner Canthus**

nǎo gài 腦蓋 BL-8   *Brain Cover**

nǎo hù 腦戶 GV-17   *Brain's Door*

nǎo kōng 腦空 GB-19   *Brain Hollow*

nào huì 臑會 TB-13   *Upper Arm Convergence*

nào jiāo 臑交 TB-13   *Upper Arm Intersection**

nào liáo 臑髎 TB-13   *Upper Arm Bone-Hole**

nào shū 臑俞 TB-13   *Upper Arm Shu**

nào shū 臑俞 SI-10   *Upper Arm Shu*

nèi guān 内關 PC-6   *Inner Pass*

nèi tíng 内庭 ST-44   *Inner Court*

nèi zì wài 内眥外 BL-1   *Outside the Inner Canthus**

ní wán gōng 泥丸宮 GV-20   *Mud Ball Palace**

nì zhù 逆注 LI-7   *Counterflow Pouring**

niào bāo 尿胞 CV-2   *Urinary Bladder**

niào shuǐ 溺水 CV-4   *Urine**

niè rú 顳顬 GB-19   *Temple Region**

páng guāng mù 膀胱募 CV-3   *Bladder Mu**

páng guāng shū 膀胱俞 BL-28   *Bladder Shu*

pí bù 皮部 BL-36   *Skin Region**

pí mù 脾募 LV-13   *Spleen Mu**

pí shè 脾舍 SP-8   *Spleen Abode**

pí shū 脾俞 BL-20   *Spleen Shu*

pí xī 皮郄 BL-36   *Skin Cleft**

piān gǔ 偏骨 LI-15   *End Bone**

piān lì 偏歷 LI-6   *Veering Passageway*

píng yì 平翳 CV-1   *Flat Screen**

píng yì 屏翳 CV-1   *Screen**

pò hù 魄戶 BL-42 (B-37)   *Po Door*

pú cān 僕參 BL-61   *Subservient Visitor*

qí mén 期門 LV-14   *Cycle Gate*

qí zhōng 臍中 CV-8   *Center of the Navel**

qì chōng 氣沖 ST-30   *Surging Qi*

qì fǔ 氣府 GB-25   *Qi Mansion**

qì hǎi 氣海 CV-4   *Sea of Qi**

qì hǎi 氣海 CV-6   *Sea of Qi*

qì hǎi shū 氣海俞 BL-24   *Sea-of-Qi Shu*

qì hé 氣合 CV-8 **Qi Union***
qì hù 氣戶 ST-13 **Qi Door**
qì jiē 氣街 ST-30 **Qi Thoroughfare***
qì shè 氣舍 CV-8 **Qi Abode***
qì shè 氣舍 ST-11 **Qi Abode**
qì shū 氣俞 GB-25 **Qi Shu***
qì xī 氣郄 GV-1 **Qi Cleft***
qì xuè 氣穴 KI-13 **Qi Point**
qì yú 氣魚 CV-3 **Qi Fish***
qì yuán 氣原 CV-3 **Qi Source***
qì zhī yīn xī 氣之陰郄 GV-1 **Yin**
qián dǐng 前頂 GV-21 **Before the Vertex**
qián gǔ 前谷 SI-2 **Front Valley**
qián guān 前關 GB-1 **Foregate***
qián tóu bǎi huì 前頭百會 GV-22

        Hundred Convergences of the Forehead*
qián zhāng mén 前章門 SP-12

        Front Camphorwood Gate*
qiáng jiān 強間 GV-18 **Unyielding Space**
qiáng yáng 強陽 BL-8 **Strong Yang***
qiào yīn (tóu) 竅陰 (頭) GB-11 **Portal Yin (head)***
qiào yīn (zú) 竅陰(足) GB-44 **Portal Yin (foot)***
qīng hào 清昊 TB-11 **Clear Sky***
qīng lěng quán 清冷泉 TB-11 **Clear Cold Spring***
qīng lěng yuān 清冷淵 TB-11 **Clear Cold Abyss**
qīng líng 青靈 HT-2 **Cyan Spirit**
qīng líng 清靈 TB-11 **Clear Spirit***
qīng líng quán 青靈泉 HT-2 **Cyan Spirit Spring***
qióng gǔ 窮骨 GV-1 **End Bone***
qiū xū 丘墟 GB-40 **Hill Ruins**
qiū xū 坵墟 GB-40 **Hill Ruins***
qū bìn 曲鬢 GB-7 **Temporal Hairline Curve**
qū chā 曲差 BL-4 **Deviating Turn**
qū chí 曲池 LI-11 **Pool at the Bend**
qū fǎ 曲髮 GB-7 **Hair Curve***
qū gǔ 曲骨 KI-11 **Curved Bone***
qū gǔ 曲骨 CV-2 **Curved Bone**
qū gǔ 屈骨 CV-2 **Crooked Bone***
qū gǔ 屈骨 KI-11 **Crooked Bone***
qū gǔ duān 曲骨端 KI-11 **Crooked Bone's End***

qū gŭ duān　曲骨端　CV-2　*Curved Bone's End**
qū gŭ duān　曲骨端　KI-11　*Curved Bone's End**
qū gŭ duān　屈骨端　CV-2　*Crooked Bone's End**
qū gŭ duān　屈骨端　KI-11　*Crooked Bone's End**
qū jié　曲節　HT-3　*Bending Joint**
qū quán　曲泉　LV-8　*Spring at the Bend*
qū yá　曲牙　ST-6　*Tooth Bend**
qū yuán　曲垣　SI-13　*Crooked Wall*
qū zé　曲澤　PC-3　*Marsh at the Bend*
quán liáo　權髎　SI-18　*Influential Bone-Hole**
quán liáo　顴髎　SI-18　*Cheek Bone-Hole*
quán yè　泉液　GB-22　*Spring Humor**
quán yè　泉腋 (涇)　GB-22　*Spring Armpit**
quē pén　缺盆　ST-12　*Empty Basin*
què shū　闕俞　BL-14　*Gate Tower Shu**
rán gŭ　然谷　KI-2　*Blazing Valley*
rán gŭ　然骨　KI-2　*Blazing Bone**
rè fŭ　熱府　BL-12　*Heat Mansion**
rè fŭ　熱府　GB-20　*Heat Mansion**
rén héng　人橫　SP-15　*Human's Horizontal**
rén yíng　人迎　ST-9　*Man's Prognosis*
rén zhōng　人中　GV-26　*Human Center*
rì yuè　日月　GB-24　*Sun and Moon*
róng zhŭ　容主　GB-3　*Generous Host**
ròu guì　肉桂　BL-57　*Fleshy Cinnamon**
ròu xī　肉郄　BL-36　*Flesh Cleft**
rŭ gēn　乳根　ST-18　*Breast Root*
rŭ zhōng　乳中　ST-17　*Breast Center*
ruì zhōng　鋭中　HT-7　*Edge**
sān fēn lú　三分閭　GV-1
　　　　　Three Fen From the Gate*
sān jiān　三間　LI-3　*Third Space*
sān jiāo mù　三焦募　CV-5　*Triple Burner Mu**
sān jiāo shū　三焦俞　BL-22　*Triple Burner Shu*
sān jié jiāo　三結交　CV-4　*Triple Intersection**
sān lĭ (shŏu)　三里(手)　LI-10　*Three Li (arm)**
sān lĭ (zú)　三里(足)　ST-36　*Three Li (leg)**
sān yáng　三陽　GV-20　*Three Yang**
sān yáng luò　三陽絡　TB-8　*Three Yang Connection*

sān yáng wǔ huì 三陽五會 (涇) GV-20
    Three Yang Fivefold Convergence*
sān yīn jiāo 三陰交 SP-6   *Three Yin Intersection*
sǎng dà 顙大 ST-8   *Forehead Large**
shāng qiū 商丘 SP-5   *Shang Hill*
shāng qiū 商坵 SP-5   *Shang Hill**
shāng qū 商曲 KI-17   *Shang Bend*
shāng shān 傷山 BL-57   *Damage Mountain**
shāng shān 傷山 GV-1   *Damage Mountain**
shāng shè 商舍 KI-17   *Shang Abode**
shāng yáng 商陽 LI-1   *Shang Yang*
shàng cí gōng 上慈宮 SP-12   *Upper Palace of Charity**
shàng guān 上關 GB-3   *Upper Gate*
shàng guǎn 上管 CV-13   *Upper Duct**
shàng jì 上紀 CV-12   *Upper Regulator**
shàng jì 上紀 CV-13   *Upper Regulator**
shàng jù xū 上巨虛 ST-37   *Upper Great Hollow*
shàng lián 上廉 ST-37   *Upper Ridge**
shàng lián 上廉 LI-9   *Upper Ridge*
shàng liáo 上髎 BL-31   *Upper Bone-Hole*
shàng mén 上門 KI-20   *Upper Gate**
shàng mén 上門 KI-21   *Upper Gate**
shàng qì hǎi 上氣海 CV-17   *Upper Sea of Qi**
shàng sān lǐ 上三里 LI-10   *Upper Three Li**
shàng tiān tī 上天梯 GV-1   *Stairway to Heaven**
shàng wǎn 上脘 CV-13   *Upper Venter*
shàng xīng 上星 GV-23   *Upper Star*
shào chōng 少沖 HT-9   *Lesser Surge*
shào chōng 少衝 HT-9   *Lesser Thoroughfare**
shào fǔ 少府 HT-8   *Lesser Mansion*
shào gǔ 少谷 LI-3   *Lesser Valley**
shào guān 少關 CV-7   *Scarce Pass**
shào hǎi 少海 HT-3   *Lesser Sea*
shào shāng 少商 LU-11   *Lesser Shang*
shào yīn xī 少陰郄 HT-6   *Shao Yin Bone-Hole**
shào yīn xī 少陰郄 HT-6   *Shao Yin Cleft**
shào zé 少澤 SI-1   *Lesser Marsh*
shé běn 舌本 CV-23   *Tongue Root**
shé běn 舌本 GV-16   *Tongue Root**
shé gēn 舌根 GV-15   *Tongue Root**

shé héng 舌橫 GV-15　*Tongue's Horizontal**
shé tóu 蛇頭 LI-7　*Snake Head**
shé yàn 舌厭 GV-15　*Tongue Repression**
shé zhǒng 舌腫 GV-15　*Tongue Swelling**
shēn mài 申脈 BL-62　*Extending Vessel*
shēn zhù 身柱 GV-12　*Body Pillar*
shén cáng 神藏 KI-25　*Spirit Storehouse*
shén dào 神道 GV-11　*Spirit Path*
shén fēng 神封 KI-23　*Spirit Seal*
shén fǔ 神府 CV-15　*Spirit Mansion**
shén guāng 神光 GB-23　*Spirit Light**
shén guāng 神光 GB-24　*Spirit Light**
shén mén 神門 HT-7　*Spirit Gate*
shén què 神闕 CV-8　*Spirit Gate*
shén táng 神堂 GV-23　*Spirit Hall**
shén táng 神堂 BL-44　*Spirit Hall*
shén tíng 神庭 GV-24　*Spirit Court*
shén zōng 神宗 GV-6　*Spirit Gathering**
shèn mù 腎募 GB-25　*Kidney Mu**
shèn qì 腎氣 SP-15　*Kidney Qi**
shèn shū 腎俞 BL-23　*Kidney Shu*
shí dòu 食竇 SP-17　*Food Hole*
shí gōng 石宮 HT-6　*Stone Palace**
shí gōng 石宮 KI-19　*Stone Palace**
shí gōng 食宮 KI-19　*Food Palace**
shí guān 石關 KI-18　*Stone Pass*
shí lǚ 食呂 KI-19　*Food Tube**
shí mén 石門 CV-5　*Stone Gate*
shí què 石闕 KI-18　*Stone Gate Tower**
shí yī jiāo zhī jiān 十
　　　Within the Eleventh Burner
shǐ guāng 始光 BL-2　*Beginning of Light**
shǒu sān lǐ 手三里 LI-10　*Arm Three Li*
shǒu tài yáng 手太陽 SI-2　*Hand Tai Yang**
shǒu wǔ lǐ 手五里 LI-13　*Arm Five Li*
shǒu xīn zhǔ 手心主 PC-7　*Hand Heart Governor**
shǒu zhī shàng lián 手之上廉 LI-9
　　　Upper Ridge of the Arm*
shǒu zhī wǔ lǐ 手之五里 LI-13
shǒu zhī xià lián 手之下廉 LI-8
　　　Lower Ridge of the Arm*

shū fǔ 俞府 KI-27 *Shu Mansion*
shū fǔ 輸府 KI-27 *Transport Mansion**
shū hé zhōng 樞合中 GB-30 *Pivot Union Center**
shū mén 俞門 CV-5 *Shu Gate**
shū zhōng 樞中 GB-30 *Pivot Center**
shǔ lèi 屬累 GV-4 *Connected**
shù gǔ 束骨 BL-65 *Bundle Bone*
shuài gǔ 率谷 GB-8 *Valley Lead*
shuài gǔ 率骨 GB-8 *Following the Bone**
shuài jiǎo 率角 GB-8 *Following the Corner**
shuài róng 蟀容 BL-8 *Cricket Container**
shuài róng 蟀容 GB-8 *Cricket Container**
shuī fēn 水分 CV-9 *Water Divide*
shuǐ dào 水道 ST-28 *Waterway*
shuǐ gōu 水溝 GV-26 *Water Trough*
shuǐ mén 水門 ST-10 *Water Gate**
shuǐ quán 水泉 LV-1 *Water Spring**
shuǐ quán 水泉 KI-5 *Water Spring*
shuǐ tiān 水天 ST-10 *Water Heaven**
shuǐ tú 水突 ST-10 *Water Prominence*
shuǐ xuè 水穴 LI-18 *Water Hole**
sī běn 思本 GV-16 *Root of Preoccupation**
sī tiān 司天 ST-24 *Celestial Manager**
sī zhú kōng 絲竹空 TB-23 *Silk Bamboo Hole*
sì bái 四白 ST-2 *Four Whites*
sì dú 四瀆 TB-9 *Four Rivers*
sì mǎn 四滿 KI-14 *Fourfold Fullness*
sù liáo 素髎 GV-25 *White Bone-Hole*
suí fǔ 髓府 GV-2 *Marrow Mansion**
suí fǔ 髓府 KI-14 *Marrow Mansion**
suí huì 髓會 GB-39 *Marrow Convergence**
suí kōng 髓孔 GB-5 *Marrow Hole**
suí kōng 髓空 GV-2 *Marrow Hole**
suí kǒng 髓孔 GV-2 *Marrow Hole**
suí kǒng 髓孔 ST-5 *Marrow Hole**
suí shū 髓俞 CV-2 *Marrow Shu**
suí zhōng 髓中 GB-5 *Marrow Center**
suí zhōng 髓中 KI-14 *Marrow Center**
suǐ shū 髓俞 GV-2 *Marrow Shu**
suǒ wén 所聞 SI-19 *Heard**

tài bái 太白 SP-3   *Supreme White*
tài cāng 太倉 CV-12   *Supreme Granary**
tài chōng 太沖 LV-3   *Supreme Surge*
tài chōng 太衝 LV-3   *Great Thoroughfare**
tài quán 太泉 LU-9   *Great Spring**
tài xī 太谿 KI-3   *Great Ravine*
tài yáng 太陽 GB-1   *Greater Yang**
tài yáng 太陽 GB-3   *Greater Yang**
tài yī 太一 ST-23   *Supreme Unity**
tài yǐ 太乙 ST-23   *Supreme Unity*
tài yin luò 太陰絡 SP-7   *Tai Yin Connection**
tài yīn 太陰 LV-6   *Supreme Yin**
tài yīn 太陰 SP-6   *Tai Yin**
tài yīn nèi shì 太陰内市 SP-11
        *Tai Yin Inner Market**
tài yuān 太淵 LU-9   *Great Abyss*
tài zhōng 太鐘 KI-4   *Great Goblet**
táo dào 陶道 GV-13   *Kiln Path*
tǐ mài 體脈 TB-18   *Corporal Vessel**
tiān bái 天白 BL-7   *Celestial White**
tiān bó 天伯 BL-7   *Celestial Lord**
tiān chí 天池 CV-24   *Celestial Pool**
tiān chí 天池 PC-1   *Celestial Pool*
tiān chōng 天沖 GB-9   *Celestial Surge**
tiān chòng 天衝 GB-9   *Celestial Hub*
tiān chuāng 天窗 SI-16   *Celestial Window*
tiān dǐng 天頂 LI-17   *Celestial Summit**
tiān dǐng 天鼎 LI-17   *Celestial Tripod*
tiān fǔ 天府 LU-3   *Celestial Storehouse*
tiān gài 天蓋 ST-12   *Celestial Cover**
tiān huì 天會 PC-1   *Celestial Convergence**
tiān jǐng 天井 TB-10   *Celestial Well*
tiān jiù 天臼 BL-7   *Celestial Mortar**
tiān jiù 天舊 BL-7   *Old as the Heavens**
tiān jú 天瞿 CV-22   *Celestial Mu**
tiān liáo 天髎 TB-15   *Celestial Bone-Hole*
tiān mǎn 天滿 GV-20   *Celestial Fullness**
tiān qú 天衢 GB-9   *Celestial Crossroads**
tiān quán 天泉 PC-2   *Celestial Spring*
tiān róng 天容 SI-17   *Celestial Countenance*

tiān shī 天濕 PC-2   *Celestial Damp**
tiān shū 天樞 ST-25   *Celestial Pivot*
tiān tīng 天聽 TB-15   *Celestial Hearing**
tiān tú 天突 CV-22   *Celestial Chimney*
tiān wēn 天溫 PC-2   *Celestial Warmth**
tiān wǔ huì 天五會 ST-9
                Celestial Fivefold Confluence*
tiān xī 天谿 SP-18   *Celestial Ravine*
tiān xiàng 天項 LI-17   *Celestial Nape**
tiān yǒu 天牖 TB-16   *Celestial Window*
tiān zhù 天柱 BL-10   *Celestial Pillar*
tiān zōng 天宗 SI-11   *Celestial Gathering*
tiáo kǒu 條口 ST-38   *Ribbon Opening*
tīng gōng 聽宮 SI-19   *Auditory Palace*
tīng hē 聽呵 GB-2   *Hearing Laughter**
tīng huì 聽會 GB-2   *Auditory Convergence*
tōng gǔ 通穀 KI-2   *Grain Connection**
tōng gǔ 通穀 KI-20   *Freeing the Grain**
tōng gǔ (fù) 通谷(腹) KI-20   *Open Valley*
tōng gǔ (zú) 通谷(足) BL-66   *Valley Passage*
tōng guān 通關 KI-19   *Free Passage**
tōng jiān 通間 TB-8   *Connect Between**
tōng lǐ 通里 HT-5   *Connecting Li*
tōng lǐ 通理 HT-5   *Connecting Grain**
tōng mén 通門 TB-8   *Connecting Gate**
tōng tiān 通天 BL-7   *Celestial Connection*
tóng xuán 童玄 LU-7   *Child Mystery**
tóng zǐ liáo 瞳子髎 GB-1   *Pupil Bone-Hole*
tóu chōng 頭沖 LI-14   *Head Surge**
tóu chōng 頭衝 LI-14   *Head Thoroughfare**
tóu lín qì 頭臨泣 GB-15   *Head Overlooking Tears*
tóu qiào yīn 頭竅陰 GB-11   *Head Portal Yin*
tóu wéi 頭維 ST-8   *Head Corner*
tuǐ dù 腿肚 KI-9   *Leg Belly**
wài gōu 外勾 ST-32   *Outer Hook**
wài guān 外關 TB-5   *Outer Pass*
wài líng 外陵 ST-26   *Outer Mound*
wài mìng 外命 KI-7   *Outer Life**
wài qiū 外丘 ST-32   *Outer Hill**
wài qiū 外丘 GB-36   *Outer Hill*

wài shū 外樞 GB-28　　*Outer Pivot**
wán gǔ 完骨 GB-12　　*Completion Bone*
wàn gǔ 腕骨 SI-4　　*Wrist Bone*
wàn láo 腕勞 LU-7　　*Wrist Taxation**
wéi dào 維道 GB-28　　*Linking Path*
wéi huì 維會 CV-8　　*Linking Convergence**
wéi huì 維會 GV-20　　*Linking Convergence**
wéi zhī 爲之 GV-1　　*That's It**
wěi cuì gǔ 尾翠骨 GV-1　　*Tail Kingfisher Bone**
wěi gǔ xià kōng 尾骨下空 GV-1
　　　　Hollow Below the Tail Bone*
wěi lǘ 尾櫚 GV-1　　*Tail Palm**
wěi qū gǔ 尾蛆骨 GV-1　　*Tail Maggot Bone**
wěi yáng 委陽 BL-39 (B-53)　　*Bend Yang*
wěi yì 尾翳 CV-15　　*Tail Screen**
wěi zhōng 委中 BL-40　　*Bend Middle*
wèi cāng 胃倉 BL-50 (B-45)　　*Stomach Granary*
wèi guǎn 胃管 CV-13　　*Stomach Duct**
wèi mù 胃募 CV-12　　*Stomach Mu**
wèi shū 胃俞 BL-21　　*Stomach Shu*
wèi wǎn 胃脘 CV-12　　*Venter**
wèi wǎn 胃脘 CV-13　　*Venter**
wèi wéi 胃維 ST-4　　*Stomach Link**
wēn liù 溫溜 LI-7　　*Warm Dwelling*
wū jiāo zhī jiān 伍焦之間 BL-15
　　　　Within the Fifth Burner*
wū yì 屋翳 ST-15　　*Roof*
wǔ chéng 五城 CV-4　　*Fifth City**
wǔ chù 五處 BL-5　　*Fifth Place*
wǔ huì 五會 GV-20　　*Fivefold Confluence**
wǔ huì 五會 ST-9　　*Fivefold Confluence**
wǔ lǐ 五里 PC-8　　*Five Li**
wǔ lǐ (shǒu) 五里 (手) LI-13　　*Five Li (arm)**
wǔ lǐ (zú) 五里 (足) LV-10　　*Five Li (foot)**
wǔ shū 五樞 GB-27　　*Fifth Pivot*
xī fēng 西風 GV-17　　*West Wind**
xī gǔ 谿谷 ST-29　　*Ravine Valley**
xī guān 膝關 LV-7　　*Knee Joint*
xī mén 郄門 PC-4　　*Cleft Gate*
xī xuè 谿穴 ST-1　　*Ravine Hole**

xī xuè 谿穴 ST-29 *Ravine Hole**
xī xuè 鼠穴 ST-1 *Mouse Hole**
xī yáng guān 膝陽關 GB-33 *Knee Yang Joint*
xī zhōng 郄中 BL-40 *Cleft Center**
xiá bái 俠白 LU-4 *Guarding White*
xiá xī 俠谿 GB-43 *Pinched Ravine*
xià dū 下都 TB-3 *Lower Metropolis**
xià guān 下關 ST-7 *Below the Joint*
xià guǎn 下管 CV-10 *Lower Duct**
xià huāng 下肓 CV-4 *Lower Huang**
xià huāng 下肓 CV-6 *Lower Huang**
xià jí 下極 CV-1 *Lower Extreme**
xià jí 下極 KI-11 *Lower Extreme**
xià jì 下紀 CV-4 *Lower Regulator**
xià jù xū 下巨虛 ST-39 *Lower Great Hollow*
xià kūn lún 下崑崙 BL-60 *Lower Kunlun Mountains**
xià lián 下廉 ST-39 *Lower Ridge**
xià lián 下廉 LI-8 *Lower Ridge*
xià liáo 下髎 BL-34 *Lower Bone-Hole*
xià líng 下陵 ST-36 *Lower Mound**
xià líng sān lǐ 下陵三里 ST-36
          Lower Mound Three Li*
xià qì hǎi 下氣海 CV-6 *Lower Sea of Qi**
xià qì hǎi 下氣海 ST-36 *Lower Sea of Qi**
xià sān lǐ 下三里 SP-6 *Lower Three Li**
xià sān lǐ 下三里 ST-36 *Lower Three Li**
xià wǎn 下脘 CV-10 *Lower Venter*
xià xū sān lǐ 下虛三里 ST-36
          Lower Hollow Three Li*
xià yīn bié 下陰別 CV-1 *Lower Yin Divergence**
xià zhī sān lǐ 下之三里 SP-6 *Lower Three Li**
xiàn gǔ 陷谷 ST-43 *Sunken Valley*
xiāo luò 消濼 TB-12 *Dispersing Riverbed*
xiāo shuò 消爍 TB-12 *Dispersing Brilliance**
xiǎo cháng shū 小腸俞 BL-27 *Small Intestine Shu*
xiǎo gǔ 小谷 LI-3 *Small Valley**
xiǎo guān 小關 CV-7 *Small Pass**
xiǎo hǎi 小海 SI-8 *Small Sea*
xiǎo jí 小吉 SI-1 *Small Propitiousness**
xié dài 鞋帶 ST-41 *Shoe Lace**

xié liáo 脅䯒 LV-13   *Lateral Costal Bone-Hole**
xié liáo 脅髎 LV-13   *Lateral Costal Bone-Hole**
xīn mù 心募 CV-14   *Heart Mu**
xīn shū 心俞 BL-15   *Heart Shu*
xīn zhī shū 心之俞 BL-15   *Heart's Shu**
xìn huì 囟會 GV-22   *Fontanel Meeting*
xìn mén 囟門 GV-22   *Fontanel Gate**
xìn shàng 囟上 GV-22   *Top of the Fontanel**
xīng xīng 惺惺 GV-16   *Clearheadedness**
xíng jiān 行間 LV-2   *Moving Between*
xiōng táng 胸堂 CV-17   *Chest Hall**
xiōng xiāng 胸鄉 SP-19   *Chest Village*
xuán jī 旋機 CV-21   *Turning Pivot**
xuán jī 璇璣 CV-21   *Jade Pivot*
xuán jiāng 懸漿 CV-24   *Suspended Sauce**
xuán lí 懸厘 GB-6   *Suspended Tuft*
xuán lú 懸顱 GB-5   *Suspended Skull*
xuán quán 懸泉 LV-4   *Suspended Spring**
xuán shū 旋俞 BL-29   *Return Shu**
xuán shū 懸樞 GV-5   *Suspended Pivot*
xuán zhōng 懸鐘 GB-39   *Suspended Bell*
xuè hǎi 血海 CV-4   *Sea of Blood**
xuè hǎi 血海 SP-10   *Sea of Blood*
xuè shì 血室 CV-4   *Blood Chamber**
xuè xī 血郄 BL-40   *Blood Cleft**
xuè xī 血郄 SP-10   *Blood Cleft**
xún jì 循際 ST-25   *Cycle Border**
yǎ mén 啞門 GV-15   *Mute's Gate*
yàn shé 厭舌 GV-15   *Repressed Tongue**
yáng bái 陽白 GB-14   *Yang White*
yáng chí 陽池 TB-4   *Yang Pool*
yáng fǔ 陽輔 GB-38   *Yang Assistance*
yáng gāng 陽綱 BL-48 (B-43)   *Yang Headrope*
yáng gǔ 陽谷 SI-5   *Yang Valley*
yáng jiāo 陽交 GB-35   *Yang Intersection*
yáng jiǎo 陽矯 BL-59   *Yang Correction**
yáng líng 陽陵 GB-33   *Yang Mound**
yáng líng 陽陵 GB-34   *Yang Mound**
yáng líng quán 陽陵泉 GB-34   *Yang Mound Spring*
yáng qiāo 陽蹺 BL-62   *Yang Motility**

yáng qiáo 陽蹻 BL-62　*Yang Motility**
yáng shǐ 羊矢 LV-12　*Goat Arrow**
yáng shǐ 羊屎 ST-30　*Sheep's Droppings**
yáng xī 陽谿 LI-5　*Yang Ravine*
yáng zé 陽澤 LI-11　*Yang Marsh**
yáng zhī líng quán 陽之陵泉 GB-34
　　　　*Yang's Mound Spring**
yǎng lǎo 養老 SI-6　*Nursing the Aged*
yàng qì 羕泣 ST-1　*Brimming Tears**
yāo hù 腰戶 GV-2　*Lumbar Door**
yāo shū 腰俞 GV-2　*Lumbar Shu*
yāo yáng guān 腰陽關 GV-3　*Lumbar Yang Pass*
yāo zhù 腰柱 GV-2　*Lumbar Pillar**
yè guāng 夜光 BL-2　*Night Light**
yè mén 掖門 TB-2　*Armpit Gate**
yè mén 液門 GB-22　*Humor Gate**
yè mén 液門 ST-27　*Humor Gate**
yè mén 液門 TB-2　*Humor Gate*
yè mén 腋門 GB-22　*Armpit Gate**
yè mén 腋門 ST-27　*Armpit Gate**
yè mén 腋門 TB-2　*Armpit Gate**
yì xī 譩譆 BL-45　*Yi Xi*
yì fēng 翳風 TB-17　*Wind Screen*
yì qián 臆前 CV-15　*Anterior Breast**
yì shè 意舍 BL-49　*Mentation Abode*
yīn bái 陰白 SP-1　*Yin White**
yīn bāo 陰包 LV-9　*Yin Bladder*
yīn bāo 陰胞 LV-9　*Yin Bladder**
yīn dǐng 陰鼎 ST-33　*Yin Tripod**
yīn dū 陰都 KI-19　*Yin Metropolis*
yīn gǔ 陰谷 KI-1　*Yin Valley**
yīn gǔ 陰谷 KI-10　*Yin Valley*
yīn guān 陰關 BL-36　*Yin Joint**
yīn guān 陰關 KI-12　*Yin Gate**
yīn jiāo 陰交 CV-7　*Yin Intersection*
yīn jīng 陰經 SP-7　*Yin Channel**
yīn lián 陰廉 LV-11　*Yin Corner*
yīn líng quán 陰陵泉 SP-9　*Yin Mound Spring*
yīn mén 殷門 BL-37 (B-51)　*Gate of Abundance*
yīn mén 瘖門 GV-15　*Loss-of-Voice Gate**

yīn qiāo 陰蹻 KI-6   *Yin Motility**
yīn qiáo 陰蹺 KI-6   *Yin Motility**
yīn shì 陰市 ST-33   *Yin Market*
yīn wéi 陰維 KI-12   *Yin Link**
yīn xī 陰郄 GV-1   *Yin Cleft**
yīn xī 陰郄 HT-6   *Yin Cleft*
yīn zhī líng quán 陰之陵泉 SP-9
        Yin's Mound Spring*
yín fèng jīn zhōng 齦縫筋中 GV-28
        Gum Crevice Sinew Center*
yín jiāo 齦交 GV-28   *Gum Intersection*
yǐn bái 隱白 SP-1   *Hidden White*
yīng chuāng 膺窗 ST-16   *Breast Window*
yīng shū 膺俞 LU-1   *Breast Shu**
yīng zhōng shū* 膺中俞 LU-1
        Breast Center Shu*
yíng gōng 營宮 PC-8   *Construction Palace**
yíng xiāng 迎香 LI-20   *Welcome Fragrance*
yǒng quǎn 涌泉 KI-1   *Gushing Spring*
yōu mén 幽門 CV-10   *Dark Gate**
yōu mén 幽門 KI-21   *Dark Gate*
yú fù 魚腹 BL-57   *Fish Belly**
yú gǔ 髃骨 LI-15   *Collarbone**
yú jì 魚際 LU-10   *Fish Border*
yú wěi 魚尾 GV-1   *Fish Tail**
yú yāo 魚腰 BL-57   *Fish's Lumbus**
yù fáng shū 玉房俞 BL-30   *Jade House Shu**
yù hù 玉戶 CV-22   *Jade Door**
yù huán shū 玉環俞 BL-30   *Jade Ring Shu**
yù quán 玉泉 CV-3   *Jade Spring**
yù táng 玉堂 CV-18   *Jade Hall*
yù yīng 玉英 CV-18   *Jade's Beauty**
yù zhěn 玉枕 BL-9   *Jade Pillow*
yù zhōng 彧中 KI-26   *Lively Center*
yù zhōng 域中 KI-26   *Within Bounds**
yuān yè 淵腋 GB-22   *Armpit Abyss*
yuán ér 元兒 CV-17   *Original Child**
yuán jiàn 元見 CV-17   *The Source**
yuán yè 淵液 GB-22   *Abyss Humor**
yuán zài 員在 BL-2   *Man Present**

yuán zhù 元柱 BL-2   *Origin Pillar**
yuán zhù 員柱 BL-2   *Pillar Border**
yuè liáo 月髎 TB-23   *Moon Bone-Hole**
yún mén 雲門 LU-2   *Cloud Gate*
zā fēng 匝風 GV-17   *Circumference Wind**
zài quán 在泉 ST-26   *At the Spring**
zǎn zhú 攢竹 BL-2   *Bamboo Gathering*
zàng zhū 臟俞 GV-11   *Visceral Shu**
zhāng mén 章門 LV-13   *Camphorwood Gate*
zhǎng zhōng 掌中 PC-8   *Center of the Palm**
zhào hǎi 照海 KI-6   *Shining Sea*
zhé jīn 輒筋 GB-23   *Sinew Seat*
zhěn gǔ 枕骨 GB-11   *Occipital Bone**
zhěn gǔ 枕骨 GB-11   *Pillow Bone**
zhèng miàn 正面 GV-25   *Center of the Face**
zhèng yíng 正營 GB-17   *Upright Construction*
zhī gōu 支溝 TB-6   *Branch Ditch*
zhī lì jiè 知利介 GV-12   *Wisdom's Advantage Armor**
zhī lì qì 知利氣 GV-12   *Wisdom's Advantage Qi**
zhī zhèng 支正 SI-7   *Branch to the Correct*
zhí cháng 直腸 BL-56   *Rectum**
zhǐ jǐng 指井 BL-67   *Digit Well**
zhì biān 秩邊 BL-54   *Sequential Limit*
zhì lì máo 智利毛 GV-12   *Wisdom's Advantage Hair**
zhì róng 至榮 GB-16   *Arriving at Splendor**
zhì shì 志室 BL-52 (B-47)   *Will Chamber*
zhì yáng 至陽 GV-9   *Extremity of Yang*
zhì yīn 至陰 BL-67   *Reaching Yin*
zhōng chōng 中衝 PC-9   *Central Hub*
zhōng dū 中都 HT-7   *Central Metropolis**
zhōng dū 中都 LV-6   *Central Metropolis*
zhōng dú 中瀆 GB-32   *Central River*
zhōng fēng 中封 LV-4   *Mound Center*
zhōng fǔ 中府 LU-1   *Central Treasury*
zhōng guǎn 中管 CV-12   *Central Duct**
zhōng jí 中極 CV-3   *Central Pole*
zhōng jiān jǐng 中肩井 LI-15
        Central Shoulder Well*
zhōng kōng 中空 BL-33   *Central Hole**
zhōng kuí 中魁 LI-5   *Central Eminence**

zhōng liáo 中髎 BL-33　**Central Bone-Hole**
zhōng lǚ 中膂 BL-29　**Central Backbone***
zhōng lǚ nèi shū 中膂內俞 BL-29
　　　　Central Backbone Inner Shu*
zhōng lǚ shū 中膂俞 BL-29
　　　　Central Backbone Shu
zhōng shǒu 中守 CV-9　**Central Guard***
zhōng shū 中樞 GV-7　**Central Pivot**
zhōng tíng 中庭 CV-16　**Center Palace**
zhōng wǎn 中脘 CV-12　**Central Venter**
zhōng xī 中郄 BL-40　**Central Cleft***
zhōng xī 中郄 LV-6　**Central Cleft***
zhōng zhǔ 中渚 TB-3　**Central Islet**
zhōng zhù 中注 KI-15　**Central Flow**
zhòng jiàng 重漿 CV-24　**Heavy Sauce***
zhōu gǔ 周谷 LI-2　**Whole Valley***
zhōu róng 周榮 SP-20　**All-Round Flourishing**
zhōu yíng 周營 SP-20　**All-Round Construction***
zhǒu jiān 肘尖 LI-12　**Tip of the Elbow***
zhǒu jiān 肘尖 LV-13　**Elbow Tip***
zhǒu liáo 肘髎 LI-12　**Elbow Bone-Hole**
zhú bīn 築賓 KI-9　**Guest House**
zhú zhàng 竹杖 GV-4　**Bamboo Stick***
zhǔ xīn 主心 PC-7　**Heart Governor***
zhuàng gǔ 壯骨 GV-27　**Bone Strengthener***
zhuī liáo 椎髎 SI-18　**Hammer Bone-Hole***
zhǔn tóu 準頭 GV-25　**Nose Tip***
zī mài 資脈 TB-18　**Supporting Vessel***
zǐ cháng 子腸 CV-4　**Infant's Intestine***
zǐ chù 子處 CV-4　**Infant's Place***
zǐ gōng 子宮 CV-4　**Infant's Palace***
zǐ gōng 紫宮 CV-19　**Purple Palace**
zǐ hù 子戶 CV-4　**Infant's Door***
zǐ hù 子戶 KI-13　**Infant's Door (right)***
zú kōng 足空 GB-35　**Leg Hollow***
zú liáo 足窌 BL-35　**Leg Bone-Hole***
zú liáo 足窌 GB-35　**Leg Bone-Hole***
zú liáo 足髎 GB-35　**Leg Bone-Hole***
zú lín qì 足臨泣 GB-41　**Foot Overlooking Tears**
zú qiào yīn 足竅陰 GB-44　**Foot Portal Yin**

zú sān lǐ 足三里 ST-36 *Leg Three Li*
zú shào yīn hé 足少陰合 KI-1 *Foot Shao Yin Union**
zú tōng gǔ 足通谷 BL-66 *Foot Valley Passage**
zú wǔ lǐ 足五里 LV-10 *Foot Five Li*
zú xià zhōng yāng zhī mài 足下中央之脈 KI-1
 Vessel in the Center of the Sole*
zú zhī shàng lián 足之上廉 ST-37
 Upper Ridge of the Leg*

Bibliography of Chinese Sources

針灸大成校釋**　　　　　　　　　啓業書局
　台北 1987
針灸歌賦校釋**　　范土生　著　　山西科學教育出版社
　山西 1987
針灸治療學**　　　范　銘　著　　文源書局
　台北 1982
針灸學**　　　上海中醫學院　編　人民衛生出版社
　北京 1974
黃帝內經**　　　　　　　　　　　聯國風出版社
　台北 1984
傷寒論新註**　　承澹盦　著　　　文光圖書公司
　台北 1979
針灸聚英**　　（明）高　武　著　武陵出版社
　台北 1983
簡明中醫字典**　　　　　　　　　貴州人民出版社
　貴州 1985
中醫難字典**　　　李　戎　編　　四川科學技術出版社
　成都 1986
中國醫學大辭典**　謝利恆　編　　商務印書館
　香港 1974
中國大辭典**　　　　　　　　　　啓業書局
　台北 1983
中醫詞典**　　　　徐元貞　等編　河南科學技術出版社
　河南 1982
針灸經穴學**　　　楊維傑　編著　樂群出版公司
　台北 1979
古漢語常用字字典**　　　　　　　商務印書館
　北京 1979
腧穴學**　　　　　楊甲三　主編　上海科學技術出版社
　上海 1987
經穴釋義匯解**　　張晟星　戚淦　編著　上海翻譯出版
公司　上海 1984
鍼灸穴名釋義**　　周楣聲　著　　安徽科學技術出版社
　安徽 1985
醫經針灸類編**　　靳　瑞　著　　西太平洋圖書出版公
司　香港 1983
中國醫籍考**　　　日．丹波元胤　編　人民衛生出版社
　北京 1983

三百種醫籍錄**　　　　　　　　啓業書局
　台北 1986
針灸腧穴圖譜**　陸瘦燕　朱汝功　著　上海科學技術
出版社　　上海 1988
針灸腧穴之命名涵義及其代號**　　黃民德　著　　中
華針灸科學研究基金會　　台北 1978
靈樞經語釋**　　張珍玉　主編　　山東科學技術出版
社　　山東 1983
黃帝内經素問語釋**　　　　周鳳梧　編　　　山
東科學技術出版社　　山東 1985
采艾編**　　蕭天石　主編　　自由出版社
　台北 1978

Chinese Language Books Cited in the Text

The Book of History 史記. Si-Ma Qian 司馬遷, Han Dynasty 漢.

The Canon of the Yellow Court 黃庭内景經. Anon., Jin Dynasty 晉.

Book of Changes 易經. Anon., Spring and Autumn 春秋時代

The Book of Prolonging Life and Preserving the Origin 壽世保元. Gong Ting-Xian Editor 龔廷賢編, 1615.

Bronze Statue Illustrated Canon of Acupuncture Points 銅人腧穴針灸圖經 (Bronze Statue). Wang Wei-Yi 王惟一, 1026

Compilation of Acupuncture and Moxibustion 針灸集成. Liao Run-Hong 廖潤鴻, 1874.

The Classic of Difficult Issues 難經. Anon., Han Dynasty 漢.

Elucidation of Characters 説文解字. Xu Shen 許愼, 120 A.D.

The Essential Book of Bian Que 扁鵲心書. Collected by Dou Cai-Zhong 竇材重, Song Dynasty 宋.

Essential Questions 素問. See Inner Canon.

The Four Books of Acupuncture 針灸四書. Collected by Dou Gui-Fang 竇桂芳, Yuan Dynasty 元.

The Gateway to Medicine (The Gateway) 醫學入門. Li Yan 李梴, 1575.

The Glorious Anthology of Acupuncture (The Glorious Anthology) 針灸聚英. Gao Wu 高武, 1529.

The Golden Mirror of Medicine (The Golden Mirror) 醫宗金鑒. Wu Qian 吳謙, 1742.

The Great Compendium of Acupuncture and Moxibustion (The Graet Compendium) 針灸大成. Yang JI-Zhou 楊繼洲, 1601.

Illustrated Supplement to the Differentiated Canon (Illustrated Supplement) 內經圖翼. Zhang Jie-Bin 張介賓, 1624.

The Inner Canon 內經 (Consisting of the Spiritual Axis and the Essential Questions.) anon., circa 100 B.C.

The Jin Classic 晉書. Fang Xuan-Ling et al. 房玄齡, Tang Dynasty 唐.

Jing-Yue's Complete Work 景岳全書. Zhang Jing-Yue 張景岳, 1624.

The Kang Xi Dictionary 康熙字典. 1716

The Life-Promoting Canon of Acupuncture and Moxibustion (Life Promoting Canon) 針灸資生經. Wang Zhi-Zhong 王執中, 1220.

Recovery from the Myriad Illnesses 萬病回春. Gong Ting-Xian 龔廷賢, 1587.

The Shen Nong Canon 神農經. Anon., Qin-Han Dynasty 秦漢.

Spiritual Axis 靈樞. See *Inner Canon.*

Supplemented Thousand Gold Piece Prescriptions 千金翼方. Sun Si-Miao 孫思邈, 682.

The Systemized Canon of Acupuncture and Moxibustion (The Systemized Canon) 針灸甲乙經. Huang Pu-Mi 皇甫謐, 282 A.D.

Tao Te Ching 道德經. Lao Tsu 老子, Warring States Period 戰國時代.

The Taoist Storehouse 道藏. A classical collection of Taoist texts.

The Thousand Gold Piece Prescriptions 千金要方. Sun Si-Miao 孫思邈, 625 A.D.

Treatise on Cold Damage 傷寒論. Zhang Zhong-Jing 張仲景, 200 A.D.

Chinese Language Odes and Songs Cited in the Text

Ode to Elucidate Mysteries 標幽賦. First recorded in the *Guide to Acupuncture and Moxibustion* 針灸指南, 1241.

Ode of a Hundred Patterns 百症賦. First recorded in the *Glorious Antholgy of Acupuncture* 針灸聚英, 1529.

Ode of the Jade Dragon 玉龍賦. First recorded in the *Glorious Antholgy of Acupuncture* 針灸聚英, 1529.

Ode of Xi Hong 席紅賦. First recorded in the *Complete Book of Acupuncture and Moxibustion* 針灸大全, 1439.

Song of the Jade Dragon 玉龍歌. First recorded in Bian Que's *Jade Canon*

Spiritual Guide to Acupuncture and Moxibustion 扁鵲神應針灸玉龍經, Yuan Dynasty元.

Song to Keep Up Your Sleeve 肘後歌. First recorded in the *Glorious Anthology of Acupuncture* 針灸聚英, 1529.

Song of Ma Dan Yang's Twelve Celestial Star Points 馬丹陽天星十二穴歌. First recorded in Bian Que's *Jade Canon Spiritual Guide to Acupuncture and Moxibustion*扁鵲神應針灸玉龍歌, Yuan Dynasty 元.

Song of Needle Practice 行針指要歌. First recorded in the *Glorious Anthology of Acupuncture* 針灸聚英, 1529.

Song of the Nine Needles for Returning Yang 回陽九針歌. First recorded in the*Glorious Anthology of Acupuncture* 針灸聚英, 1529.

Song of Point Applications for Miscellaneous Disease 雜病穴法歌. First recorded in the *Gateway to Medicine* 醫學入門, 1557.

Bladder

BL-1:	143	BL-50:	179
BL-2:	144	BL-51:	179
BL-3:	145	BL-52:	180
BL-4:	146	BL-53:	181
BL-5:	147	BL-54:	182
BL-6:	147	BL-55:	182
BL-7:	148	BL-56:	183
BL-8:	149	BL-57:	184
BL-9:	150	BL-58:	185
BL-10:	150	BL-59:	186
BL-11:	151	BL-60:	188
BL-12:	152	BL-61:	189
BL-13:	153	BL-62:	190
BL-14:	154	BL-63:	191
BL-15:	155	BL-64:	192
BL-16:	155	BL-65:	193
BL-17:	156	BL-66:	194
BL-18:	157	BL-67:	195
BL-19:	157		
BL-20:	158		
BL-21:	159		
BL-22:	159		
BL-23:	160		
BL-24:	161		
BL-25:	161		
BL-26:	162		
BL-27:	163		
BL-28:	163		
BL-29:	164		
BL-30:	165		
BL-31:	166		
BL-32:	167		
BL-33:	167		
BL-34:	168		
BL-35:	168		
BL-36:	169		
BL-37:	170		
BL-38:	171		
BL-39:	171		
BL-40:	172		
BL-41:	173		
BL-42:	173		
BL-43:	174		
BL-44:	175		
BL-45:	175		
BL-46:	176		
BL-47:	177		
BL-48:	177		
BL-49:	178		

Conception Vessel

CV-1:	303
CV-2:	304
CV-3:	305
CV-4:	306
CV-5:	308
CV-6:	309
CV-7:	310
CV-8:	311
CV-9:	312
CV-10:	312
CV-11:	313
CV-12:	314
CV-13:	315
CV-14:	316
CV-15:	317
CV-16:	318
CV-17:	319
CV-18:	320
CV-19:	321
CV-20:	322
CV-21:	323
CV-22:	324
CV-23:	325
CV-24:	326

Gallbladder

GB-1:	252
GB-2:	253
GB-3:	253
GB-4:	254
GB-5:	255
GB-6:	256
GB-7:	257
GB-8:	258
GB-9:	259
GB-10:	260
GB-11:	261
GB-12:	262
GB-13:	262
GB-14:	263
GB-15:	264
GB-16:	265
GB-17:	266
GB-18:	267
GB-19:	267
GB-20:	268
GB-21:	269
GB-22:	270
GB-23:	271
GB-24:	272
GB-25:	273
GB-26:	274
GB-27:	275
GB-28:	276
GB-29:	277
GB-30:	277
GB-31:	278
GB-32:	279
GB-33:	280
GB-34:	280
GB-35:	281
GB-36:	282
GB-37:	283
GB-38:	284
GB-39:	284
GB-40:	285
GB-41:	286
GB-42:	287
GB-43:	288
GB-44:	289

Governing Vessel

GV-1:	327
GV-2:	329
GV-3:	330
GV-4:	331
GV-5:	332
GV-6:	332
GV-7:	333
GV-8:	334
GV-9:	334
GV-10:	335
GV-11:	336
GV-12:	336
GV-13:	337
GV-14:	338
GV-15:	339
GV-16:	340
GV-17:	341
GV-18:	342
GV-19:	343
GV-20:	343
GV-21:	345
GV-22:	345
GV-23:	346
GV-24:	347
GV-25:	348
GV-26:	349
GV-27:	350
GV-28:	351

Heart

HT-1:	120
HT-2:	121
HT-3:	122
HT-4:	122
HT-5:	123
HT-6:	124
HT-7:	125
HT-8:	126
HT-9:	127

Kidney

KI-1:	196
KI-2:	197
KI-3:	198
KI-4:	199
KI-5:	200
KI-6:	201
KI-7:	202
KI-8:	204
KI-9:	205
KI-10:	206
KI-11:	206
KI-12:	207
KI-13:	208

KI-14: 209	LU-11: 35	SI-17: 140	ST-22: 75
KI-15: 210		SI-18: 141	ST-23: 76
KI-16: 211		SI-19: 142	ST-24: 77
KI-17: 212	**Liver**		ST-25: 78
KI-18: 213	LV-1: 291		ST-26: 80
KI-19: 214	LV-2: 292	**Spleen**	ST-27: 81
KI-20: 215	LV-3: 292	SP-1: 100	ST-28: 82
KI-21: 216	LV-4: 293	SP-2: 101	ST-29: 83
KI-22: 217	LV-5: 294	SP-3: 102	ST-30: 84
KI-23: 218	LV-6: 295	SP-4: 103	ST-31: 85
KI-24: 219	LV-7: 296	SP-5: 104	ST-32: 86
KI-25: 220	LV-8: 297	SP-6: 105	ST-33: 86
KI-26: 220	LV-9: 297	SP-7: 106	ST-34: 87
KI-27: 221	LV-10: 298	SP-8: 107	ST-35: 89
	LV-11: 299	SP-9: 108	ST-36: 90
	LV-12: 299	SP-10: 109	ST-37: 91
Large	LV-13: 300	SP-11: 110	ST-38: 92
Intestine	LV-14: 302	SP-12: 111	ST-39: 93
LI-1: 36		SP-13: 112	ST-40: 94
LI-2: 37		SP-14: 112	ST-41: 95
LI-3: 38		SP-15: 113	ST-42: 96
LI-4: 39	**Pericardium**	SP-16: 114	ST-43: 97
LI-5: 40	PC-1: 223	SP-17: 115	ST-44: 98
LI-6: 41	PC-2: 224	SP-18: 116	ST-45: 98
LI-7: 42	PC-3: 225	SP-19: 116	
LI-8: 43	PC-4: 226	SP-20: 117	
LI-9: 44	PC-5: 226	SP-21: 118	**Triple**
LI-10: 45	PC-6: 227		**Burner**
LI-11: 46	PC-7: 228		TB-1: 231
LI-12: 47	PC-8: 229	**Stomach**	TB-2: 232
LI-13: 48	PC-9: 230	ST-1: 56	TB-3: 233
LI-14: 49		ST-2: 57	TB-4: 234
LI-15: 50		ST-3: 58	TB-5: 235
LI-16: 51	**Small**	ST-4: 59	TB-6: 235
LI-17: 52	**Intestine**	ST-5: 60	TB-7: 236
LI-18: 53	SI-1: 128	ST-6: 61	TB-8: 237
LI-19: 54	SI-2: 129	ST-7: 62	TB-9: 238
LI-20: 55	SI-3: 130	ST-8: 63	TB-10: 239
	SI-4: 131	ST-9: 64	TB-11: 240
	SI-5: 131	ST-10: 65	TB-12: 240
	SI-6: 132	ST-11: 66	TB-13: 242
Lung	SI-7: 133	ST-12: 67	TB-14: 243
LU-1: 23	SI-8: 133	ST-13: 68	TB-15: 243
LU-2: 24	SI-9: 134	ST-14: 69	TB-16: 244
LU-3: 26	SI-10: 135	ST-15: 70	TB-17: 245
LU-4: 27	SI-11: 136	ST-16: 71	TB-18: 245
LU-5: 28	SI-12: 136	ST-17: 71	TB-19: 246
LU-6: 29	SI-13: 137	ST-18: 72	TB-20: 247
LU-7: 30	SI-14: 138	ST-19: 72	TB-21: 248
LU-8: 32	SI-15: 138	ST-20: 73	TB-22: 249
LU-9: 33	SI-16: 139	ST-21: 74	TB-23: 250
LU-10: 34			